To Dear Dr. Chen

Compliments

Z.Y. Tang
汤钊猷

Subclinical Hepatocellular Carcinoma

Edited by Tang Zhao-you

With 136 Figures and 144 Tables

China Academic Publishers Beijing

Springer-Verlag
Berlin Heidelberg New York Tokyo 1985

Tang Zhao-you, M. D.

Professor of Surgery
Chairman, Liver Cancer Research Unit
Zhong Shan Hospital
Shanghai First Medical College
Shanghai 200032
The People's Republic of China

ISBN 3-540-12664-3 Springer-Verlag Berlin Heidelberg New York Tokyo
ISBN 0-387-12664-3 Springer-Verlag New York Heidelberg Berlin Tokyo
CSBN W 14262.006 China Academic Publishers Beijing

Library of Congress Cataloging in Publication Data. Main entry under title: Subclinical hepatocellular carcinoma. Bibliography: p. Includes index. 1. Liver-Cancer. I. T'ang, Zhao-you. [DNLM: 1. Liver Neoplasms. 2. Hepatoma. WI 735 S941] RC280.L5S83 1985 616.99'436 84-17887

Typesetting. printing and bookbinding: G. Appl. Wemding
2124/3140-543210

To my Teachers
To the Peoples of the World

Foreword

Hepatocellular carcinoma is a relatively rare malignancy in the Western world, but one of the most frequent fatal tumors in the Far East and in sub-Saharan Africa, that means, in the areas where the majority of mankind lives. Until a few decades ago it was mainly detected at autopsy or, far less frequently, at operation. The improvement of imaging methods and the widespread use of liver biopsy have subsequently permitted earlier recognition. Still, it has only been detected when the process was far advanced and frequently only when a palpable mass or dramatic clinical symptoms encouraged thorough clinical investigation. This detection during life led to attempts at surgical removal. Nevertheless, these often far advanced tumors were usually associated with a bad prognosis and a relatively low rate of cure or prolonged survival after operation.

Several factors are responsible for the greater clinical interest in hepatocellular carcinoma in the past decade. The reproduction of the carcinoma in experimental animals has contributed greatly to the increasing interest in the understanding of carcinogenesis in general, although the extensive experimental investigations of these animal carcinomas have had relatively little impact on the clinical management of the tumor. Advancements in surgical techniques have improved the prognosis; transplantation of the liver, however, has so far proven to be of only limited therapeutic value. Chemotherapy of hepatocellular carcinoma with various drugs and various routes of administration has also resulted in some success, though it is so far barely convincing as a widely useful therapeutic modality. The interest in hepatocellular carcinoma has been conspicuously enhanced by the recognition of its relation to hepatitis B virus infection; carriers, of which there are 200 million worldwide, are at particular risk to develop the carcinoma. Cell lines established from hepatocellular carcinoma produce some specific viral antigens, particularly the surface antigen, and integration of hepatitis B viral DNA into the genome of the host has been demonstrated in the tumor, in the surrounding liver, and in carrier livers, but the oncogenicity of the hepatitis B virus is so far not established. Nevertheless, the hope exists that elimination of hepatitis B virus infection by administration of the vaccine and/or hyperimmune globulin may prevent the tumor, thus establishing the causal relation. The relation is also supported by the observation of hepatitis and hepatocellular carcinoma in animals infected by a virus related to, but different from, the hepatitis B virus. This holds true for the woodchuck and – especially in China – for the duck. However, factors other than hepatitis B virus infection are also incriminated in hepatocellular carcinoma. They include alcohol abuse – particularly in the Western world – and, worldwide aflatoxin, though at present it cannot be excluded that even in these instances, hepatitis B infection plays a contributory role. Other chemical agents that are potent hepatocarcinogens in animals or incriminated in tumors other than the liver seem not to cause hepatocellular carcinoma, whereas sex hormones, metabolic diseases, and the Budd-Chiari syndrome seem to be infrequent causes, and a carcinogenic role of hepatitis non-A, non-B is problematic. Hepatitis B virus infection is therefore the most common factor today in hepatocellular carcinoma, particularly in the Orient and in Africa.

Probably the most compelling reason for the rising clinical interest in hepatocellular carcinoma, however, is the discovery of more or less specific serum markers, some of them oncofetal proteins, with alpha-fetoprotein the most important in practical use today. Although moderate serum elevations may accompany unrelated diseases, for instance those referable to yolk sac disorders, otherwise conspicuous and sustained elevations have permitted screening for hepatocellular carcinoma in earlier stages even if it is not necessarily present in all cases and if some elevations are found in chronic hepatitis. While this screening takes place in many locations, the most extensive and successful such attempt has been made in China. Such screening, together with or supplemented by various imaging techniques (particularly angiography and sonography), has led to the clinical detection of hepatocellular carcinoma in an early stage, before any clinical or even other laboratory abnormalities are evident. This detection of the small tumors in the early stages in Japan, but particularly in China and predominantly in Shanghai, has been rewarded with excellent chances of survival and possibly cure by surgical removal of the carcinoma, at this stage often still single.

These observations and successes have completely altered the clinical outlook in hepatocellular carcinoma and have led to the concept of subclinical hepatocellular carcinoma by the authors of this monograph. This concept represents major progress in the understanding, and particularly the management, of hepatocellular carcinoma, permitting "secondary prevention" at a time when primary prevention by immunization techniques such as vaccine and hyperimmune globulin is still a goal of the future. However, it has not yet been established whether the experiences in the Far East hold true for other parts of the world; in Africa there seems to be a tendency for more rapid growth of the hepatocellular carcinoma with less development of cirrhosis. Sufficient observational data are not yet available for us to know whether or not this geographical difference is real, or to determine the predominant pattern in Western countries, aside from that in Oriental immigrants.

Nevertheless, this monograph, based on the study of an unusually large amount of material and its thorough laboratory evaluation, and supplemented by Chinese experiences with the basic aspects of the disease, should be of major interest to clinicians as well as to basic science-oriented physicians and other scientists all over the world, including the Western countries. It should assist them in understanding the problem and encourage them to repeat these studies in their own countries. The scientific community is indebted to Dr. Tang for making this information widely available.

New York, November 1984 Hans Popper, MD, PhD

Contents

Contributors

Cao Yun-zhen (Cao Y. Z.), Lecturer in Internal Medicine, Liver Cancer Research Unit, Zhong Shan Hospital, Shanghai First Medical College, Shanghai, P. R. China

Chen Hui-li (Chen H. L.), Associate Professor, Department of Biochemistry, Shanghai First Medical College, Shanghai, P. R. China

Chen Rui-ming (Chen R. M.), Senior Research Scientist (Professor), Ph. D., Head of Cancer Research Laboratory and Member of Scientific Council, Shanghai Institute of Cell Biology, Academia Sinica, Shanghai, P. R. China

Gu Tian-Jue (Gu T. J.), Professor and Head, Department of Biochemistry, Shanghai First Medical College, Shanghai, P. R. China

He Kai-ling (He K. L.), Associate Professor, Department of Biochemistry, Shanghai First Medical College, Shanghai, P. R. China

Li Mao-shen (Li M. S.), Associate Professor, Department of Biochemistry, Shanghai First Medical College, Shanghai, P. R. China

Lin Zhi-ying (Lin Z. Y.), Lecturer of Internal Medicine, Vice-Chairman of Liver Cancer Research Unit, Zhong Shan Hospital, Shanghai First Medical College, Shanghai, P. R. China

Shen Ding-wu (Shen D. W.), Research Associate (Assistant Professor), Cancer Research Laboratory, Shanghai Institute of Cell Biology, Academia Sinica, Shanghai, P. R. China

Tang Zhao-you (Tang Z. Y.), Professor of Surgery, Chairman of Liver Cancer Research Unit, Zhong Shan Hospital, Shanghai First Medical College, Shanghai, P. R. China

Wang Hen-wen (Wang H. W.), Senior Research Scientist (Professor), Group Leader of Environmental Carcinogenesis, Laboratory of Cancer Biology, Shanghai Institute of Cell Biology, Academia Sinica, Shanghai, P. R. China

Wen Yu-mei (Wen Y. M.), Associate Professor and Chairman of Department of Microbiology, Shanghai First Medical College, Shanghai, P. R. China

Xu He (Xu H.), Research Associate (Assistant Professor), Member of Environmental Carcinogenesis Group, Shanghai Institute of Cell Biology, Academia Sinica, Shanghai, P. R. China

Xu Zhi-zhang (Xu Z. Z.), Associate Professor and Chairman, Laboratory of Ultrasonic Diagnosis, Zhong Shan Hospital, Shanghai First Medical College, Shanghai, P. R. China

Yang Bing-hui (Yang B. H.), Lecturer in Internal Medicine, Liver Cancer Research Unit, Zhong Shan Hospital, Shanghai First Medical College, Shanghai, P. R. China

Yao Zhen (Yao Z.), Senior Research Scientist (Professor), Deputy Director of the Institute, Head of Department of Cancer Cell Biology, Shanghai Institute of Cell Biology, Academia Sinica, Shanghai, P. R. China

Ye Sheng-long (Ye S. L.), Doctor (Masters Degree), Liver Cancer Research Unit, Zhong Shan Hospital, Shanghai First Medical College, Shanghai, P. R. China

Ying Yue-ying (Ying Y. Y.), Professor and Vice-Chairman of Department of Pathology, Shanghai First Medical College, Shanghai, P. R. China

Yu Shun-zhang (Yu S. Z.), Associate Professor, Department of Epidemiology, Shanghai First Medical College, Shanghai, P. R. China

Yu Ye-qin (Yu Y. Q.), Associate Professor of Surgery, Vice-Chairman of Liver Cancer Research Unit, Zhong Shan Hospital, Shanghai First Medical College, Shanghai, P. R. China

Zhai Wei-rong (Zhai W. R.), Lecturer in Pathology, Department of Pathology, Shanghai First Medical College, Shanghai, P. R. China

Zhang Yu-yan (Zhang Y. Y.), Associate Scientist (Associate Professor), Shanghai Institute of Cell Biology, Academia Sinica, Shanghai, P. R. China

Zhen Qing-yi (Zhen Q. Y.), Research Associate (Assistant Professor), Head of the Division of Cancer Biochemistry, Shanghai Institute of Biochemistry, Academia Sinica, Shanghai, P. R. China

Zhou Xin-da (Zhou X. D.), Lecturer in Surgery, Liver Cancer Research Unit, Zhong Shan Hospital, Shanghai First Medical College, Shanghai, P. R. China

Zhou Yi-zhong (Zhou Y. Z.), Research Associate (Assistant Professor), Division of Cancer Biochemistry, Shanghai Institute of Biochemistry, Academia Sinica, Shanghai, P. R. China

Abbreviations

AFP	Alpha fetoprotein
AGD	Agar gel diffusion
ALD	Active-stage liver disease
ALP	Alkaline phosphatase
ALT	Alanine aminotransferase
anti-HBc	Antibody to hepatitis B core antigen
anti-HBe	Antibody to hepatitis B "e" antigen
anti-HBs	Antibody to hepatitis B surface antigen
CHCC	Clinical hepatocellular carcinoma
CIEP	Countercurrent immunoelectrophoresis
CT	Computed tomography
γ-GTP	Gamma glutamyl transpeptidase
HA	Hepatic angiography
HBcAg	Hepatitis B core antigen
HBeAg	Hepatitis B "e" antigen
HBsAg	Hepatitis B surface antigen
HBV	Hepatitis B virus
HCC	Hepatocellular carcinoma
LDH	Lactate dehydrogenase
OT	Skin delayed hypersensitivity reaction to old tuberculin
PLC	Primary liver cancer
RIA	Radioimmunoassay
RN	Radionuclide imaging
RPHA	Reverse passive hemagglutination
RREA	Radiorocket electrophoresis autography
SCHCC	Subclinical hepatocellular carcinoma
US	Ultrasound, ultrasonography

Acknowledgements

The editor wishes to express his appreciation to Dr. Zhou X. D. and Dr. Ye S. L. for their help with the manuscripts.

The editor is also sincerely grateful to the following people for their contribution in clinical and research work at the Liver Cancer Research Unit, Zhong Shan Hospital, Shanghai First Medical College, Shanghai; Dr. Zhou N. Q., Dr. Lu J. Z., Dr. Tang C. L., Dr. Ma Z. C., and others.

The English of this manuscript has been improved by Professor Yang Chang-yi and Associate Professor Yao Zi-ran of the Department of Foreign Languages, Shanghai First Medical College, Shanghai, P.R. China.

1 Subclinical Hepatocellular Carcinoma – Historical Aspects and General Considerations

Tang Zhao-you

Hepatocellular carcinoma has long been regarded as a hopeless illness, owing to the great difficulties in early detection and effective treatment. The discovery of subclinical HCC in the early 1970s, however, has opened a new scope in clinical research of HCC. The facts that serum AFP is detectable in the majority of HCC cases and that it is applied in serosurvey, either in high-risk areas or in populations with chronic hepatitis and cirrhosis, are responsible for this progress. New concepts involving early diagnosis, surgical management of SCHCC, the natural history of HCC, and the theory of unicentric or multicentric origin also deserve to be mentioned (Tang et al. 1982b). It is especially worth noting that the 5-year survival rate of 72.9% has been achieved after resection of tumor in SCHCC patients, thus showing a hopeful future and sparking a lively interest in this particular neoplasm and greater research endeavors in the field.

I. Definition

A. Subclinical Hepatocellular Carcinoma

A patient with SCHCC was arbitrarily defined as one without obvious HCC symptoms and signs (Tang et al. 1980), while CHCC exhibits both symptoms and signs.

Asymptomatic SCHCC is detected principally by AFP survey or serial AFP monitoring in subjects with a background of liver disease; however, CHCC is discovered in the majority of cases in patients who seek medical care because of the appearance of symptoms.

B. Small or Minute Hepatocellular Carcinoma

Small or minute HCC was also arbitrarily defined with minor variations in the literature. Minute HCC was defined by Okuda as a single nodule with the longest diameter not exceeding 4.5 cm, or as a few nodules (less than four), the biggest one smaller than 3.5 cm (Okuda et al. 1977). Akin to the definition of minute HCC, the authors defined small HCC as a single nodule HCC ⩽5 cm, or as two nodules totaling 5×5×5 cm (Tang et al. 1979a).

C. Relationship Between SCHCC and Small HCC

Both SCHCC and small HCC have been acknowledged as relatively early stage HCC, mimicking each other substantially. It has been reported that in operated cases of SCHCC up to 81.6% (40/49) of the tumor nodules measured smaller than 5 cm (Tang et al. 1979b). On the other hand, up to 76.7% (23/30) of patients with surgically proven small HCC were asymptomatic (Tang et al. 1979a). In small HCC tumor size can be more accurately defined, thus facilitating a more accurate comparative study of large tumors and closer representation of early-stage HCC. However, SCHCC has facilitated the study of the natural history as well as the early evolution and behavior of HCC; moreover, SCHCC includes patients receiving treatment other than surgery. This is why we tend to analyze our material of early-stage HCC in terms of SCHCC.

II. Historical Aspect

A. General History

Nearly a century has gone by since the pathological basis of primary liver cancer was first established; a great deal of research work has been done in both clinical and basic aspects. Unfortunately, the grave prognosis of this particular neoplasm is not remarkably altered, the difficulty in early detection being acknowledged as one of the major deterrents.

In recent years, it has been universally accepted that early detection and early treatment of subclinical cancer may be an important approach to rescuing the patient, until breakthroughs are made in the research on basic as well as etiological aspects. A special lecture entitled "Subclinical Cancer – Concepts and Management" was delivered by Leffall at the 12th International Cancer Congress in 1978, representing a landmark of growing interest in this particular field. Subclinical cancer was defined as "cancer that produces no symptoms in patients and that is not detected on routine physical examination" (Leffall 1979). A dramatic ultimate outcome has been achieved, with 5-year survival around 90% after resection of minute or small cancers in the breast, esophagus, stomach, and colorectum, as well as early treatment of in situ cervical cancer, etc. As a matter of fact, subclinical cancer was proven surgically to be minute cancer in the majority of cases. These encouraging results have stimulated research endeavors in the early detection of subclinical cancer in high-risk populations, in the study of new tumor markers, and in innovations of early treatment. The rapidly increasing knowledge in the field of subclinical cancer has been accepted as one of the major advances in clinical oncology in the 1970s.

Owing to the deep location of liver in the abdomen and to the lack of specific diagnostic tools, early-stage HCC patients were seldom encountered in clinical practice in past decades. According to the analysis of 3254 cases of primary liver cancer, up to 52.6% of clinically diagnosed patients had jaundice, ascites, or distant metastases, SCHCC amounting to only 0.4% of the accidental findings in the overall series during operation (Tang et al. 1974). Fortunately, advances in enzymology, nuclide imaging technique, ultrasonography, and selective arteriography, and particularly the discovery of tumor marker AFP have raised the diagnostic level of HCC from "postmortem diagnosis," through "clinical (symptomatic) diagnosis," to the present stage of "subclinical diagnosis." A steady rise in the rate of accurate diagnosis has been recorded during the past decades – 11.3% (Gustafson 1937), 23.6% (Rosenberg and Oshsner 1948), 36% (MacDonald 1957), 40% (San Jose et al. 1965), and 86% (Alpert et al. 1969).

B. History of Study of SCHCC and Small HCC Abroad

The history of the study of SCHCC and small HCC represents the true history of early detection and early diagnosis of HCC. As mentioned above, SCHCC patients were seldom seen in clinical practice. Patients with small HCC were also scarcely encountered, small HCC amounting to only 5.5% (7/127) (Foster and Berman 1977) – 6.8% (6/88) (Tang et al. 1979a) of the resection cases in symptomatic clinical patients. As is well known, less than 10% (6.1%) (Tang et al. 1974) of all patients with HCC underwent successful resection. Therefore, it is estimated that SCHCC and small HCC were encountered in less than 1% of the overall series of clinical HCC. However, the discovery of AFP and its application in mass screening has opened the way for marked changes in the clinical staging pattern.

The value of AFP as a useful marker for HCC has been widely accepted since its discovery in 1956 and its detection in HCC (Tatarinov 1964, reviewed by Abelev 1971). In 1972 Purves and Geddes reported on the discovery of a 0.5-cm HCC during an autopsy of a patient who had 300 ng/ml serum AFP before he died.

In the same year, Malt (1972) anticipated that detection of SCHCC might be achieved by AFP examination. However, the value of AFP in detection of SCHCC was not widely accepted on account of the dismal results of an AFP survey in Africa. Leblance et al. (1973) studied almost 10000 male adults in Senegal at intervals of 4 months for 2 years, and only one of the nine identified cases of HCC could be regarded as asymptomatic at the time when the AFP became positive (reviewed by Purves 1976). On the other hand, in Japan, Okuda et al. (1977) analyzed 20 cases of minute HCC, including 16 autopsies and four resections. Ishikawa (1976) summarized data collected in Japan from 1960 to 1974 and found 20 (6.2%) of 324 resected cases of HCC to be minute HCC. In the United States, Foster (1977) collected data on the resected cases of primary liver cancer during the period 1960–1974; minute tumors occurred in seven (5.5%) of the 127 cases.

C. History of Study of SCHCC and Small HCC in China

In China, advances in early detection of SCHCC have been made since the application of AFP examination in a mass survey in 1971. As a result of employing an assay of relatively low sensitivity – AGD and CIEP assay – for the initial AFP screening during 1971–1973, the value of early detection was not satisfactory. However, unquestionable results were shown in 1972, after AFP screening of 343999 people with AGD and CIEP assay; 147 asymptomatic patients had positive AFP, 88.4% of whom were subsequently proved to have HCC during 2–10 months of follow-up study. A preliminary result concerning the value of AFP in early detection was reported in the 11th International Cancer Congress (The Coordinating Group for Research on Liver Cancer, China, 1974). More impressive early detection of SCHCC has been achieved by using an even more sensitive assay – passive reverse hemagglutination assay – and radiorocket electrophoresis autography since 1974 (Sun et al. 1979). The earlier report concerning small HCC in a high-risk area – Qidong County of Jiangsu Province – was made in 1975 (Yu and Sang 1975). Two years later, 48 cases of SCHCC during a 5-year period (1972–1976) were reported in the same area, and resection was done in 33 of them, the resectability rate accounting for 68.7%, the operative mortality being 0%, and a 2-year survival rate of 77.0% being recorded (Tang and Qian 1977). In Shanghai, during the period 1971–1976, 1967511 persons were screened; 134 (44.7%) of the 300 cases of HCC detected were SCHCC and a 3-year survival of 57.1% after resection was reported (Tang et al. 1979b). This material was presented at the 12th International Cancer Congress. From 1967 to 1978, data on 30 cases of small HCC were collected in the author's hospital, the 3-year survival after resection being reported to be as high as 70.5% (Tang et al. 1979a). In Qidong County of Jiangsu Province 1223912 persons were screened during 1974–1977, cases of SCHCC amounting to 35.2% (167/475) and the 2-year survival rate after resection of SCHCC being 69.0% (Zhu 1981).

The value of AFP examination in early detection of SCHCC has been debated since the 1970s. The great difference between detection rates of SCHCC in Africa and in China has been blamed upon the difference in the growth rate of HCC in different geographical areas (Purves 1976); however, the possible value of AFP in early detection was noted quite recently by Johnson and William (1980).

D. Present Status and Latest Trend

The number of cases of small (or minute) HCC resected worldwide is around 200 (Table 1); more than 100 of these patients were operated on in China. Small HCC amounted to only 5.5% (7/127) (Foster and Berman 1977), 6.2% (20/324) (Ishikawa 1976), and 6.8% (6/88) (Tang et al. 1979) of the overall CHCC resected; however, the proportion increased to 56.8% (25/44) (Tang et al. 1979b) and 72.7% (16/22) (Tang et al. 1979a) in resection of mass-survey patients. The discovery of patients with small HCC was realized principally by AFP survey in China, by AFP monitoring of chronic liver disease in Japan, and by accidental findings during surgery in the United States. It is worth noting that an extremely low operative mortality (2.3%) has been recorded in a major series (Tang 1982a). An encouraging ultimate outcome has been achieved, with 5-year survival rates of 49.3% (Huang et al. 1980), 59.6% (Li GC et al. 1980), and 66.4% (Tang 1982a). Table 1 summarizes the results of small HCC after resection. Their extremely low operative mortality as well as the dramatic 5-year survival rates mimic those for SCHCC in Table 2.

It seems, therefore, that AFP survey or AFP follow-up monitoring in chronic liver diseases remains the best approach for early detection of SCHCC, as well as of small HCC. The incidence of SCHCC and small HCC detected with AFP was about ten times that in clinically symptomatic patients undergoing resection. Resection of SCHCC or small HCC has resulted in large-scale prolongation of survival and low operative mortality; it may thus play an important role in the improvement of the overall ultimate outcome of HCC.

Table 1. Selective data on resection of small (or minute) HCC

Year / Author	Country	Cases	Op. death	Survival
1975 Yu and Sang[a]	China–Qidong 1972–1974	13	0	–
1976 Ishikawa	Japan 1960–1974	20	–	–
1977 Okuda et al.	Japan–Chiba 1970–1975	4	2	1+[d], 2.5 yrs
1977 Foster and Berman	USA 1960–1974	7	2	mean 42 mos
1979 Tang et al.[b]	China–Zhongshan 1967–1978	22	0	3-yr 70.5%
1979 Chen and Wu[c]	China–Shanghai 1965–1977	15	0	–
1980 Huang et al.[a]	China–Qidong 1971–1979	38	0	5-yr 49.3%
1980 Li et al.	China–Guangdong 1968–1980	15	1	5-yr 59.6%
1980 Shimoyama et al.	Japan–Nagasaki 1961–1979	4	1	3+, 7+, 15 mos
1981 Okita et al.	Japan	3		
1981 Munehisa et al.	Japan–Nagasaki	11		
1982a Tang[a]	China–Zhongshan 1967–1981	43	1	5-yr 66.4%
1982 Chen et al.	China (Taiwan) 1979–1981	10	0	–
1982 Yamasaki et al.	Japan–Natl. Cancer Inst.	29	2	–
1982 Wu et al.[c]	China–Shanghai 1960–1981	38	–	5-yr 53.8%

[a, b, c] Represent the same series
[d] + means "still alive"

Table 2. Resection of SCHCC

Author	Cases	Op. death	Survival
1977 Tang and Qian (China-Qidong 1972–1976)	33	0	2-yr 77.0%
1979 Tang et al. (Shanghai) 1971–1976	31	0	3-yr 57.1%
1983 This series (Zhongshan 1971–1982)	60	1	5-yr 72.9%

III. Aim of Studying SCHCC

Primary liver cancer has been regarded as an incurable disease, and no remarkable change in mean survival has been recorded in the past decades – 3.2 months (Gustafson 1937), 2.8 months (Rosenberg and Oshsner 1948), 5.6 months (Ervasti 1964), and 5.74 months (Tang et al. 1974). The overall 5-year survival rate has seldom exceeded 3%: the United States 1955–1964, 913 cases = 3% (Axtell et al. 1972); Japan 1968–1977, HCC 1424 cases = 2.4% (Okuda et al. 1980); China (data from author's hospital) 1970–1974, 277 cases = 2.5% (Tang et al. 1983). In China, the standarized mortality of primary liver cancer has been reported to be as high as 14.52/100000 in men and 5.61/100000 in women (Li and Li 1980). The disease ranks third in malignancies in men and fourth in those in women. It is estimated that nearly 100000 people die of PLC in China annually; moreover, HCC amounted to 89.9% of overall PLC (Tang et al. 1974). It is therefore urgent that every endeavor be made to rescue the patient, the relatively specific HCC marker AFP having been proven to be a source of hope for this particular problem.

The aim of this study is to elucidate the following questions:

1. Can HCC be detected early?
2. How can SCHCC or small HCC be diagnosed early?
3. What measurement provides accurate information for localization of small HCC?
4. Can survival be prolonged after early treatment of SCHCC?
5. What modality of treatment provides the best ultimate outcome?
6. How can the surgeon increase the resectability rate, decrease the operative mortality, and reduce the blood loss in SCHCC surgery?
7. What modality of treatment would be preferred in nonresectable SCHCC?
8. Can subclinical recurrence be detected early, and what is the treatment of choice?
9. If early resection does prolong survival of SCHCC, is there any theoretical basis from a pathological as well as an immunological point of view?
10. Are there any new concepts concerning the natural history of HCC, its early evolution, principles in management, etc?
11. How closely is HCC related to hepatitis B virus?
12. What are the problems concerning basic aspects, and what are the future prospects of HCC?

IV. Materials and Methods

A. Patients

From January 1971 to December 1982, 100 cases of SCHCC were grouped in the Zhong Shan Hospital of the Shanghai First Medical College for this study, 466 cases of CHCC being grouped in the same period for comparative study. Disease was established pathologically in 95% and 99.6% of patients in the SCHCC group and the CHCC group respectively (for histological types refer to Chap. 29); the remaining cases were diagnosed on the strength of positive AFP and angiography.

B. Assays Employed for Laboratory Examinations

Serum AFP was measured by RIA, RREA, CIEP, and AGD; serum ALT activity was examined simultaneously, and γ-GTP and ALP were measured periodically.

C. Measurements of Immunostatus of Host

Skin delayed hypersensitivity reaction on old tuberculin (OT) was employed as the parameter of the cell-mediated immunostatus of host; serial monitoring was carried out every 1–2 months, and a skin reaction >5 cm in diameter was assessed as positive. The lymphocyte transformation test was employed as an in vitro index, and transformation equal to or higher than normal ($>50\%$) was assumed as positive. Other measurements were carried out in individual cases.

D. Calculation of Survival Rate

The 1, 3, and 5-year survival rates were calculated according to the life-table method.

E. Storage, Analysis, and Statistical Treatment of Data

An extended Apple II Plus microcomputer (RAM 64K, ROM 12K) was used for storage, analysis, and statistical treatment of clinical data, with Applesoft Basic as the programming language. Each patients's record comprised 61 items of data, with random text file employed for storage. Analyses were made of those records with corresponding items.

V. Brief Outline of Study

The extremely high mortality of HCC has pressed the authors to seek new approaches. As true knowledge comes from practice, the members of the author's Liver Cancer Research Unit each took part in field work for 1 year during the period 1971–1977, in Qidong County of Jiangsu Province, which was acknowledged as a predominant high-risk area for HCC in China, with mortality reaching around 50/100000.

The first problem is – can HCC be detected early? A mass survey by AFP detection has been carried out in both Qidong County of Jiangsu Province and in Shanghai since 1971. Conservative treatment was employed in the majority of SCHCC cases detected by AFP survey at the very beginning, owing to lack of experience; however, follow-up study within 2–10 months revealed that 88.4% of the asymptomatic, AFP-positive subjects who had normal ALT proved to have HCC and subsequently died. This preliminary observation has shown that SCHCC can be detected an average of 3.1 months prior to the appearance of symptoms by using AGD or CIEP assay as the initial AFP survey (The Coordinating Group for Research on Liver Cancer, China 1974).

Can SCHCC be detected early enough to be resected? More aggressive therapeutic strategy was expedited by the survey mentioned above. Exploratory laparotomy has repeatedly confirmed that the majority of subjects with positive AFP and normal ALT suffer from HCC with small tumor and high resectability (Yu and Sang 1975).

Is there any change in concept for early diagnosis of SCHCC? Our knowledge of SCHCC, involving diagnostic, therapeutic, and basic aspects, is based principally on accumulated experience in surgical intervention with asymptomatic SCHCC patients. The diagnostic level improved especially after 1974 with the employment of more sensitive assays (RPHA or RREA) for initial AFP survey. It was estimated that diagnosis could be made as early as 8 months before symptoms occurred. It was impressive that the lower the AFP level, the smaller the tumor size. The diagnostic criterion for SCHCC progressed from a relatively high AFP level (AFP ⩾

500 ng/ml, or positive CIEP persisting for 1 month with normal ALT), which was universally accepted, to a relatively low AFP level (AFP ⩾200 ng/ml lasting for over 2 months with normal ALT). As the positivities of conventional measurements, including enzymology and liver scintiscan, were too low to be employed for diagnosis of SCHCC, the method of early diagnosis has been changes from combined analysis of symptoms, signs, enzymological findings, and scintiscan to that of AFP, ALT level, and its serial change (Tang et al. 1979b).

How can the site of small HCC be determined? Where is the tumor located? This problem is of prime importance for surgical intervention. Nuclide imaging and type-A sonography have proven to be useless for the localization of small HCC; transumbilical hepatography has been employed since 1973 and proved useful in showing occupying lesions as small as 2 cm in the left lobe (Zhou et al. 1975). Selective celiac or hepatic arteriography, however, has been subsequently confirmed to be superior, with a discrimination limit of 1 cm (Tang et al. 1978). In recent years, real-time B sonography has been tested and is an acceptable noninvasive measurement, especially good for initial screening for localization of small HCC larger than 2 cm (Tang et al. 1982a).

Can early treatment effectively save life? The longer the follow-up study, the clearer the answer. In 1977, a 2-year survival of 77.0% was achieved after resection of SCHCC (Tang and Qian 1977); in 1978, the 3-year survival for resectable cases was reported as 57.1% (Tang et al. 1979b). In this series, a 5-year survival of 72.9% after resection was observed, being four times higher than that obtained in CHCC after resection (16.1%). It is concluded that early resection of SCHCC does effectively save life.

Should some principles concerning surgical treatment of HCC be revised in the management of SCHCC? As mentioned, resection provides the best ultimate result; therefore, increasing resectability, decreasing operative mortality, and prolonging survival even further may be the key task. With the accumulation of experience, it seems that local resection instead of lobectomy means higher resectability, lower operative mortality, and a similar ultimate outcome in resection of small HCC located at the right lobe, with coexistent cirrhosis (Tang et al. 1982b). Bloodless operation with hypothermic perfusion is one of the effective approaches to resection of a tumor near the hepatic portal area or the inferior vena cava (Yu et al. 1980). Reoperation for subclinical recurrence or solitary lung metastasis seems acceptable, having increased 5-year survival from 56.2% (Tang et al. 1981) to 66.4% (Tang 1982a) after resection of small HCC. This may lead to a revision of some surgical principles: local resection rather than classical lobectomy seems acceptable in the management of small HCC; cancer recurrence is no longer a contraindication for surgery if early detection in the subclinical stage can be achieved.

What modality of treatment would be preferred in nonresectable SCHCC? Cryosurgery of liver cancer was started experimentally in 1973 and clinically in 1974 (Zhou et al. 1979). A radical cure can be obtained if adequate cryosurgery is applied to small HCC. High-power YAG laser vaporization of small HCC has also proven to be of value; it was started experimentally in 1975 (Zhou et al. 1980) and applied to clinical practice in 1980 (Yu et al. 1981).

Are there any changes in concepts in the field of HCC? Based on 10 years' study of SCHCC, a new concept of the natural history of HCC has been developed (Tang 1981). A unicentric origin of HCC has been postulated as an important basis for the favorable ultimate outcome of SCHCC after resection (Tang 1982b). Some new findings in immunology (Lin and Tang 1979) and pathology have also been observed (Ying and Chai 1978).

To sum up, a nearly completely new theory of SCHCC has been formed on the basis of the observation of 100 cases of SCHCC with more than 10 years' follow-up; however, a number of problems remained to be solved.

VI. Significance of the Study of SCHCC

The study of SCHCC has shown hope for the treatment of HCC, which is of both practical and theoretical significance. This may prove to be an important approach to saving the patient and improving the overall survival for HCC before breakthroughs are made in all basic aspects of research. The worldwide literature covering the period from 1905 to 1970 reviewed by Curutchet et al. (1971), and only 77 cases of PLC were documented with 3-year survival after resection. However, 47 patients of the present series have survived over 3 years.

The study of SCHCC has greatly promoted research endeavors involving diagnostic and therapeutic aspects. The problems of early diagnosis in AFP-negative HCC, and differential diagnosis of AFP-positive HCC with abnormal ALT and active chronic hepatitis with abnormal AFP have stimulated the search for new tumor markers; the problem of localization of small HCC with a diameter of less than 1 cm has enhanced the investigation of positive scanning by using radioimmunodetection and thus stimulated the search for the relatively specific substance of HCC.

Development of new modalities in conservative treatment is also required, owing to coexistent severe cirrhosis in some patients. Many concepts have to be changed and some principles may have to be revised; these changing concepts may be of importance to the entire field of HCC study in the 1980s. The study of SCHCC may provide valuable information elucidating the early evolution of HCC, and the correlation of cirrhosis with HCC, as well as its mode of origin in HCC. This study also touches on the precancerous stage of HCC. The study of the high-risk population for HCC will also stimulate research into the etiology, with particular attention paid to viral hepatitis. We predict, therefore, that the nature and theory of SCHCC will be established in the 1980s.

References

Abelev GI (1971) Alpha fetoprotein in ontogenesis and its association with malignant tumors. Adv Cancer Res 14: 295–358

Alpert ME, Hutt MSR, Davidson CS et al. (1969) Primary hepatoma in Uganda – a prospective clinical and epidemiologic study of forty-six patients. Am J Med 46: 794–802

Axtell IM, Cutler SJ, Myers MH (1972) End results in cancer – report No4. US Department of Health, Education and Welfare, Public Health Service, NIH, NCI, Bethesda, pp 72–76
Chan KT (1967) The management of primary liver carcinoma. Ann R Coll Surg Engl 41: 235–282
Chen H, Wu MC (1979) Resection of primary liver cancer with diameter smaller than 5 cm. Shanghai Med J 2: 136–138[1]
Chen DS, Sheu JC, Sung JL et al (1982) Small hepatocellular carcinoma – A clinicopathological study in thirteen patients. Gastroenterology 83: 1109–1119
Curutchet HP, Terz JJ, Kay S et al (1971) Primary liver cancer. Surgery 70: 467–479
Ervasti J (1964) Primary carcinoma of the liver – a pathologic and clinical study of 100 cases. Acta Chir Scand [Suppl] 334: 1–65
Foster JH, Berman MM (1977) Solid liver tumors. Saunders, Philadelphia, pp 62–104
Gustafson EG (1937) An analysis of 62 cases of primary carcinoma of the liver based on 24000 necropsies at Bellevue Hospital. Ann Intern Med 11: 889–900
Huang XY, Sha YW et al (1980) Diagnosis, surgical resection and prognosis of 38 cases of small hepatocellular carcinoma. Tumor Prevent Treat Study 8: 7–9[1]
Ishikawa K (1976) Follow-up study of patients with primary liver cancer. Report 3. Acta Hepatol Jpn 17: 460–465
Johnson PJ, William R (1980) Serum alpha fetoprotein estimation and doubling time in hepatocellular carcinoma – influence of therapy and possible value in early detection. J Natl Cancer Inst 64: 1329–1332
Leffall LD (1979) Subclinical cancer – concepts and management. In: Fox M (ed) Advances in medical oncology, research and education, vol 4. Pergamon, London, pp 269–283
Li B, Li JY (1980) National survey of cancer mortality in China. Chin J Oncol 2: 1–10[1]
Li GC, Li GH, Liu GS et al (1980) Resection of minute hepatocellular carcinoma – analysis of 15 cases. Cancer Control (Guangdong, China) (4): 24–29[1]
Lin ZY, Tang ZY (1979) Delayed hypersensitivity reaction to old tuberculin and the prognosis of primary carcinoma of the liver. Acta Acad Med Primae Shanghai 6: 103–110[1]
MacDonald RA (1957) Primary carcinoma of the liver – a clinicopathologic study of one hundred eight cases. Arch Intern Med 99: 266–279
Malt RA (1972) Manifestations and prognosis of carcinoma of the liver. Surg Gynecol Obstet 135: 361–364
Munehisa T, Nakata K, Furahori A et al (1981) Clinical study on minute hepatocellular carcinoma. Jpn J Gastroenterol 78: 2376–2383
Okita K, Ando K, Tsubota W et al (1981) The fate of 7 cases with minute hepatoma followed by selective coeliac angiography. Acta Hepatol Jpn 22: 1004–1008
Okuda K, Kotoda K, Obata H et al (1975) Clinical observations during a relatively early stage of hepatocellular carcinoma, with special reference to serum alpha fetoprotein levels. Gastroenterology 69: 226–234
Okuda K, Nakashima T, Obata H, Kubo Y (1977) Clinicopathological studies of minute hepatocellular carcinoma. Analysis of 20 cases, including 4 with hepatic resection. Gastroenterology 73: 109–115
Okuda K et al. The Liver Cancer Study Group of Japan (1980) Primary liver cancer in Japan. Cancer 45: 2663–2669
Purves LR (1976) Alpha fetoprotein and the diagnosis of liver cell cancer. In: Cameron HM, Linsell DA, Warwick GP (eds) Liver cell cancer. Elsevier, Amsterdam, pp 61–69
Purves LR, Geddes EW (1972) A more sensitive test for alpha fetoprotein. Lancet 1: 47–48
Rosenberg DML, Oshsner A (1948) Primary carcinoma of the liver – an analysis of fifty-five autopsied cases, the record of a case with resection, and a review of the recent literature. Surgery 24: 1036–1068
San Jose D, Cady A, West M et al (1965) Primary carcinoma of the liver – analysis of clinical and biochemical features of 80 cases. Am J Digest Dis 10: 657–674
Schreiber WM, Kato H, Robertson JD (1970) Primary carcinoma of the liver in Hiroshima and Nagasaki, Japan. Cancer 26: 69–75
Shimoyama T, Kitasato S, Fujitomi Y et al (1980) A study of minute hepatocellular carcinoma – clinicopathologic observation on 4 resected cases. Acta Hepatol Jpn 21: 1008–1015
Sun TT, Wrn LC, Chang YL et al (1979) Radiorocket electrophoresis autography (RREA) through labelled antigen for AFP assay and its application in sero-epidemiological investigation on primary hepatocellular carcinoma. Chin Med J [Engl] 92: 17–22

Tang ZY (1981) A new concept on the natural course of hepatocellular carcinoma. Chin Med J [Engl] 94: 585–588

Tang ZY (1982a) Resection of minute hepatocellular carcinoma. Postgraduate Course in IASL-APASL meeting, Hong Kong

Tang ZY (1982b) Clinical evidence of unicentric origin in hepatocellular carcinoma. VI. International Congress of Liver Diseases – Liver in metabolic diseases. (Poster abstract No 191) Basel

Tang ZY, Qian SQ (1977) Surgical treatment of primary liver cancer. Jiangsu Med 3: 501–505[1]

Tang ZY, Yang BH (1974) Primary liver cancer – clinical analysis of 3254 cases (from 11 provinces, 21 hospitals, in China). Tumor Prevent Treat Study 2: 207–215[1]

Tang ZY, Yu YQ, Zhou XD et al (1978) Small hepatocellular carcinoma. IV. Diagnosis of small hepatocellular carcinoma. Acta Acad Med Primae Shanghai 5: 118–125[1]

Tang ZY, Yu YQ, Lin ZY et al (1979a) Small hepatocellular carcinoma – clinical analysis of 30 cases. Chin Med J [Engl] 92: 455–462

Tang ZY, Yu EX, Wu CE, Gu XY (1979b) Diagnosis and treatment of primary hepatocellular carcinoma in early stage – report of 134 cases. Chin Med J [Engl] 92: 801–806

Tang ZY, Yang BH, Tang CL et al (1980) Evaluation of population screening for hepatocellular carcinoma. Chin Med J [Engl] 93: 795–799

Tang ZY, Cao YZ, Yu YQ, Lin ZY (1981) Small hepatocellular carcinoma. V. Prognosis and factors influencing prognosis of small HCC. Acta Acad Med Primae Shanghai 8: 203–207[1]

Tang ZY, Lu JZ, Zhou NQ, Yu YQ (1982a) Small hepatocellular carcinoma (HCC). VI. Value of hepatoarteriography, B-scan ultrasonography and liver scintiscan in the localization of small HCC – a comparative study based on operative findings. Acta Acad Med Primae Shanghai 9: 101–105[1]

Tang ZY, Ying YY, Gu TJ (1982b) Hepatocellular carcinoma – changing concepts in recent years. In: Popper H, Schaffner F (eds) Progress in liver diseases, vol 7. Grune and Stratton, New York pp 637–647

Tang ZY, Yu YQ, Lin ZY et al (1983) Clinical research of primary liver cancer – A 10-year (1970–1979) survey. Chin Med J [Engl] 96: 247–250

Tatarinov Y (1964) Detection of embryo-specific-globulin in the blood sera of patients with primary liver tumors. Vopr Med Khim 10: 90–91

The Coordinating Group for Research on Liver Cancer, China (1974) Alpha fetoprotein assay in primary hepatocellular carcinoma mass survey and follow-up studies. Tumor Prevent Treat Study 2: 277–286[1]

Wu MC, Zhang XH, Chen H, Wu BW (1982) Experiences in hepatectomies of 467 cases. Chin J Digest 2: 190–193[1]

Yamasaki S, Hasegawa H, Makunchi M (1982) Pathological and surgical consideration on minute liver cancer, analysis of 29 resected cases. APASL meeting, Hong Kong (abstract No 18)

Ying YY, Chai WY (1978) Small hepatocellular carcinoma. III. Pathology of small hepatocellular carcinoma. Acta Acad Med Primae Shanghai 5: 111–118[1]

Yu YQ, Sang LA (1975) Early diagnosis and resection of primary liver cancer. Tumor Prevent Treat Study 3: 1–5[1]

Yu YQ, Tang ZY, Zhou XD et al (1980) Bloodless hepatectomy. Chin J Surg 18: 146–147[1]

Yu YQ, Tang ZY, Zhou XD et al (1981) Treatment of primary hepatic cancer by YAG laser, a preliminary report. Acta Acad Med Primae Shanghai 8: 29–31[1]

Zhou XD, Tang ZY, Yu YQ et al (1975) Transumbilical hepatography for diagnosis of primary liver cancer. Natl Med J China 55: 265–269[1]

Zhou XD, Tang ZY, Yu YQ et al (1979) Cryosurgery for liver cancer – experimental and clinical study. Chin J Surg 17: 480–483[1]

Zhou XD, Yu YQ, Tang ZY et al (1980) Experimental study of laser hepatic surgery. Acta Acad Med Primae Shanghai 7: 216–221[1]

Zhu YR (1981) AFP serosurvey and early diagnosis of liver cell cancer in the Qidong area. Chin J Oncol 3: 35–37[1]

---

1 in Chinese

2 Early Detection of Subclinical Hepatocellular Carcinoma

Tang Zhao-you, Yang Bing-hui

Primary liver cancer causes 100000 deaths annually in China, attacking mainly men 30–59 years old (Li and Li 1980). It is most urgent to seek effective ways to lower the incidence and to save those afflicted. Thanks to basic research, particularly regarding HBV and AFP, there is hope for primary and secondary prevention of HCC in the future. Based on the close relationship between HBV and HCC, more effective results could be obtained for primary prevention by using HB vaccine; nevertheless, this will take 40–50 more years before intervention in the newborn is possible and 10–20 years to prepare for adult vaccination. Preventive measures against chemicals such as aflatoxin also need further investigation. Fortunately, the results of early aggressive treatment of survey HCC are encouraging; thus, early detection of SCHCC becomes the key to secondary prevention (Tang 1980).

I. Discovery of Small HCC and SCHCC

Small HCC and SCHCC have been reported in autopsy findings, operative findings, serial monitoring of AFP in chronic liver diseases, and AFP surveys of natural populations.

A. Autopsy Findings

In 1972, Purves and Geddes observed a case with an AFP level of 300 ng/ml and found a 0.5-cm HCC during autopsy. In 1977, Okuda et al. reported on 154 HCC autopsies, in 16 of which (10.4%) the finding was small HCC. Pathological examinations revealed single nodules which were well encapsulated and differentiated, the majority of which coexisted with cirrhosis. A total of 39 autopsy findings with small HCC were collected in Japan (Ishikawa 1976); however, only individual cases were reported in the west (Mahmood and Schatzki 1976).

B. Clinical Findings During Operation

According to data on liver cancer collected from 98 hospitals in the United States over 15 years (1960–1974), only seven (5.5%) of 127 resections were found to be small HCC (Foster and Berman 1977), and according to data collected in Japan from 1960 to 1974, 20 (6.2%) of 324 resections of HCC proved to be small HCC (i.e.

a single nodule <5 cm and a few nodules, the biggest of which is <4 cm) (Ishikawa 1976). The incidence of small HCC in resections of CHCC accounted for 6.8% (6/88) (Tang et al. 1979) and 8.2% (4/49) (Shimoyama et al. 1980).

C. Serial Monitoring of AFP and/or Arteriography in Subjects with Background of Liver Disease

In Japan, small HCC was found chiefly by serial monitoring of AFP and/or selective celiac or hepatic arteriography in subjects with chronic hepatitis or cirrhosis. Early in 1975, Okuda reported five cases in a relatively early stage of HCC, detected mainly by AFP and selective celiac angiography, which suggested that AFP might be a useful tool for early detection of HCC (Okuda et al. 1975). In 1976, Hiroshi discovered four cases of HCC in a prospective study of 59 cases of liver cirrhosis; they were diagnosed by means of AFP (RIA assay) monitoring and confirmed by means of celiac angiography. Two of the patients underwent resection and presented with small HCC measuring around 2 cm and AFP levels of 307 and 1060 ng/ml respectively (Hiroshi et al. 1976). In 1981, Ando reported follow-up angiographic findings in 68 cases of chronic liver disease, 42 of which were detected to be HCC, including ten small HCC. This suggested that follow-up selective celiac angiography might be of value for early detection of HCC in patients with a background of chronic liver disease (Ando et al. 1981).

D. AFP Survey in Natural and High-Risk Populations

In China, SCHCC and small HCC patients were discovered principally by AFP survey in natural as well as high-risk populations (Table 1). In Qidong County of Jiangsu Province, a high-risk area, 1310871 persons were screened during the period 1974–1980, with SCHCC constituting 35.5% of cases (Zhu and Lu 1983), while

Table 1. Selective data from AFP serosurvey

Population/survey	Population screened (*n*)	Cases of HCC detected	Discovery rate 1/100000
Natural population			
Shanghai (1971–1976)	1967511	300	15.3
Qidong (1974–1980)	1310871	499	38.1
Author (1972–1980)	305997	51	16.7
With liver disease			
Shanghai and Qidong	76660	253	330.0
Qidong	4875	48	984.6
Author	22300	15	67.3
With serum HBsAg			
Chen	3454	31[a]	897.5

[a] AFP survey for 5 years

in Shanghai, 1976511 persons of the natural population were screened, 44.7% of 300 cases of HCC detected being SCHCC (Tang et al. 1979b). The latest trend is to confine AFP survey to high-risk populations. In a prospective study to estimate the risk of HCC in 3454 HBsAg carriers by means of annual serum-AFP screening with RIA, nine patients with HCC not larger than 3 cm were detected (Chen et al. 1982).

E. Measurements Employed for Early Detection

As a screening method, AFP remains the best assay. Sensitive assays such as RPHA, RREA, and RIA were emphasized to be employed for initial AFP screening. However, owing to the fact that some HCC patients had normal AFP levels, and that a good proportion of patients with hepatitis or cirrhosis had abnormal AFP levels, adjunct measurements were required. Unfortunately, none of the tumor markers other than AFP has been of value for early detection of SCHCC as yet. On the other hand, localization measurements, including hepatic angiography (HA), computed tomography (CT), real-time ultrasound (US), and radionuclide imaging (RN) were employed as adjuncts. It was accepted that lesions larger than 3 cm could be detected by all of these methods and that those between 2 and 3 cm were generally shown by US, CT, and HA but not by RN. Only HA was of value for diagnosis of lesions less than 2 cm; therefore AFP and US were recommended to minimize expense and radiation exposure, and HA was indicated in questionable cases (Takashima et al. 1982; Tang et al. 1982a).

II. General Data from Authors' Series of SCHCC

From January 1971 to December 1982, 100 patients with SCHCC were admitted to Zhong Shan Hospital. Of the entire series, 76 cases were discovered by AFP detection during a mass survey, 22 cases by AFP monitoring in subjects with a history of hepatitis, and only two cases clinically. It is worth noting that following an educational campaign many people with histories of hepatitis came of their own accord to have AFP checked. During the period from 1971 to 1976, large-scale screening was performed among the natural population of Shanghai (Tang et al. 1979b); only 23 patients with SCHCC were admitted to our hospital. In contrast, AFP survey among the natural population was less frequently performed from 1977 to 1982, but 77 cases of SCHCC were diagnosed.

A global comparison between 100 cases of SCHCC and 466 cases of CHCC revealed that despite similar patterns in age and coexisting cirrhosis, there were great differences in tumor size, incidence of solitary tumor, and the 5-year survival rate (Table 2).

III. Significance of AFP Survey

A comparison between survey HCC and nonsurvey HCC during the 1972–1978 period has strongly indicated the advantage of AFP survey (Tang et al. 1980). With longer follow-up study and more aggressive treatment, the picture was even clearer.

Table 2. Comparison of general data on SCHCC and CHCC

Items		SCHCC ($n=100$)	CHCC ($n=466$)
Discovery	Mass survey %	76.0 (76/100)	7.3 (34/466)
	Clinical %	2.0 (2/100)	89.9 (419/466)
	AFP monitoring %	22.0 (22/100)	2.8 (13/466)
Median age		47.5 (20–65)	46.0 (13–82)
Male: female		15.7:1	8.3:1
Coexistent cirrhosis %		85.7 (78/91)	80.5 (231/287)
Tumor size (cm)[a]		4.5 (0.8–16)	10.0 (1–35)
Solitary tumor %		66.7 (60/90)	39.3 (118/300)
5-year survival % (life table method)		43.9	4.2

[a] Expressed in median (range)

Table 3. Comparison of stage patterns in survey and nonsurvey group

Clinical stage		Survey HCC		Nonsurvey HCC	
		Cases	%	Cases	%
Subclinical	(I)	98	67.6	2	0.5
Moderate	(II)	35	24.1	300	71.2
Late	(III)	12	8.3	119	28.3
Total		145	100.0	421	100.0

Of the series of 566 patients treated in Zhong Shan Hospital from 1971 to 1982, 145 cases were survey patients and 421 cases nonsurvey patients. The AFP survey is significant in changing patterns of staging, therapy, and prognosis.

A. Marked Change in Clinical Staging Pattern

Criteria for clinical staging were arbitrarily defined as: Stage I (subclinical) – without obvious HCC symptoms or signs, Stage II (moderate) – between criteria for Stages I and III, and Stage III (late) – with obvious cachexia, jaundice, ascites, or distant metastases.

As shown in Table 3, 67.6% of survey patients have SCHCC, but only 0.5% of nonsurvey patients. On the other hand, the proportion of late-stage patients decreases markedly with the survey. The proportion of SCHCC in survey patients was reported to be from 35.5% (177 of 499) in Qidong data (Zhu and Lu 1983) to 44.7% (134 of 300) in Shanghai data (Tang et al. 1979b).

B. Marked Change in Therapy Pattern

Surgical resection has been acknowledged as a principal approach which may lead to long survival. The proportions of both resection and local resection in the survey group were double those in the nonsurvey group (Table 4).

C. Marked Change in Prognostic Pattern

It was noted that the 5-year survival rate was nearly ten times higher in survey patients. Moreover, resection made the 5-year survival rate for survey patients four times higher than that for nonsurvey HCC patients (Table 5).

D. The Role of Mass Survey in the Overall Series

A comparison was made between the periods 1971–1976 and 1977–1982. As a result of the much higher proportion of SCHCC during the latter period, a nearly twofold increase of resection in the whole series was noted. It is particularly noteworthy that the prognosis for HCC patients overall has remained unchanged for decades, with

Table 4. Comparison of therapy patterns in survey and nonsurvey group

		Survey HCC	Nonsurvey HCC
Resection in whole series	%	53.8 (78/145)	23.3 (98/421)
Local resection in resection group	%	57.7 (45/78)	23.5 (23/98)
Operative mortality	%	2.6 (2/78)	6.1 (6/98)

Table 5. Comparison of prognostic patterns in survey and nonsurvey group

Survival (life table method) [%]	Survey HCC (n=145)	Nonsurvey HCC (n=421)
Whole series	(n=145)	(n=421)
1-year	64.4 (73)[a]	22.8 (75)
3-year	40.2 (30)	7.3 (17)
5-year	34.7 (11)	3.7 (7)
Resection	(n=78)	(n=98)
1-year	79.9 (51)	59.8 (44)
3-year	68.3 (27)	22.6 (13)
5-year	63.1 (11)	15.1 (7)
Nonresection	(n=67)	(n=323)
1-year	43.6 (22)	11.5 (31)
3-year	5.2 (3)	2.1 (4)
5-year	– (0)	– (0)

[a] Figures in parentheses represent number of survivors

Table 6. Comparison of pathologically proven HCC in the periods 1971–1976 and 1977–1982 (Zhong Shan Hospital)

[%]	1971–1976 ($n=250$)	1977–1982 ($n=316$)
Subclinical HCC	9.2 (23/250)	24.4 (77/316)[a]
Small HCC	8.0 (22/250)	13.3 (42/316)[b]
Resection in whole series	24.4 (61/250)	36.1 (114/316)
Resective mortality	8.2 (5/61)	2.6 (3/114)
Survival of whole series (life table method)		
1-year %	26.5	38.5
3-year %	10.4	21.7
5-year %	6.5	20.6

[a] $P<0.01$ [b] $P<0.05$

the 5-year survival rate seldom exceeding 3.0% (Axtell et al. 1972; Okuda et al. 1980). However, as a result of the increase in diagnosis of SCHCC and the higher resection rate, the 5-year survival has increased from 6.5% to 20.6% in the whole series (Table 6).

IV. Factors Influencing Detection Rate in AFP Survey

A. Subjects Screened

As shown in Table 1, the rate of HCC detection was much higher when screening was performed in populations with a background of liver disease (chronic hepatitis, cirrhosis, or a history of hepatitis) than when performed in natural populations. It was four times higher in the authors' material, the discovery rate being 67.3/100000 versus 16.7/100000. In Qidong County of Jiangsu Province, it was 984.6/100000 versus 44.7/100000; nevertheless, the proportion of SCHCC was lower in the former group (25.0% versus 37.0%) (Zhu and Lu 1983).

B. Assays Employed

It has been well documented that the proportion of SCHCC was higher when RPHA assay was employed rather than CIEP and AGD (The Coordinating Group for the Research of Liver Cancer, China 1978; Tang 1980, Tang et al. 1980) (Table 7).

C. Interval of AFP Serosurvey

As shown in Table 8, after periodic AFP serosurveys at 6-month intervals in the same population, the number of HCC patients, as well as of those with moderate or late-stage disease, decreased remarkably. It is suggested that, theoretically, the AFP serosurvey should be performed every 6 months in high-risk areas (The Coordinating Group for the Research of Liver Cancer, China 1978).

Table 7. Proportion of SCHCC found according to assay employed

Series	Assay employed	Population screened (*n*)	Cases of HCC detected	SCHCC (*n*)	SCHCC [%]
Coordinating Group for Res. Liver Cancer China	AGD	13881	43	2	4.7
	CIEP	66832	105	31	29.5
	RPHA	31231	28	17	60.7
Author	CIEP	21292	3	1	33.3
	RPHA	221619	36	19	52.8

Table 8. Results of periodic AFP serosurvey in the same population

Date of AFP survey	Population screened (*n*)	Cases of HCC detected	Cases in stages II, III (*n*)
September 1975	13224	19	4
March 1976	6825	5	2
October 1976	11182	1	0

V. Key Links in Early Detection of SCHCC

A. AFP Serosurvey and Follow-up Study

Periodic AFP serosurvey was suggested in high-risk populations by using a sensitive, but not an expensive assay for the initial screening. RPHA was proved to be an ideal assay for initial AFP screening. If the AFP level was abnormal, repeated examinations were needed at 2-week intervals. If the AFP level was markedly increased (> 500 ng/ml), HCC was highly suspected, and further examinations were required to exclude pregnancy, teratoma of gonads, and particularly hepatitis or cirrhosis in the active stage. If the AFP level was slightly increased, follow-up monitoring of AFP was recommended at monthly intervals.

B. Nature of Low and Gradually Increasing AFP

From the viewpoint of early detection of SCHCC, patients with an initial slight elevation of the AFP level were even more important than those with markedly increased AFP. The so-called low, persistent AFP was arbitrarily defined as "AFP persisting over 2 months at a level between 50 and 200 ng/ml and without evidence of pregnancy, teratoma of gonads, and hepatitis or cirrhosis in active stage." The detection rate of "low, persistent AFP" was reported to be 1‰ (772 of 743459) with AFP serosurvey in Qidong County; after a follow-up study for 1 year in 476 of the 772 subjects, HCC appeared in 18.5% (88 of 476). A higher proportion of SCHCC was noted, as compared with the survey in a natural population (56.8% versus 35.5%) (Zhu and Lu 1983). In our series, 31 of the 100 patients with SCHCC had low, persistent AFP at the very beginning.

C. Renewing Diagnostic Concept

Current diagnostic concepts of symptomatic HCC must be altered for the diagnosis of SCHCC. As will be described in the following chapter, combined analyses of AFP and serum ALT activity are emphasized, rather than symptoms, signs, and complex biochemical findings (Tang et al. 1979a, 1982b). If doctors hold to an old diagnostic concept, they will miss all the SCHCC in AFP survey.

VI. Problem Concerning Cost-Effect Relationship

A. Pros and Cons

The problem concerning cost versus effect has been debated for years. It is worthwhile to perform the AFP survey from the viewpoint of early detection, but the high cost makes it impossible to do in the entire natural population in the long run.

In order to make a more accurate assessment, the problem of cost versus effect in a group surveyed by our research unit was discussed. The discussion covered an AFP survey of 305997 persons during the period 1973–1980, in which 51 cases of HCC were detected, while 11 patients refused treatment. Of the remaining 40 patients, eight survived more than 5 years (25.0%), which meant that medical expenses for four other patients and the cost of the AFP survey were needed to save one patient. However, the 5-year survival rate in the clinical group of the same period was 2.5%, which meant that the cost for 40 patients was needed to save one patient. As shown in Table 9, the cost for detecting one patient from screening a natural population was four times higher than that in a population with a background of liver disease; however, a fivefold cost was needed to save a clinically symptomatic patients as compared with a survey patient from the high-risk population (¥ 24000 versus ¥ 4800). Furthermore, if sickbed facilities were adequate to treat 100 cases of HCC per year, according to the data of this series, 34.7 patients could be saved per year, provided all were survey (SCHCC) patients; however, only 3.7 clinical (CHCC) patients could be saved per year. In other words, it would take 9.4 years and five times as much money to save 34.7 patients at the clinical level. In conclusion, AFP survey in a high-risk population combined with aggressive treatment has remarkable effects compared with the treatment of clinical patients.

Table 9. Comparison of cost for detecting and saving a HCC patient

	Cost for detecting a HCC patient (RMB)	Cost of saving a HCC patient (RMB)*
Survey HCC from natural population	¥ 2400	¥ 19000
Population with hepatitis history	¥ 600	¥ 4800
Clinical HCC		¥ 24000

* With 5-year survival
RMB, Renminbi yuan (Chinese dollar)

B. High-risk Population – Factors Involved

In our SCHCC patients the median age was 47.5, the male to female ratio being 15.7 : 1; 63% of the patients had a history of hepatitis, 77.8% of these for over 5 years (median, 10 years); abnormal ALT and clinical (not pathological) evidence of cirrhosis were observed in only 10% and 7% respectively. The overall rate of exposure to HBV markers (mainly HBsAg and/or anti HBc) was 93.5%. From the viewpoint of trying to detect HCC early enough for a curative procedure with an acceptable cost-effect ratio, it is suggested that people – especially men aged 30–59 years – who have had a history of hepatitis for over 5 years, and/or with positive serum HBsAg or anti HBc, and/or with cirrhosis but compensated liver function, and without a marked elevation of ALT are candidates for AFP serosurvey.

VII. Suggestions and Problems to Be Solved

Our suggestion is to perform an AFP survey annually in high-risk populations as mentioned above, or to encourage such people, through an intensive educational campaign, to have AFP checked. It should be noted that AFP survey is an important means of discovering SCHCC. Ultrasound is of value for early detection of AFP-negative SCHCC. However, the majority of occupying lesions without AFP and liver disease background detected by ultrasonography were proved surgically to be hemangiomas.

Endeavors should be made to investigate the following: new tumor markers for early detection of AFP-negative HCC; positive scanning by using isotope-labeled specific antibody for localization of small HCC; effective conservative treatment of small HCC with noncompensated cirrhosis; and measures for preventing the recurrence of small HCC after radical resection.

References

Ando K, Okita K, Watanabe S et al (1981) A proposal of high-risk group for the early diagnosis of hepatocellular carcinoma. Acta Hepatol Jpn 22: 1162–1170

Axtell IM, Cutler SJ, Myers MH (1972) End results in cancer – report No 4. US Department of Health, Education and Welfare, Public Health Service, NIH, NCI, Bethesda, pp 72–76

Chen DS, Sheu JC, Sung JL et al (1982) Small hepatocellular carcinoma – a clinicopathological study in thirteen patients. Gastroenterology 83: 1109–1119

Foster JH, Berman MM (1977) Solid liver tumors. Saunders, Philadelphia, pp 62–104

Hiroshi O, Makoto T, Nadaki H et al (1976) Development of hepatocellular carcinoma on the ground of chronic liver diseases – prospective study in 59 cases of liver cirrhosis. Acta Hepatol Jpn 17: 335–347

Ishikawa K (1976) Follow-up study of patients with primary liver cancer. Report 3. Acta Hepatol Jpn 17: 460–465

Li B, Li JY (1980) National survey of cancer mortality in China. Chin J Oncol 2: 1–10

Mahmood K, Schatzki PF (1976) Solitary small hepatocellular carcinoma. Am J Digest Dis 21: 496–502

Okuda K, Kotoda K, Obata H et al (1975) Clinical observations during a relatively early stage of hepatocellular carcinoma, with special reference to serum alpha fetoprotein levels. Gastroenterology 69: 226–234

Okuda K, Nakashima T, Obata H, Kubo Y (1977) Clinicopathological studies of minute hepatocellular carcinoma – analysis of 20 cases, including 4 with hepatic resection. Gastroenterology 73: 109–115

Okuda K, Kasai Y, Sugawara K et al (1980) Primary liver cancers in Japan. Cancer 45: 2663–2669

Purves LR, Geddes EW (1972) A more sensitive test for alpha fetoprotein. Lancet 1: 47–48

Shimoyama T, Kitasato S, Fujitomi Y et al (1980) A study of minute hepatocellular carcinoma – clinicopathologic observation on 4 resected cases. Acta Hepatol Jpn 21: 1008–1015

Takashima T, Matsui O, Suzuki M, Ida M (1982) Diagnosis and screening of small hepatocellular carcinoma – comparison of radionuclide imaging, ultrasound, computed tomography, hepatic angiography, and α-fetoprotein assay. Radiology 145: 635–638

Tang ZY (1980) Screening and early treatment of primary liver cancer – with special reference to the eastern part of China. Ann Acad Med Singapore 9: 234–239

Tang ZY, Yu YQ, Lin ZY et al (1979a) Small hepatocellular carcinoma – clinical analysis of 30 cases. Chin Med J [Engl] 92: 455–462

Tang ZY, Yu EX, Wu CE, Gu XY (1979b) Diagnosis and treatment of primary hepatocellular carcinoma in early stage – report of 134 cases. Chin Med J [Engl] 92: 801–806

Tang ZY, Yang BH, Tang CL et al (1980) Evaluation of population screening for hepatocellular carcinoma. Chin Med J [Engl] 93: 795–799

Tang ZY, Lu JZ, Zhou NQ et al (1982a) Small hepatocellular carcinoma (HCC). VI. Value of hepatoarteriography, B-scan ultrasonography, and liver scintiscan in the localization of small HCC – a comparative study based on operative findings. Acta Acad Med Primae Shanghai 9: 101–105[1]

Tang ZY, Ying YY, Gu TJ (1982b) Hepatocellular carcinoma – changing concepts in recent years. In: Popper H, Schaffner F (eds) Progress in liver disease, vol VII. Grune and Stratton, New York, pp 637–647

The Coordinating Group for the Research of Liver Cancer, China (1978) Further investigation on alpha fetoprotein in mass survey and follow-up studies of primary hepatocellular carcinoma. Natl Med J China 58: 586–588[1]

Zhu YR, Lu BX (1983) Clinical implication of AFP serosurvey. Chin J Oncol 5: 38–40[1]

[1] in Chinese

3 New Concepts of Diagnosis of Subclinical Hepatocellular Carcinoma

Tang Zhao-you, Yang Bing-hui

The diagnosis of hepatocellular carcinoma has long been acknowledged as one of the most difficult tasks in cancer diagnosis; however, great advances have been made during the past decades. The diagnosis of HCC has progressed from "postmortem diagnosis" in the 1930s, through "clinical diagnosis", to "subclinical diagnosis" in the 1970s. In the process, the concept involved in early diagnosis of HCC has been changed from combined analyses of symptoms, signs, enzymologic findings, and nuclide imaging to that of AFP and ALT levels, their serial change and interrelationship.

I. Brief History of Diagnosis of HCC

A. Postmortem Diagnosis

In 1937, Gustafson reported 62 cases of PLC. Of the 62, accurate clinical diagnosis was obtained in only seven cases (11.3%); the remaining were diagnosed postmortem. The extremely late disease stage was also notable because of its frequent association with jaundice (51.6%) and ascites (45.2%) (see Table 1). In 1948, 55 cases were reported by Rosenberg and Oshsner, accurate clinical diagnosis being made in only 13 (23.6%). A mean survival of 2.8 months strongly indicated that PLC was indeed an incurable disease.

B. Clinical Diagnosis

With the advances made in hepatic enzymology, ultrasonography (type A), nuclide imaging, and hepatic angiography, diagnostic accuracy has increased by 36% (MacDonald 1957), 30% (Ervasti 1964), and 40% (San Jose et al. 1965) to 86% (Alpert et al. 1969). However, no remarkable changes in disease stage at diagnosis could be observed either in China or in the West.

C. Subclinical Diagnosis

Thanks to research in the field of AFP, the diagnosis of HCC has progressed from the clinical to the subclinical stage since the 1970s. The discovery of AFP in the serum of HCC patients (Tatarinov 1964), its application in mass survey (Shanghai Coordinating Group on Research of Liver Cancer 1973), and monitoring in chronic

Table 1. Incidence of jaundice and ascites in primary liver cancer patients during past decades

Series	No. of cases	With	
		Jaundice (%)	Ascites (%)
1930 Wu and Kang	11	63.7	72.8
1937 Gustafson	62	51.6	45.2
1948 Rosenberg and Oshsner	55	44	54
1956 Zhong and Chan	107	37.3	38.3
1964 Ervasti	100	43	23
1974 Tang and Yang	3254	37.5	43.3
1976 Okuda	134	29.9	49.3

liver disease (Okuda et al. 1975) have resulted in great advances in the diagnosis of SCHCC. Selective celiac or hepatic arteriography, the superselective technique using a twist catheter, infusion hepatic arteriography, and real-time ultrasonography are responsible for advances in the localization of small HCC.

II. Comparison of Clinical and Laboratory Findings in SCHCC and CHCC

In an analysis of 387 cases of PLC from 1961 to 1970 in Zhong Shan Hospital of the Shanghai First Medical College, the incidences of symptoms were as follows: upper abdominal pain constituting 60.1%, anorexia 59.8%, weight loss 49.0%, weakness 44.6%, abdominal mass 38.1%, fullness in the epigastrium 28.0%, and fever 21.5%. The liver was firm, irregular, and enlarged in the majority of cases (Yang and Tang 1982a). However, no obvious HCC symptoms or signs were presented clinically in 100 cases of SCHCC.

Marked differences were also noted in comparing laboratory findings, as well as in medical imaging of SCHCC and CHCC (Tables 2 and 3). It should be mentioned that many conventional measurements which had provided valuable information for diagnosis of CHCC, such as γ-GTP, ALP, scintigraphy, etc. were of little value in the diagnosis of SCHCC. Of those markers and imaging measurements available, only AFP, angiography and real-time ultrasonography seemed to be acceptable for diagnosis of SCHCC.

Table 2. Comparison of laboratory findings in SCHCC and CHCC patients

Items (%)	SCHCC	CHCC
γ-GTP > 10 units	24.7 (22/ 89)	77.0 (315/409)[a]
ALP > 13 units	22.5 (20/ 89)	56.9 (235/413)[a]
5′-NPDase V (+)	60.0 (15/ 25)	62.9 (39/ 62)
ALT > 40 units	10.0 (10/100)	20.7 (96/464)
OT test > 5 mm	79.0 (64/ 81)	59.7 (184/308)[a]
X-ray diaphragm sign (+)	7.8 (6/ 77)	35.7 (112/314)[a]

[a] $P < 0.01$

Table 3. Comparison of angiography, ultrasonography, and scintigraphy in SCHCC and CHCC

(%)	SCHCC	CHCC
Angiography (+)	86.5 (32/37)	86.4 (19/ 22)
B-ultrasonography (+)	59.5 (22/37)	94.2 (98/104)[a]
A-ultrasonography (+)	8.3 (7/84)	70.5 (284/403)[a]
Scintigraphy (+)	32.0 (31/97)	88.8 (362/430)[a]

[a] $P<0.01$

III. Diagnosis of SCHCC by AFP

Of the 100 cases of SCHCC, 98 were initially diagnosed by AFP test; the remaining two were detected by real-time ultrasonography. Only a limited number of patients in this series had positive findings with γ-GTP and ALP tests, angiography, ultrasonography, and/or scintigraphy (Tables 2 and 3). Diagnosis was based mainly on AFP findings in a good number of SCHCC cases. Experience gained during the past 10 years or more has indicated that combined analysis of levels of AFP and ALT, their kinetic patterns, and the interrelationship of AFP and ALT curves are of prime importance (Tang et al. 1978, Tang and Yang 1981).

A. AFP Level

It has long been documented that AFP is produced by fetal liver and the yolk sac, with small amounts also produced by the gastrointestinal tract, resulting in the appearance of AFP in some patients with hepatitis, cirrhosis, teratoma of gonads, GI-tract cancers, etc. (Abelev 1971). However, the AFP level seldom exceeded 500 ng/ml in the above disorders (Bagshawe and Cameron 1976). In contrast, 90.5% of CHCC patients in a series of HCC patients with abnormal AFP had levels ≥ 500 ng/ml. Consequently, the AFP level of 500 ng/ml was universally accepted as the diagnostic level of HCC. If a patient had an AFP level ≥500 ng/ml, HCC was strongly indicated, and if the AFP level did not exceed 500 ng/ml, hepatitis or cirrhosis in the active stage had to be excluded first. As shown in Table 4, of the 98 patients with SCHCC who showed abnormal AFP levels, 22 (22.4%) had AFP < 500 ng/ml, the lowest level being 150 ng/ml with the tumor measuring 1.5 × 1.0 cm. It is our opinion that the patient with AFP around 200 ng/ml is a candidate to be carefully studied.

Table 4. Comparison of AFP levels in SCHCC and CHCC patients

	CHCC	SCHCC
Median AFP (ng/ml)	2000	4750
Median tumor size (cm)	98.0 (98/100)	10.0
AFP > 20 ng/ml %	4.5	70.1 (317/452)
AFP < 500 ng/ml in patients with abnormal AFP %	22.4 (22/ 98)	9.5 (30/317)[a]

[a] $P<0.01$

B. Serial Change in AFP

Three principal types of AFP kinetic curves were observed in this series: (a) Low (around 50 ng/ml) but gradually rising – amounting to 10.2% (10/98); (b) persistent moderate level (around 200 ng/ml) – 21.4% (21/98); (c) persistent high level (> 500 ng/ml) – 67.3% (66/98). A saddle curve was observed in only one case. It deserves to be mentioned here that relatively small HCC was observed in those with "low but rising" and "persistent moderate level" curves, as compared with those with "persistent high level" curves (see Fig. 1). To sum up, those patients who show persistent or rising AFP curves are most likely to be HCC cases, and the majority of those who show declining AFP will eventually prove to be hepatitis or cirrhosis cases.

C. Alanine Aminotransferase Level

It is necessary to emphasize that the diagnosis of SCHCC should be combined with an analysis of the ALT level and its serial change, which is especially important in regard to the differential diagnosis of hepatitis and cirrhosis in active-stage liver disease (ALD). Generally, ALD should be more seriously considered than HCC when the value of ALT is several times the normal; however, HCC should not be excluded in cases with a slight elevation of ALT.

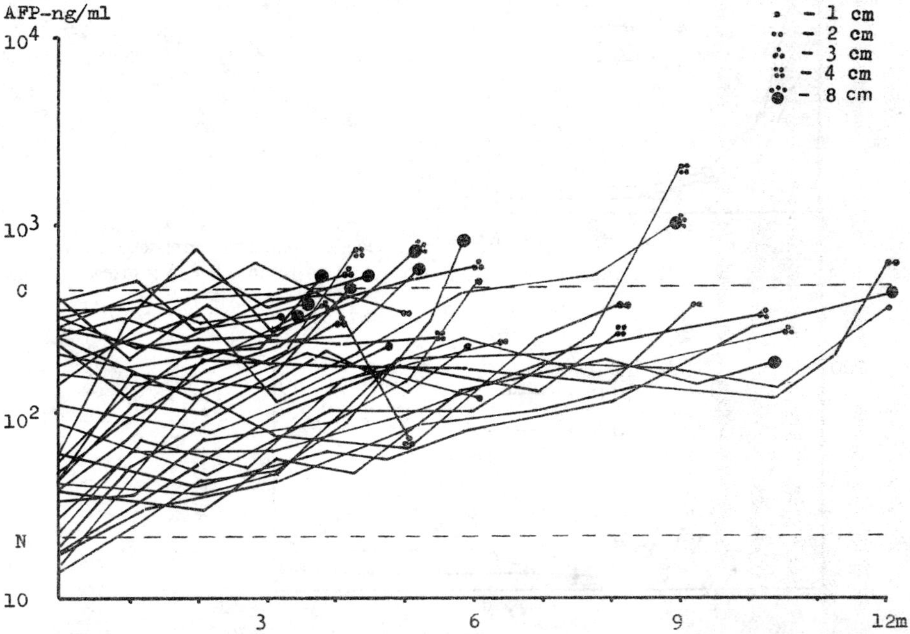

Fig. 1. Serial change of AFP level in 33 SCHCC patients undergoing surgical resection, showing tumor size and AFP level

D. *Interrelationship Between AFP and ALT Curves*

In cases where abnormal ALT is determined, serial observation of AFP and ALT curves is of prime importance. Generally, ALD often produces similar or correlated curves of AFP and ALT in serial monitoring; however, the divergence of the two curves suggests that SCHCC is likely to be present (Figs. 2 and 3).

E. *Diagnostic Criteria of AFP*

Several diagnostic criteria of AFP have been established in China. One of the widely accepted is positive CIEP or AFP ⩾500 ng/ml persisting over 1 month, with pregnancy, ALD, and teratoma of gonads excluded (National Conference for Liver Cancer Control 1977).

However, it has been mentioned with regard to this series that if diagnostic criteria are set at a level of AFP ⩾500 ng/ml, at least 22.4% of SCHCC cases will be missed; therefore, the diagnosis of SCHCC at a relatively low AFP level is made with positive CIEP persisting over 3 weeks, or AFP ⩾200 ng/ml for more than 8 weeks, provided ALT is normal and pregnancy and gonad teratoma can be excluded. The period between AFP diagnosis and appearance of symptoms in 15

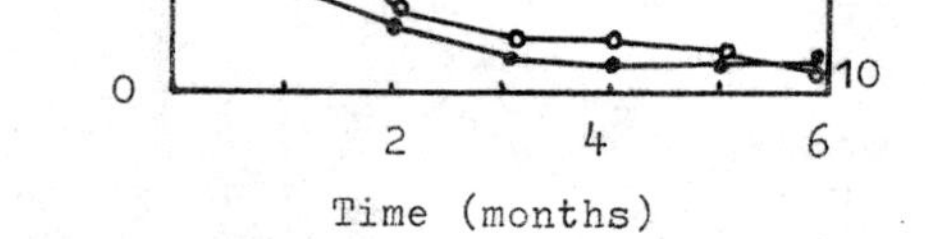

Fig. 2. Similar or correlated AFP and ALT curves in active liver diseases

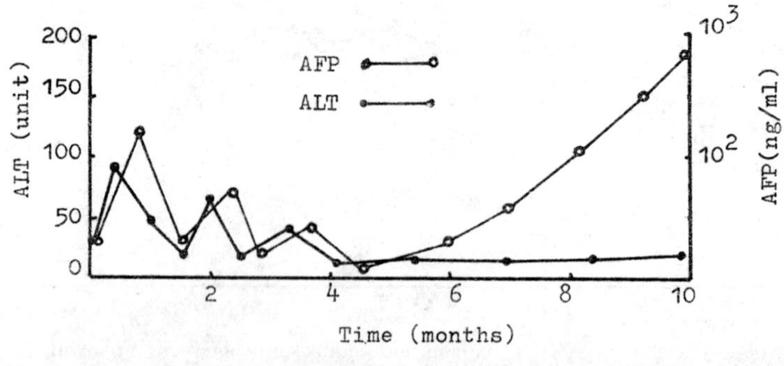

Fig. 3. Divergence of AFP and ALT curves usually suggests SCHCC

pathologically proven SCHCC cases treated conservatively ranged from 2 to 18 months, averaging 7.9 months. The accuracy rate has been reported to be as high as 98% (Tang et al. 1978, 1979a).

F. Key Link to Further Improvement in Diagnostic Level of SCHCC

The median size of SCHCC tumors in this series was 4.5 cm (range 0.8–16 cm) – not very small compared with other subclinical cancers, such as those of the esophagus, stomach, breast, cervix, etc. (around 1 cm). Therefore, further improvement in the diagnostic level of SCHCC is necessary. In contrast to the earlier report that tumor size in CHCC (with huge tumors) was not related to AFP level (Purves 1976), the authors have demonstrated, on the basis of operative findings, a general correlation between AFP level and median tumor size in SCHCC (Tang et al. 1983a; Table 5) as well as between tumor size and median AFP level in small HCC (Tang 1982; Table 6). It should be noted that the median AFP level in HCC ⩽2.0 cm was 385 ng/ml, and that the median tumor size was 1.75 cm at AFP levels ⩽300 ng/ml. It seems that the key link to further improvement in the diagnostic level of SCHCC is to establish the diagnosis at a relatively low AFP level (around 200 ng/ml), especially in those patients with "low but gradually rising" and "persistent moderate" AFP curves. In the meantime, superselective infusion hepatic arteriography will be of great value in the diagnosis. However, it must be kept in mind that the lower the AFP level, the less the specificity to HCC, and ALD is one of the major possibilities to be excluded, particularly in those patients with abnormal serum ALT, bilirubin, prothrombin time, and γ-GTP.

Table 5. AFP level and median tumor size

AFP (ng/ml)	Median tumor size (cm)
⩽300	1.75
⩽500	2.75
501– 5000	3.0
5001–10000	5.0
10001–30000	5.5
>30000	7.5

Table 6. Tumor size and median AFP level

Tumor size (cm)	AFP (ng/ml)	
	Median	Range
⩽2.0	385	190– 1500
2.1–3.0	1500	400– 6000
3.1–4.0	1500	250–30000
4.1–5.0	4000	290–25000

IV. Role of Other Markers in Diagnosis of SCHCC

Some markers other than AFP have been claimed to be of value in the diagnosis of HCC, including γ-glutamyl transpeptidase isozyme (Sawabu et al. 1980), 5′-nucleotide phosphodiesterase isozyme V (5′-NPDase V; Tsou and Lo 1980; Lu et al. 1981), α_1-antitrypsin (Oon et al. 1980), and ferritin (Kumada et al. 1981; Chapman et al. 1982). Some have been reported to be useful in the diagnosis of AFP-negative HCC, but unfortunately none of them have proved to be helpful in the early diagnosis of

SCHCC. Kaneto et al. (1980) reported that abnormal serum ferritin was detectable in four out five small HCC cases, thus giving a clue to the diagnosis of SCHCC. As shown in Table 2, the authors demonstrated comparable positivity of abnormal serum 5′-NPDase V in SCHCC and CHCC (60.0% and 62.9% respectively); however, this isozyme was also positive in 45.5% of patients with various benign hepatobiliary diseases or tumors other than HCC (Yang and Tang 1982b). Of those tumor markers tested, AFP remains the best for early diagnosis of SCHCC (Tang et al. 1983b).

V. Localization of SCHCC

A. Hepatic Angiography

The hepatic arteriographic features of 190 cases of HCC were reviewed by Okuda (1978); tumors as small as 1 cm could be detected (Okuda 1976; Tang et al. 1978). The smallest tumor detected by transumbilical hepatography and confirmed by op-

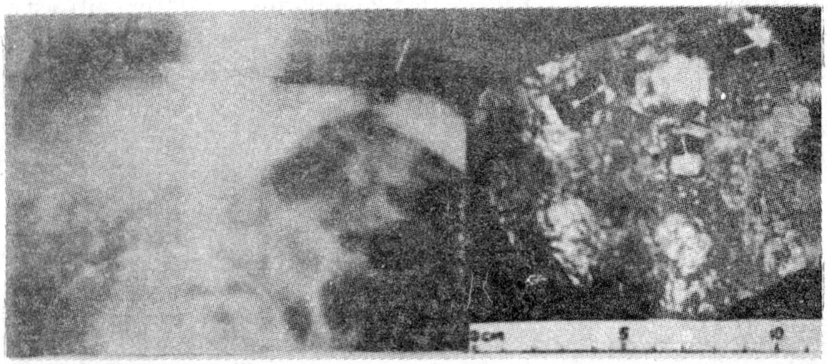

Fig. 4. Transumbilical hepatography showing a filling defect in left lateral segment, confirmed surgically to be a small HCC (2.5 × 2.5 cm)

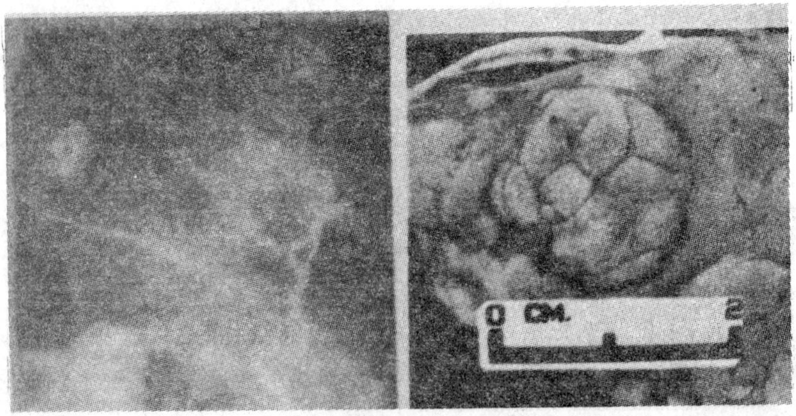

Fig. 5. A 1.2-cm small HCC confirmed by surgery was shown as tumor stain in selective arteriography

eration was found to be 2.5 × 2.5 cm (Fig. 4); however, this procedure produced negative shadow and failed to show small HCC in the right lobe in the majority of cases (Zhou et al. 1975). Selective celiac or hepatic arteriography was accepted as the modality of choice for localization of small HCC. Similar positivity rates were obtained with SCHCC and CHCC (86.5% and 86.4% respectively). Superselective hepatic arteriography using the twist catheter (Ando et al. 1980) and the infusion technique (Takashima and Matsui 1980) were claimed to be of importance in localization of HCC with a diameter smaller than 2 cm. Tumors as small as 1 cm were

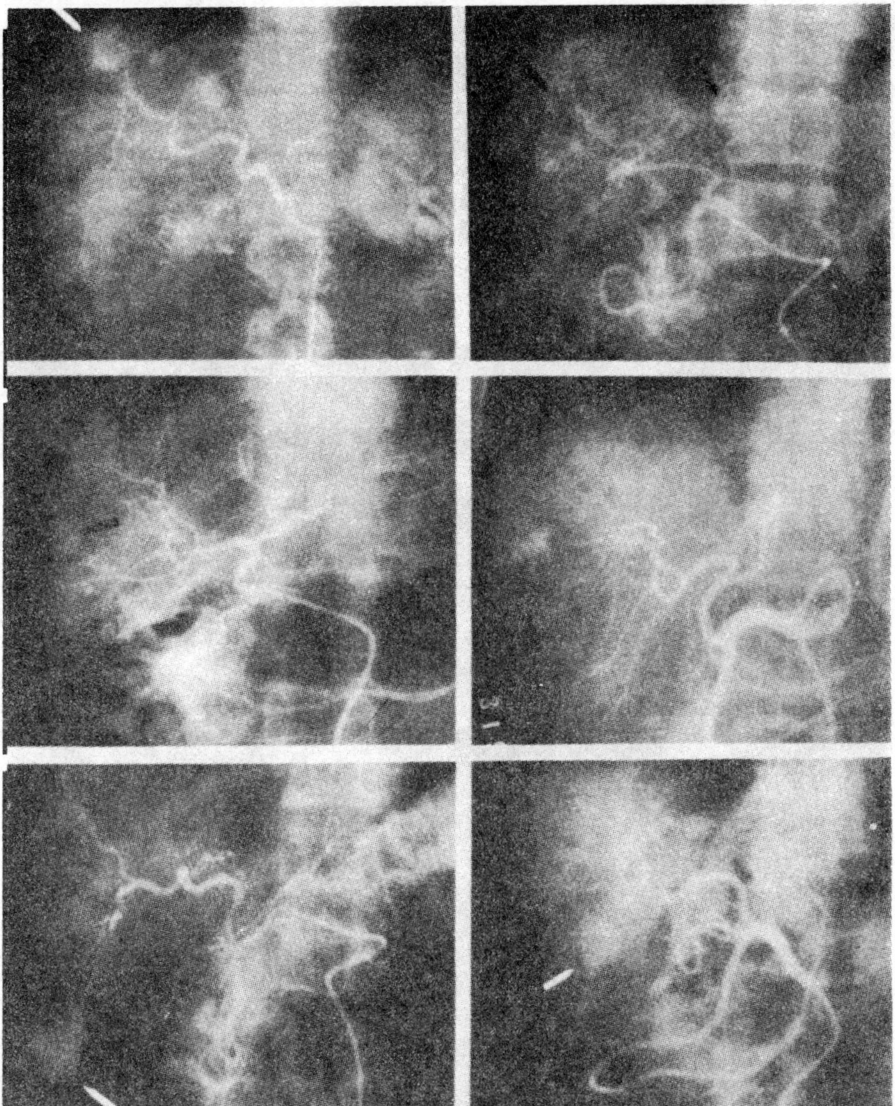

Fig. 6. Several pictures showing tumor vessels and tumor stain of small HCC

shown to be of the hypervascular type (Fig. 5). Tumor vessels and tumor stain were the two distinctive features of small HCC in selective arteriography (Fig. 6). "Ring-like" tumor vessels were often seen as a special feature of early-phase arteriography in HCC of 1–2 cm (Fig. 7). The smallest diameter detectable by this technique was considered to be 1 cm; for tumors of the hypovascular type and those located in the left lobe it was found to be unsatisfactory.

B. Ultrasonography

Real-time US has been acknowledged as an ideal noninvasive approach for localization of hepatic tumors and is less expensive than CT. Echo patterns correlated with histological findings have been thoroughly studied (Shinagawa et al. 1981). In our series, the positivity rate of US in CHCC (94.2%) was as high as that of other imaging measurements; although it was lower (59.5%) in SCHCC, it was still much higher than that of nuclide imaging (32.0%; Table 3). The detection limit with US was considered to be 2 cm (Tang et al. 1982a; Fig. 8).

To our knowledge, the value of US in SCHCC patients can be summarized as follows: (a) US is an ideal noninvasive initial screening procedure for localization, and

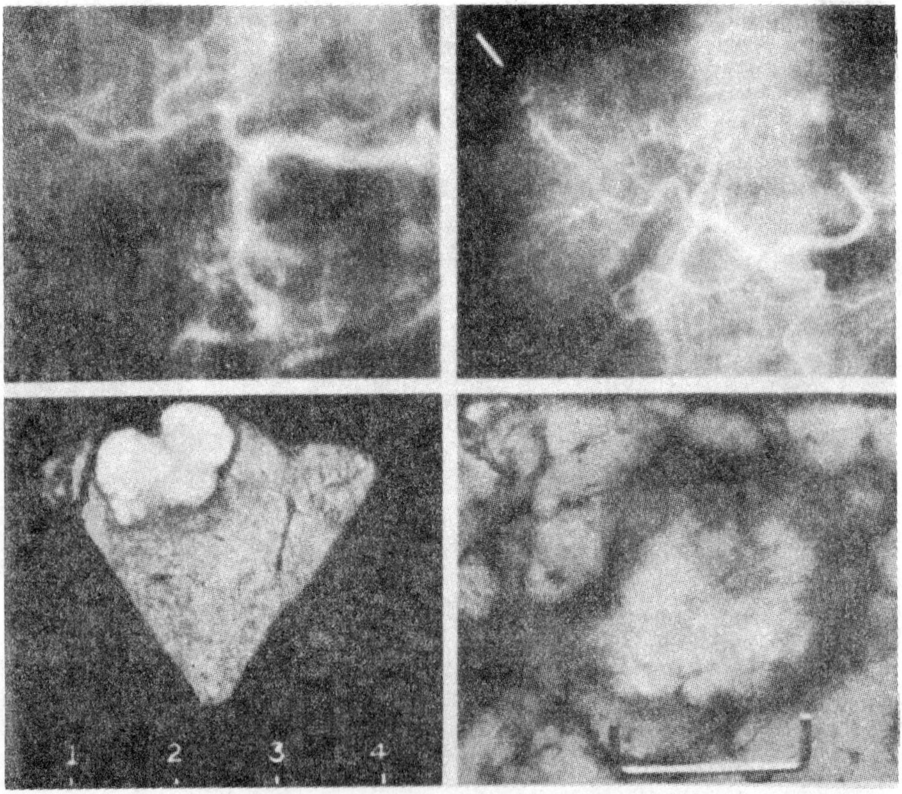

Fig. 7. "Ring-like" tumor vessels (arrows) in small HCC of 1–2 cm in early-phase arteriography

thus of help in diagnosing SCHCC. (b) US is of value in determining tumor emboli in the portal vein, and can be employed as a guide for selecting the mode of therapy. (c) US is less expensive than CT, avoids much exposure to radiation, and is of value in repeated monitoring after conservative treatment. (d) US may be an effective approach for early detection of AFP-negative SCHCC. However, we have encountered only two cases of AFP-negative SCHCC detected by US; the majority of space-occupying lesions detected by US without association of AFP and HBV markers (mainly HBsAg and anti-HBc) proved to be hepatic hemangiomas under surgery.

C. Computed Tomography

Another noninvasive measure for localization of HCC is CT. It was noted that in the majority of HCC cases, the difference in density between the tumor and the surrounding parenchyma was so small that the relatively lucent area might easily be overlooked (Yeh 1979). Dynamic CT using a bolus injection of contrast medium

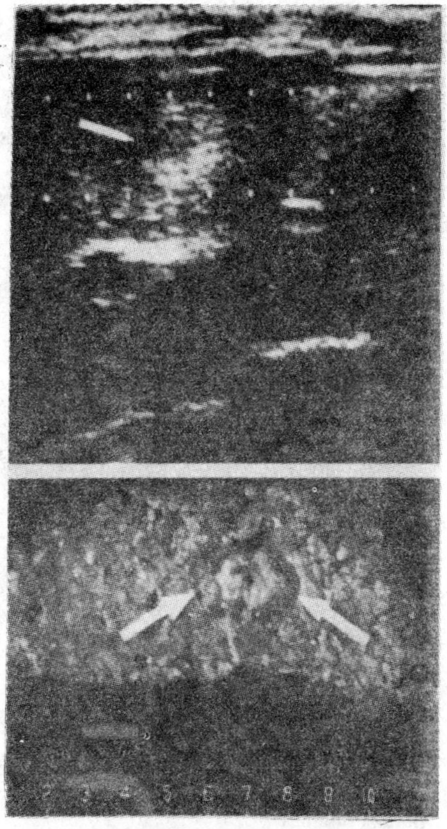

Fig. 8. A hyperecho shadow was confirmed surgically to be a small HCC measuring 2 cm in diameter

was claimed to be helpful (Araki et al. 1980). In a series of 47 cases of HCC, 37 were definitely identified, with results equivocal in five cases and negative in the other five (Itai et al. 1979). The detection rate was reported to be as high as 94% (15/16) (Kunstlinger et al. 1980). In China, in a series comprising 38 cases of pathologically proven HCC, positive findings were made in 37 cases; 62.2% of these presented low-density areas, including four cases with HCC smaller than 5 cm (Su et al. 1982).

D. Radionuclide Imaging

Radionuclide imaging remains a valuable tool for the localization of CHCC; unfortunately, its use for the localization of SCHCC has been disappointing. As shown in Table 3, the positivity rate of RN for detecting SCHCC was much lower than that obtained for CHCC (32.0% versus 88.8%), its detection limit is considered to be 3 cm. Radioimmunodetection, however, presents a hopeful means for localizing small HCC in the future. ^{131}I-labeled goat IgG against human AFP was reported to be of value in detecting and localizing AFP-containing tumors in vivo (Goldenberg et al. 1980), small HCC being also detected in three of four cases (Munehisa et al. 1981).

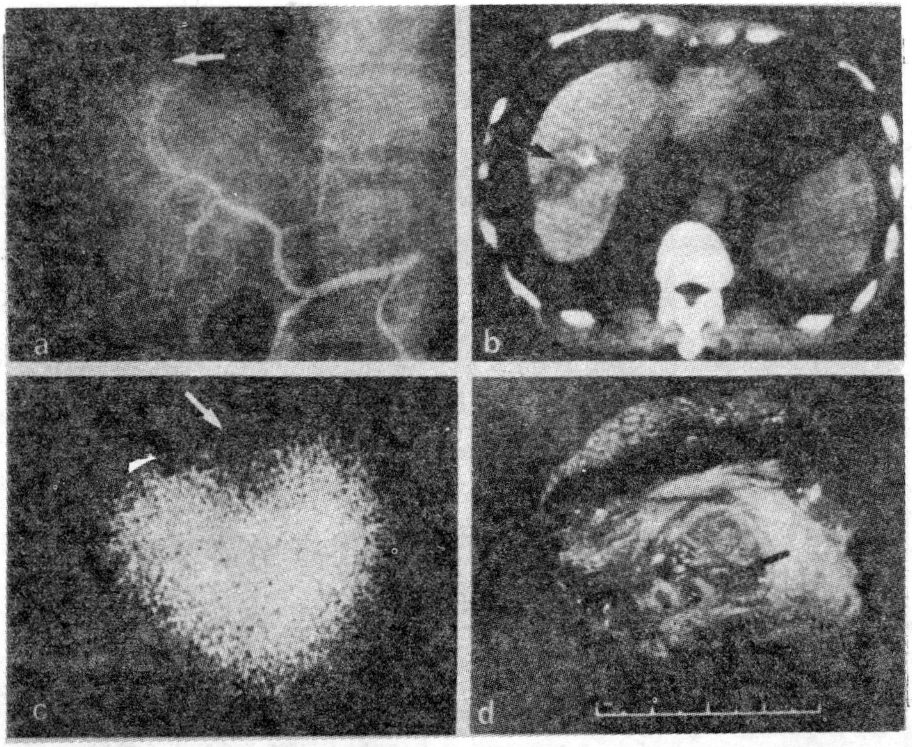

Fig. 9 a–d. Localization of small HCC by (**a**) angiography, (**b**) computed tomography, and (**c**) nuclide imaging in AFP-negative patient, compared with (**d**) surgical specimen. *Arrows* indicate important findings

Table 7. Tumor size and positivity rates of various imaging procedures[a]

Tumor size (cm)	Angiogram (+) %	Sonogram (+) %	Scintigram (+) %
≤3.0	85.7 (12/14)	37.5 (3/ 8)	10.0 (2/20)
3.1– 5.0	87.5 (7/ 8)	66.7 (10/15)	53.8 (14/26)
5.1–10.0	88.9 (8/ 9)	94.4 (17/18)	79.6 (39/49)
>10.0	100.0 (4/ 4)	100.0 (9/ 9)	100.0 (25/25)

[a] All rates in box are acceptable levels of positivity

E. Comparison of Localization Procedures

The findings in a series of pathologically proven HCC cases by means of HA, US, and RN, verified by surgery, demonstrated that the positivity rates of HA, US, and RN were all acceptable (92.3%, 96.3%, and 86.5% respectively) in HCC with a diameter >5 cm; however, great differences were shown in HCC 3.1–5.0 cm (87.5%, 66.7%, and 53.8%) and in HCC ≤3 cm (85.7%, 37.5%, and 10.0%) (see Table 7). Moreover, only 93.0%, 66.7% and 60.0% of the actual tumor size could be demonstrated by these methods respectively. Data showed that the smallest HCC size for differentiation was 1.2 cm with HA, 2 cm with US, and 3 cm with RN. Results indicated that meticulous US detection by a good hand was useful as noninvasive initial screening and follow-up monitoring for SCHCC. Angiography remained the best method for localization of SCHCC, but it should be used selectively when US and RN have failed, RN being promising only for large tumors (Tang et al. 1982a; Fig. 9).

Similar results were also reported by Takashima et al., sensitivity being 39% with RN, 50% with US, 56% with CT, and 94% with infusion HA. Lesions larger than 3 cm could be detected by all of these methods; those between 2 and 3 cm were generally shown by US and CT but not by RN. Infusion HA was essential for diagnosis of lesions smaller than 2 cm. AFP and US were recommended to minimize expense and radiation exposure, and infusion HA was performed only in questionable cases (Takashima et al. 1982).

VI. Problems with Diagnosis of SCHCC

Problems to be worked on include early diagnosis of AFP-negative HCC; differential diagnosis of AFP-positive HCC with abnormal ALT or other markers representing ALD, and ALD with abnormal AFP; and noninvasive localization of HCC <2 cm. Therefore, research is necessary on tumor markers other than AFP and on radioimmunodetection with specific antibody or monoclonal specific antibody.

References

Abelev GI (1971) Alpha fetoprotein in ontogenesis and its association with malignant tumors. Adv Cancer Res 14: 295–358

Alpert ME, Hutt MSR, Davidson CS, et al (1969) Primary hepatoma in Uganda – a prospective clinical and epidemiologic study of forty-six patients. Am J Med 46: 794–802

Ando K, Kodama T, Okita K, et al (1980) Simplification of superselective hepatic arteriography by "twist catheter." Acta Hepatol Jpn 21: 999–1007

Araki T, Itai Y, Furui S, Tasaka A (1980) Dynamic computed tomography densitometry of hepatic tumors. AJR 135: 1037–1043

Bagshawe A, Cameron HM (1976) The clinical problem of liver cell cancer in a high-incidence area. In: Cameron HM, Linsell DA, Warwick GP (eds) Liver cell cancer. Elsevier, Amsterdam, pp 45–60

Chapman RW, Bassendine MF, Lanlicht M, et al (1982) Serum ferritin and binding of serum ferritin to concanavalin A as a tumor marker in patients with primary liver cell cancer and chronic liver disease. Digest Dis Sci 27: 111–116

Ervasti J (1964) Primary carcinoma of the liver – a pathologic and clinical study of 100 cases. Acta Chir Scand 334: 1–65

Goldenberg DM, Kim EE, Deland F, et al (1980) Clinical studies on the radioimmunodetection of tumors containing alpha-fetoprotein. Cancer 45: 2500–2505

Gustafson EG (1937) An analysis of 62 cases of primary carcinoma of the liver based on 24000 necropsies at Bellevue Hospital. Ann Intern Med 11: 889–900

Itai Y, Nishikawa J, Tasaka A (1979) Computed tomography in the evaluation of hepatocellular carcinoma. Radiology 131: 165–170

Kaneto A, Kubo Y, Nagasak Y, et al (1980) Clinical evaluation of serum ferritin in hepatocellular carcinoma and liver cirrhosis. Acta Hepatol Jpn 21: 745–753

Kumada T, Nakano S, Ohta H, et al (1981) Clinical evaluation of serum ferritin on the diagnosis for hepatocellular carcinoma. Jpn J Gastroenterol 78: 2367–2375

Kunstlinger F, Federle MP, Moss AA, et al (1980) Computed tomography of hepatocellular carcinoma. AJR 134: 431–437

Lu HM, Chen J, Jiang KL, et al (1981) The value of serum 5′-nucleotide phosphodiesterase isozyme in the diagnosis of primary liver cancer. Natl Med J China 61: 219–221[1]

MacDonald RA (1957) Primary carcinoma of the liver – a clinicopathologic study of one hundred eight cases. Arch Intern Med 99: 266–279

Munehisa T, Nakata K, Furahori A, et al (1981) Clinical studies on minute hepatocellular carcinoma. Jpn J Gastroenterol 78: 2376–2383

National Conference for Liver Cancer Control, China (1977) Criteria for diagnosis, clinical staging, and typing, and assessment of therapeutic response of primary liver cancer. Shanghai Bull Cancer Control 4: 125–126[1]

Okuda K (1976) Clinical aspects of hepatocellular carcinoma – analysis of 134 cases. In: Okuda K, Peter RL (eds) Hepatocellular carcinoma. New York, John Wiley & Sons, pp 387–436

Okuda K, Kotoda K, Obata H, et al (1975) Clinical observations during a relatively early stage of hepatocellular carcinoma, with special reference to serum alpha fetoprotein levels. Gastroenterology 69: 226–234

Okuda K, Obata H, Kubo Y, Nakashima T (1978) Early diagnosis and angiographic features of hepatocellular carcinoma. In: Remmer H, Bolt HM, Bannasch P, Popper H (eds) Primary liver tumors. MTP Press, Lancaster, pp 149–164

Oon CJ, Yo SI, Chio LF, et al (1980) The evaluation of tumor marker proteins in the diagnosis of primary hepatocellular carcinoma. Ann Acad Med Singapore 9: 228–233

Purves LR (1976) Alpha-fetoprotein and the diagnosis of liver cell cancer. In: Cameron HM, Linsell DA, Warwick GP (eds) Liver cell cancer. Elsevier, Amsterdam, pp 61–80

Rosenberg DML, Oshsner A (1948) Primary carcinoma of the liver – an analysis of fifty-five autopsied cases, the record of a case with resection, and a review of the recent literature. Surgery 24: 1036–1068

San Jose D, Cady A, West M, et al (1965) Primary carcinoma of the liver – analysis of clinical and biochemical features of 80 cases. Am J Digest Dis 10: 657–674

Sawabu N, Nakagen M, Ozaki K, et al (1980) Novel γ-GTP isoenzyme as diagnostic tool for hepatocellular carcinoma. Ann Acad Med Singapore 9: 206–209

Shanghai Coordinating Group for Research on Liver Cancer (1973) AFP serosurvey in diagnosis and screening of hepatocellular carcinoma. Natl Med J China 53: 455–457[1]

Shinagawa T, Ohto M, Kimura K, et al (1981) Real-time ultrasonographic diagnosis of hepatocellular carcinoma – correlation of echograms and histopathological findings. Jpn J Gastroenterology 78: 2402–2411

Su XZ, Li GZ, Jin FL (1982) Computed tomography in diagnosis of hepatocellular carcinoma. Chin Med J [Engl] 95: 543–547

Takashima T, Matsui O (1980) Infusion hepatic angiography in the detection of small hepatocellular carcinoma. Radiology 136: 321–325

Takashima T, Matsui O, Suzuki M, Ida M (1982) Diagnosis and screening of small hepatocellular carcinoma – comparison of radionuclide imaging, ultrasound, computed tomography, hepatic angiography, and α-fetoprotein assay. Radiology 145: 635–638

Tang ZY (1980) Screening and early treatment of primary liver cancer – with special reference to the eastern part of China. Ann Acad Med Singapore 9: 234–239

Tang ZY (1982) Resection of minute hepatocellular carcinoma. Postgraduate Course in IASL-APASL Meeting, Hong Kong

Tang ZY, Yang BH (1974) Primary liver cancer – clinical analysis of 3254 cases (from 11 provinces, 21 hospitals, in China). Tumor Prevent Treat Study 2: 207–215[1]

Tang ZY, Yang BH (1981) Clinical evaluation of alpha-fetoprotein as tumor marker for hepatocellular carcinoma. Chin J Oncol 3: 205–209[1]

Tang ZY, Yu YQ, Zhou XD, et al (1978) Small hepatocellular carcinoma. VI. Diagnosis of small hepatocellular carcinoma. Acta Acad Med Primae Shanghai 5: 118–125[1]

Tang ZY, Yu YQ, Lin ZY, et al (1979a) Small hepatocellular carcinoma – clinical analysis of 30 cases. Chin Med J 92: 455–462

Tang ZY, Yang BH, Zhou XD (1979b) Advances in early diagnosis of primary liver cancer in China. Chin J Oncol 1: 233–235[1]

Tang ZY, Yang BH, Tang CL, et al (1980) Evaluation of population screening for hepatocellular carcinoma. Chin Med J 93: 795–799

Tang ZY, Lu JZ, Zhou NQ, et al (1982a) Small hepatocellular carcinoma (HCC). VI. Value of hepatoarteriography, B-scan ultrasonography, and liver scintiscan in the localization of small HCC – a comparative study based on operative findings. Acta Acad Med Primae Shanghai 9: 101–105[1]

Tang ZY, Ying YY, Gu TJ (1982b) Hepatocellular carcinoma – changing concepts in recent years. In: Popper H, Schaffner F (eds) Progress in liver diseases, vol VII. Grune and Stratton, New York, pp 637–647

Tang ZY, Yu YQ, Zhou XD, et al (1982c) Research on small hepatocellular carcinoma. Chin Sci and Technical Literature Publishers, Beijing, pp 7–11[1]

Tang ZY, Yu YQ, Lin ZY, Yang BH (1983a) Subclinical hepatocellular carcinoma. Chin J Oncol 5: 226–228[1]

Tang ZY, Yu YQ, Lin ZY, et al (1983b) Clinical research of primary liver cancer – A 10-year (1970–1979) survey. Chin Med J [Engl] 96: 247–250

Tatarinov Y (1964) Detection of embryo-specific α-globulin in the blood sera of patients with primary liver tumors. Vopr Med Khim 10: 90–91

Tsou KC, Lo KW (1980) Serum 5′-nucleotide phosphodiesterase isozyme for human liver cancer. Cancer 45: 209–213

Wu CJ, Kang HJ (1930) Primary carcinoma of the liver. Natl Med J China 16: 234–243[1]

Yang BH, Lin ZY, Tang ZY (1981) Diagnosis of subclinical hepatocellular carcinoma. Chin J Digest 1: 101–103[1]

Yang BH, Tang ZY (1982a) Improvement in diagnosis and treatment of primary liver cancer – an analysis of 1045 cases. Chin J Oncol 4: 279–282[1]

Yang BH, Tang ZY (1982b) Evaluation of 5′ nucleotide phosphodiesterase isozyme V for the diagnosis of primary liver cancer. Acta Acad Med Primae Shanghai 9: 275–278[1]

Yeh HC (1979) Ultrasonography and computed tomography of the liver. In: Popper H, Schaffner F (eds) Progress in liver diseases, vol VI. Grune and Stratton, New York, pp 519–537

Zhong XL, Chan HJ (1956) Primary liver cancer – analysis of 107 cases. Chin J Int Med 4: 169–171[1]

Zhou XD, et al (1975) Transumbilical hepatography for diagnosis of primary liver cancer. Natl Med J China 55: 265–269[1]

Zhou XD, Tang ZY, Yu YQ, et al (1975) Transumbilical hepatography for diagnosis of primary liver cancer. Natl Med J China 55: 265–269[1]

---

1 In Chinese

4 Real-Time B-Mode Ultrasonography in Localization of Subclinical Hepatocellular Carcinoma

Xu Zhi-zhang

Since 1959 the attempt to detect liver carcinoma by means of A-mode ultrasound has met with some success in China (Shanghai Ultrasonic Medical Research Group 1961 a). It was found that the wave patterns in liver carcinoma were different from those in normal liver and other hepatic diseases (An et al. 1962); 90.2% of 132 cases of hepatic carcinoma produced the typical echogram. In 1960, ultrasonotomography was performed with the ultrasound compound B-scanner, named the BP-mode, and produced at the Shanghai First Medical College. Several kinds of abnormal sonograms were noted in patients with hepatic carcinoma (Shanghai Ultrasonic Medical Research Group 1961 b); however, the method was not sensitive enough, since the machine performance was rather inferior in the early stage, with only a bi-stable display for sonograms (term "bi-stable" used by Wells 1977).

Since the introduction of the gray scale B-scanner in the 1970s (Taylor et al. 1973, 1974; Sample et al. 1975; Cosgrove 1978), the ultrasonic imaging technique for hepatic carcinoma has made great progress. Furthermore, some important improvements have been made in machine performance, such as quantitative gain setting, dynamic focusing, image memory capacity, image processing and some advanced recording techniques. All of these improvements have made the quality of the sonogram better and the diagnostic procedure easier and more efficient.

Real-time ultrasound scanners increase the sonogram frame rate – generally 24–30 frames/s – so that the ultrasound images are displayed on a screen when the ultrasound probe is placed on the body surface of a patient. The best advantage of the real-time scanner is that the space relationship between the local lesion and intrahepatic structures or extrahepatic organs can be shown by moving or tilting the probe; it is therefore very useful for localization of space-occupying lesions in the segments or lobes of the liver.

I. Equipment

It is necessary that equipment be selected for obtaining the best sonograms on ultrasound examination. Some important characteristics of hepatic sonography are as follows:

A. High Sensitivity and Low Noise

Since low-level backscattered echoes originate from the fine internal tissues of liver just above the level of electronic noise of the equipment (generally −100 to

– 120 dB), a low-noise (or good signal-to-noise ratio) amplifier must be selected. For the lowest echo display, a high-sensitivity (or high-gain) amplifier is needed (usually 60 to 100 dB).

B. Sufficient Gray Scales

The total range of reflected hepatic echoes containing low, medium, and high level signals may be divided into several degrees for display from black to white, called the "gray scales", on the TV oscilloscope. The higher the echo level, the brighter the display. Consequently, the greater the number of gray scales, the better the echo differentiation. Because many of the hepatic tumors to be detected have acoustic properties differing only slightly from those of normal liver (Cosgrove 1978), 16 gray scales are sufficient for optimal display on a hepatic sonogram, and 32–64 gray scales are still more efficient for tumor detection.

C. Dynamic Focused Beam Characteristics

In the electronic linear scanner, a focused beam improves lateral resolution efficiently, facilitating detection of smaller space-occupying lesions. Furthermore, a focused beam concentrates the ultrasonic energy along the beam axis so that it can penetrate more deeply in ultrasound examination. The best lateral resolution point is just at the focused area, generally 1 cm distant, and 3–4 focused points at distinct depths on the sound beam path are called dynamic focused beams, which are more suitable for improving the lateral resolution on the entire beam path from surface to deep areas.

D. Freeze Frame

With a freeze frame it is easy to capture the appointed sonogram which is always changing during the examination. A freeze frame also saves time and has excellent recording quality.

E. Gain Quantification and Decibel Display

The echo level of some hepatic tumors differs from that of normal liver tissue by as little as 2 dB. Gain quantification is useful in adjusting for optimal identification. It may be displayed as the dB value on TV screen, and is found to be advantageous for follow-up study. A complete function of gain quantification comprises three settings, namely, total gain, near gain (suppression), and far gain control.

F. Types of Real-Time B-Scan

A real-time B-scan produced by rapid sequential movement of the ultrasound beam may illuminate the underlying soft tissues. Two different forms of beam movement may be employed: linear scanning, which means that the sound beam moves in parallel form to obtain a sonogram of a rectangular section, and sector scanning, which means that the sound beam moves in sequential angle displacement form to obtain an arc section or sector view. The linear scan displays an isometric figure and gives similar lateral resolution from superficial to deep areas, contributing substantially to hepatic examination. Especially when the liver is enlarged, the linear scanning process is convenient for a subcostal approach with the transducer placed beneath the costal margin. The sector scan is suitable only for small acoustic windows (through intercostal space), where the liver is not enlarged.

II. Liver Scanning Techniques

A. Preparation and Posture

In general, no preparation is necessary. However, when colon distention is present the gas content in the transverse colon and the hepatic flexure prevents ultrasound penetration and may make the examination very difficult. An enema may be employed to improve the situation.

The patient should be lying in a horizontal or left lateral position during ultrasonic scanning.

B. Ultrasound Approaches (Taylor and Hill 1975; Shen et al. 1983)

Subcostal approach. With the multicrystal transducer tucked under the costal margin and tilted cephalad, a series of subcostal oblique sections can be obtained. The gall bladder, the main portal vein, the left portal vein with its umbilical portion, and the inferior vena cava (IVC) are displayed. A line joining the long axis of the gall bladder to the IVC separates the right hepatic lobe from the left (Fig. 1); another line connecting the ligamentum teres to the ligamentum venosum through the umbilical portion of the left portal vein separates the lateral segment of the left hepatic lobe from its medial segment (Fig. 2). When the scanning plane is tilted slightly upwards, the hepatic veins and IVC can be found. Generally, the right and the middle hepatic veins, and the IVC can be displayed simultaneously, whereas the left hepatic vein should often be displayed on another scanning plane. The middle hepatic vein separates the right lobe from the left; the right hepatic vein separates the cephalic portion of anterior segment from the posterior segment of the right hepatic lobe; and the left hepatic vein separates the cephalic portion of the lateral segment from the medial segment of the left hepatic lobe (Fig. 3).

Sagittal sections. When the transducer is placed on the right lower thoracic wall, down to the epigastrium parallel to the middle line, several pictures of the sagittal

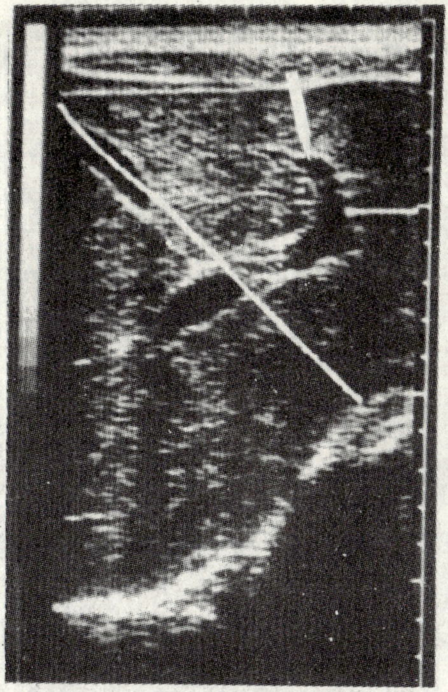

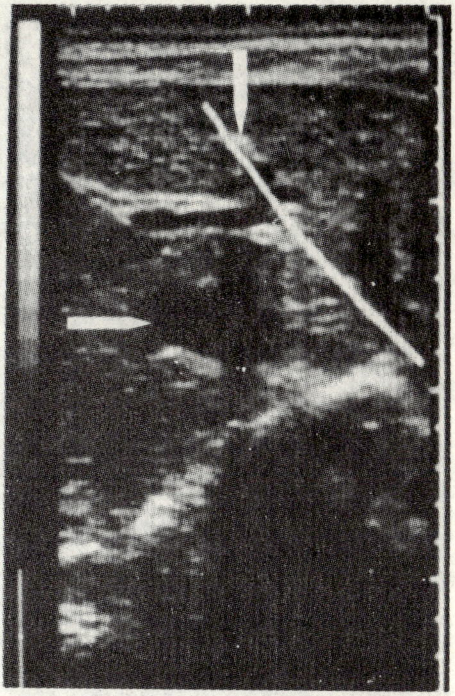

Fig. 1 *(left)*. Subcostal sonogram through the gallbladder, main portal vein, and IVC. The left portal branch with its umbilical portion *(arrow)* is also displayed. An oblique line joining the long axis of the gallbladder to the IVC divides right lobe and left lobe

Fig. 2 *(right)*. Subcostal sonogram tilted slightly cephalad from the plane of Fig. 1. A line joining the ligamentum teres *(vertical arrow)* to the ligamentum venosum through the umbilical portion of the left portal branch separates the medial and lateral segments of the left lobe. A *transverse arrow* indicates oblique section of the IVC

section can be made, from lateral to medium. On the more lateral sagittal section through the right kidney, the long section of the long branch of the right hepatic vein can be displayed, which separates the anterior segment from the posterior segment of the right hepatic lobe (Fig. 4), and a second level of the right portal vein may be found under this long branch. A vertical line drawn through this right portal second-level branch separates the upper portion from the lower portion of the right hepatic posterior segment (Fig. 4).

When the transducer is placed on the middle clavicular line, the middle hepatic vein, the common bile duct, the main portal vein, and IVC may be shown (Fig. 5). On the upper portion of this view the gallbladder, and sometimes the common hepatic duct, can be seen.

Oblique sections. These sections are made approximately near the right angles to the right costal margin; they help to show the whole path of the main portal vein and the common bile duct. Part of the IVC long section may also be displayed (Fig. 6).

These sub-costal, sagittal, and oblique sections are valuable for visualizing the intrahepatic vascular systems and biliary tracts, as well as their relationship to the sur-

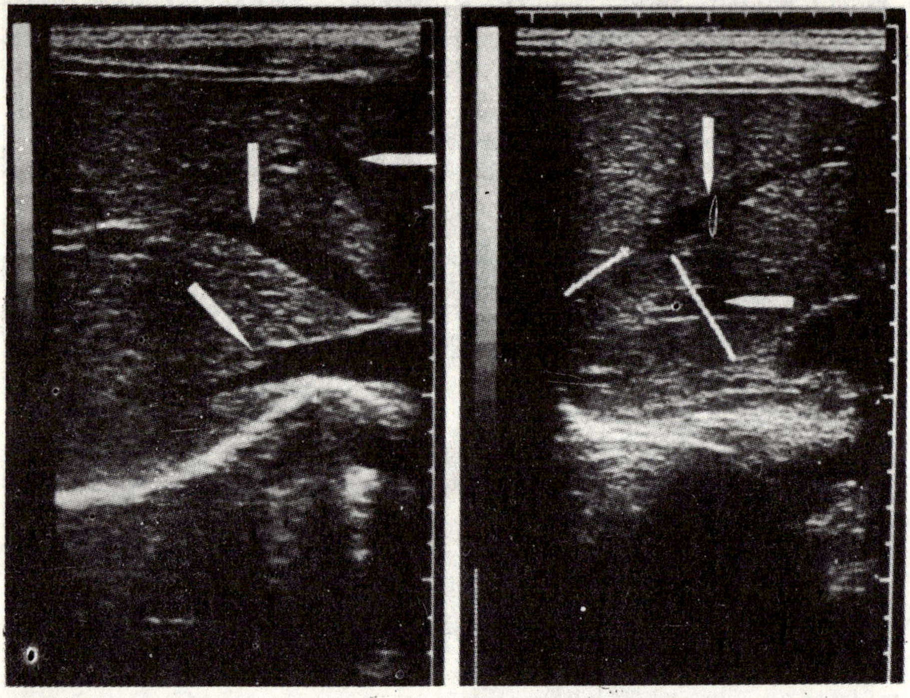

Fig. 3 *(left).* Subcostal sonogram tilted more cephalad from the plane of Fig. 1, demonstrating three branches of the hepatic vein. The middle hepatic vein *(vertical arrow)* separates the right lobe from the left. The left hepatic vein *(transverse arrow)* and right hepatic vein *(oblique arrow)* are also displayed

Fig. 4 *(right).* Longitudinal sonogram of the right lobe displays the long branch of the right hepatic vein *(vertical arrow),* which divides the anterior and posterior segments of the right lobe *(short oblique line). Another line (long, oblique)* through the second level of the right portal branch *(transverse arrow)* and perpendicular to the long branch of the right hepatic vein separates the upper portion from the lower portion of the posterior segment of the right lobe

rounding organs such as the right kidney and pancreas in tumor localization. Other sections such as transverse ones can also be selected for hepatic ultrasonic examination (Carlsen and Filly 1976; Marks et al. 1979).

III. Normal Hepatic Ultrasonogram

Ultrasonograms of normal liver are natural in shape, with the smooth edge bounded by the adjacent organs and structures. The liver is rather soft, and its shape may be deformed by the pulsating of the heart and the abdominal aorta, diaphragmatic breath movement, and changing of posture; it may also be influenced by the location of the right kidney and by distension of the transverse colon, the duodenum, or the stomach. Congenital variation of the liver, such as Riedel's, or caudate, lobe anomaly, must be identified in order to avoid false interpretation of these as neoplasms.

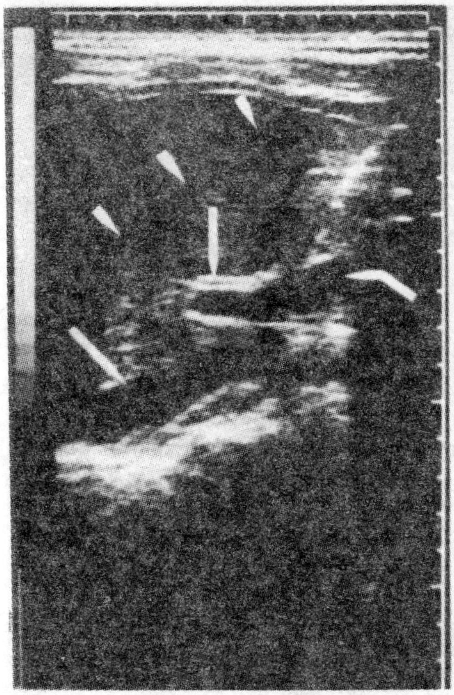

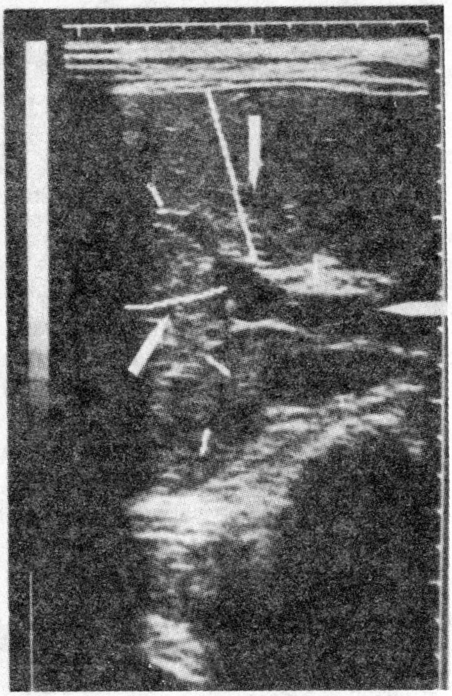

Fig. 5 *(left).* Longitudinal sonogram of the right lobe through the main portal vein *(transverse arrow),* the common bile duct *(vertical arrow),* and the IVC *(oblique arrow).* The entire path of the long branch of the right hepatic vein can also be defined *(small arrows)*

Fig. 6 *(right).* Intercostal sonogram of the right lobe displays the common bile duct, the main portal vein *(transverse arrow),* and the IVC. The *long horizontal line* from the bifurcation of the portal vein through the right hepatic vein *(oblique arrow)* divides the anterior and posterior segments of the right lobe. A *vertical line* from the bifurcation of portal vein through the middle hepatic vein *(vertical arrow)* divides the medial segment of the left lobe and the anterior segment of the right lobe

Reflections from hepatic parenchyma are displayed on the TV screen as diffused uniform bright spots. Care must be taken to adjust for the appropriate gain setting, the near gain suppression, and the far gain compensation. Gain settings should not be constant for all subjects, but should differ according to whether they are thin or obese. Though the normal hepatic sonograms are not standardized owing to different gain settings in different subjects and equipment, recent advances of dynamic beam focusing and gray-scale display techniques have greatly improved the search for space-occupying lesions in hepatic carcinoma.

The portal vein, the hepatic veins, and the biliary tract are three different intrahepatic structures. Generally, the portal vein and its branches have highly reflective walls and can be traced to the hepatic hilum; the hepatic veins and their branches have thin walls, and the right, middle, and left hepatic veins point towards the diaphragm, draining into the IVC; the intrahepatic portions of the biliary tract are small and not obvious, being usually less than 2 mm in diameter, except for the common hepatic duct just above the main portal vein, with its internal diameter of less than 6 mm.

Neither a focal region of echogenic or echo-poor patterns nor discontinuity or compression of the intrahepatic vessel can be found in normal hepatic parenchyma (Figs. 1–6).

IV. Ultrasonograms of Hepatocellular Carcinoma

A. General Presentation of HCC

Echographic presentation of HCC varies and the various patterns may be interpreted as acoustical properties of the individual tumors.

Boundary reflections are the first important phenomenon produced by variations in elasticity of pathological tissues with regard to the contour display of the tumor. Most tumors have regular contours separated from the normal surrounding tissues, but some present deformation of the tumor edge. Sometimes there is a sonolucent halo image around the tumor edge, owing to the loop configuration of the hepatic vein caused by growth of the tumor.

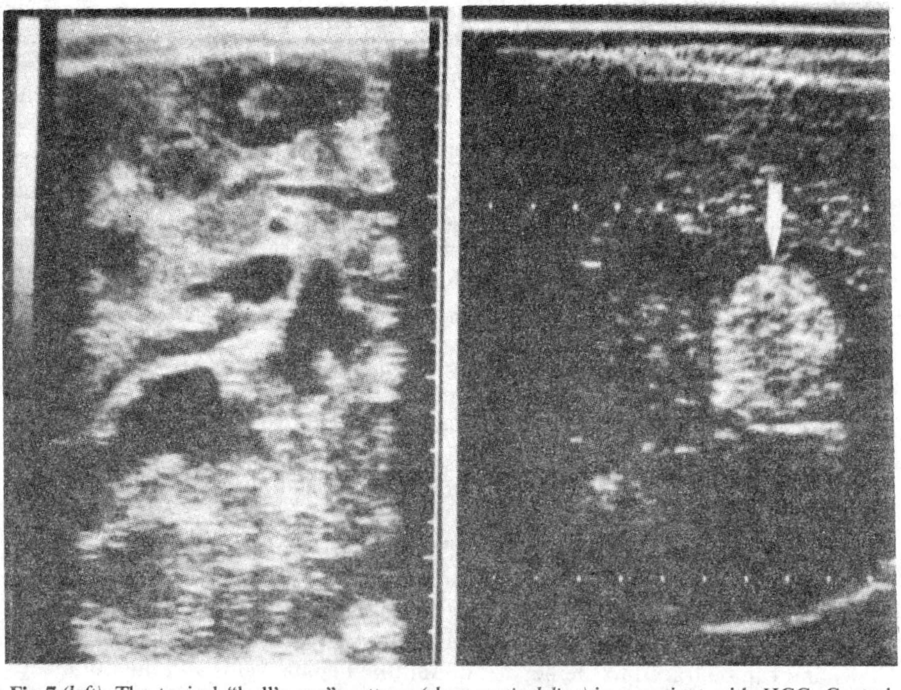

Fig. 7 *(left)*. The typical "bull's eye" pattern *(short vertical line)* in a patient with HCC. Central echogenic region is surrounded by the echo-poor zones, and sometimes another small echo-poor areas appear in the center of the echogenic region

Fig. 8 *(right)*. Echogenic type of HCC. An increased echo nodule with its boundary is well defined *(arrow)*. The internal scattered echoes of the nodule are nonuniform. The acoustical shadow is present in the posterior region

Intratumor scattering echoes are another characteristic of echo patterns, which can be quite complicated in some cases. As compared with those of the adjacent normal parenchyma, the internal patterns may be classified as "echogenic," "echo-poor," "cystic-like," "diffused echo," and "combined type"; however, the precise contribution of these factors has not been established. The presence of fibrous tissue and a small amount of fluid will form the interfaces in a tumor, producing echo-rich reflections. Tumor growth with vascularization, fibrosis, small foci of necrosis, and hemorrhage may result in echogenicity. Echogenicity in a central area with echo-poor reflections arranged around the central echogenic region is termed a "target", or "bull's eye" appearance (Fig. 7). It may be that the surrounding echo-poor region is the result of tissue atrophy produced by an increase in pressure due to the rapid growth of the tumor (Cosgrove 1981).

The third phenomenon is the attenuation effect. In many cases of HCC, increased absorption against the incident ultrasound has been revealed. Tumors with homogeneous structures and normal attenuation will cause low-level echo reflections, presenting echo-poor patterns. In a few cases, a tumor with homogeneous structures and very low attenuation properties will have a cystic-like appearance.

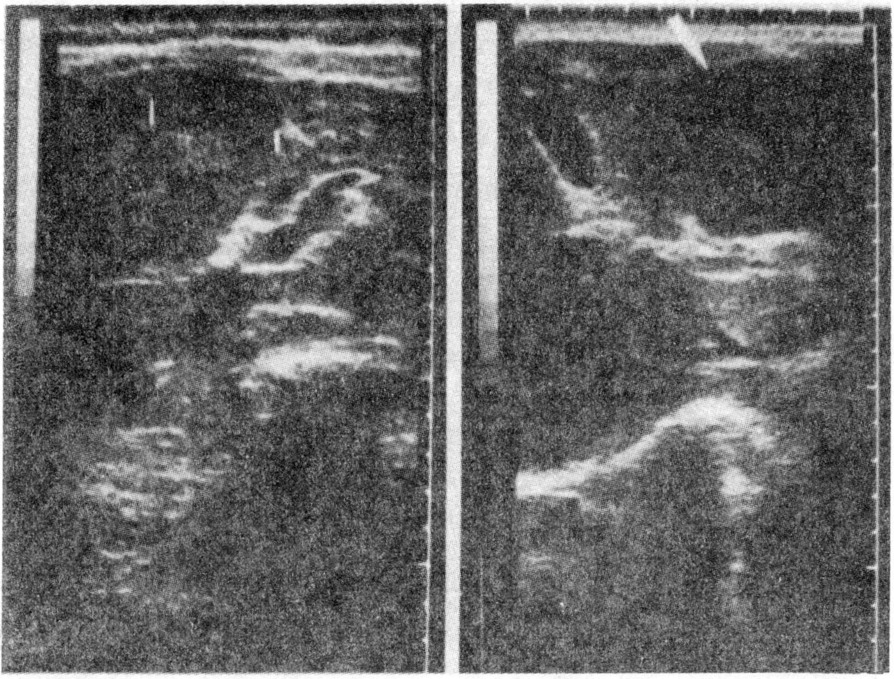

Fig. 9 *(left)*. Echogenic type of HCC with halo image. There are two nodules on the sonogram; both big and small nodules *(vertical lines)* have halo image due to the loop configuration of hepatic vein
Fig. 10 *(right)*. The echo-poor type of HCC. A space-occupying lesion is present with its ill-defined margin *(arrow)*. The anterior surface of the liver is deformed, and the structures of common bile duct *(CBD)* and portal vein are displaced posteriorly. The internal scattered echoes are very poor, with low amplitude, and heterogeneous

"Posterior detail" also serves as a measure of attenuation properties. High-attenuation tumors have fewer echo reflections behind the occupying mass, and this may be termed the "shadowing effect." Conversely, low-attenuation tumors display "posterior enhancement." In other cases there is normal attenuation of the tumor so that neither posterior shadowing nor enhancement can be seen. In the cystic-like type, or in central necrosis of echogenic HCC, posterior enhancement can often be displayed clearly, and should be differentiated from liquid lesions such as hepatic abscesses or cysts.

Our experience showed that in 148 cases of HCC, proved by surgery and pathological examination, echo patterns could be classified into six types:

1. echogenic,
2. echogenic with halo image,
3. echo-poor,
4. combined,
5. diffused echo, and
6. central necrotic (Table 1, Figs. 7–13).

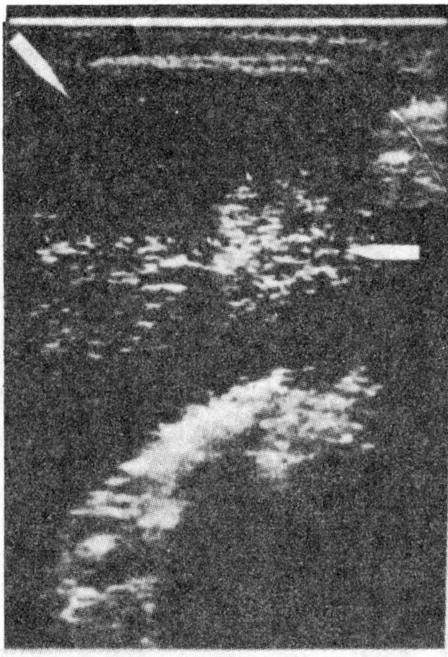
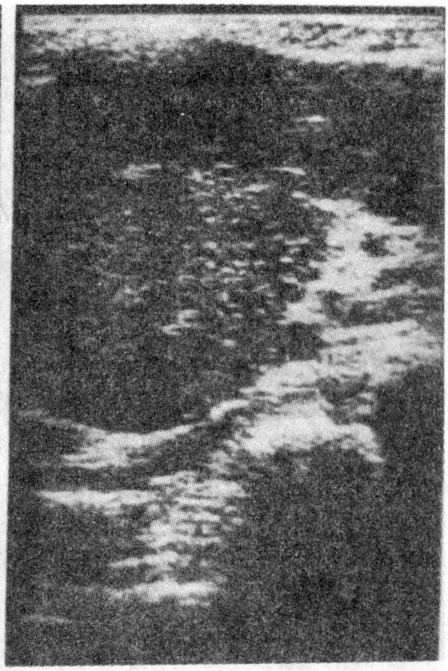

Fig. 11 *(left)*. The combined type of HCC. Two space-occupying lesions are displayed on the echogram. Bull's eye pattern is demonstrated on the upper left *(oblique arrow)*, and the echogenic nodule is displayed on the right *(transverse arrow)*

Fig. 12 *(right)*. The diffused type of HCC. The liver is enlarged, with diffused, coarse echoes. These echoes seem to be more homogeneous than those in other types of HCC

The diagnostic accuracy of US in HCC ranged from 66% to 96.3% (Xu et al. 1982; Kuwajima et al. 1980; Sakaguchi et al. 1979), depending on the different methods of adjusting different types of apparatus, the respective experience of sonographers, and the varying location of space-occupying lesions from patient to patient (Table 2).

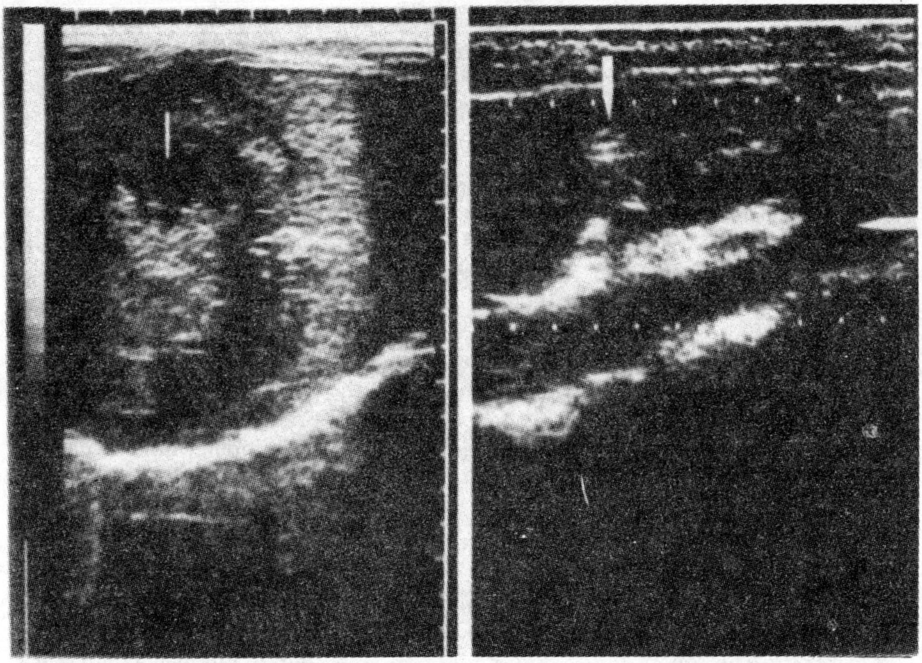

Fig. 13 *(left).* Central necrosis of HCC. There are 4 echogenic nodules on the sonogram. There is central necrosis in the large one with its liquid content *(echo-free region),* and posterior enhancement is present *(vertical line)*

Fig. 14 *(right).* A small nodule of HCC. Near the anterior surface of the liver, a small echogenic nodule is found (11 mm × 11 mm) in the lateral segment of the left lobe *(vertical arrow). Transverse arrow* indicates abdominal aorta

Table 1. Sonographic features of HCC in 148 proven cases (author)

Sonographic patterns	No. of cases	%
Echogenic	63	42.57
Echogenic with halo image	12	8.11
Echo-poor	33	22.30
Combined	11	7.43
Diffused echo	4	2.70
Central necrotic	5	3.38
Undectable	20	13.51

Table 2. Diagnostic accuracy of ultrasound in HCC

Reference	No. of cases	True positive (%)	Overall accuracy (%)
Kuwajima A et al. 1980	–	74.0	89.0
Sakaguchi S et al. 1979	77 (primary) 72 (metastatic)		76.0
Xu et al. 1982	50		66.0
Xu et al. 1982	50	86.2	
Xu et al. 1982	63	88.8	
Xu et al. 1982	54	83.3[a]	
Xu et al. 1982	50	78.0	
Xu and Yang 1983	148	86.49	

[a] From a group of patients who underwent ultrasonically guided hepatic puncture for aspiration biopsy

B. Sonograms of Small HCC

Small HCC means that the tumor is smaller than 5 cm. We have found small HCC in 46 of 169 HCC patients. The echo presentation in the small HCC group included three patterns described above: (a) echogenic in 16, (b) echogenic with halo image in seven, and (c) echo-poor in three; in 20 cases tumors were undetectable by ultrasound.

The smallest echogenic nodule, 11 mm by 11 mm, was found in the lateral segment of the left hepatic lobe and was proved by surgery to be HCC (Fig. 14). This was a special case, in which the abdominal wall was thin and the tumor was situated rather near the transducer. However, a small tumor with a diameter of less than 2 cm is generally rather difficult to detect.

Small HCC with echo-poor presentation is even more difficult to detect than that with an echogenic pattern, because the small region of decreased echo is not visible on the screen, and it simulates the blood vessels in hepatic parenchyma.

There are other difficulties in detecting a small tumor when the nodule is situated in the region of gallbladder, the porta hepatis, the upper lateral part of the right hepatic lobe, or near the upper pole of the right kidney.

The diagnostic accuracy of US in small HCC was 56.5% when the tumor was less than 5 cm in diameter and 37.5% when the tumor was less than 3 cm in diameter (Xu et al. 1982).

No diffused echo pattern was found in the small HCC group, and no central echo-free region in an echogenic figure was displayed in tumors less than 3 cm in diameter.

C. Tumor Localization

Tumor localization is most important for diagnosis and for therapeutic planning. Real-time sonograms are of great help in locating space-occupying lesions situated in the liver lobes and segments. According to the "hepatic sonographic sectional anatomy" described in Sect. II B above, the accuracy of tumor localization was 79.3% (Xu and Yang 1983).

D. Comparison with Other Studies

The different echographic patterns may be correlated to the LDH and AFP blood levels. It has been found that LDH and AFP were higher with solid (echogenic) patterns than with combined or cystic-type patterns (Ito et al. 1980). Some investigators state that the diagnostic accuracy of ultrasound is lower than that of angiography, but higher than that of the radionuclide method, especially in patients with small HCC (Tang et al. 1982; Sakaguchi et al. 1979; Table 3).

E. Ultrasonically Guided Percutaneous Liver Aspiration Biopsy in the Diagnosis of HCC

The real-time B scanner with its specially designed puncture probe is more suitable for percutaneous liver aspiration biopsy. A 22- or 23-gauge fine puncture needle should be selected to avoid complications. With the help of sonographic monitoring, a fine needle can be inserted through the skin and subcutaneous tissues and the needle tip advanced into the space-occupying lesion; a specimen can then be aspirated for cytologic examination. The true positive rate of HCC has been reported at 83.3% (Xu et al. 1982). This method is of great value for differentiating HCC from other space-occupying liver lesions.

F. Portal Vein Invasion

The portal vein may be displayed efficiently on oblique or sagittal sections. When the long axis of the main portal vein is found, the position of the transducer is changed, the main portal vein is traced to the bifurcation of the right and left portal branches, and echo abnormalities are searched for carefully in the portal lumen. Tumor cell thrombi in the portal vein often show echographic content, with regular or irregular contours (Fig. 15); this was found in three of 148 patients in our study, but

Table 3. Comparison of ultrasonography, radionuclide imaging, computed tomography, and angiography for accuracy in the diagnosis of HCC

Reference	Tumor size (cm)	US (%)	RN (%)	CT (%)	HA (%)
Sakaguchi S, et al. 1979	–	75.32 (58/77)	91.67 (55/60)	78.95 (15/19)	96.97 (32/33)
Tang, et al. 1982	>5 cm	96.3	81.5	–	92.3
	⩽5 cm	56.5	34.8	–	86.4
	⩽3 cm	37.5	10.0	–	85.7

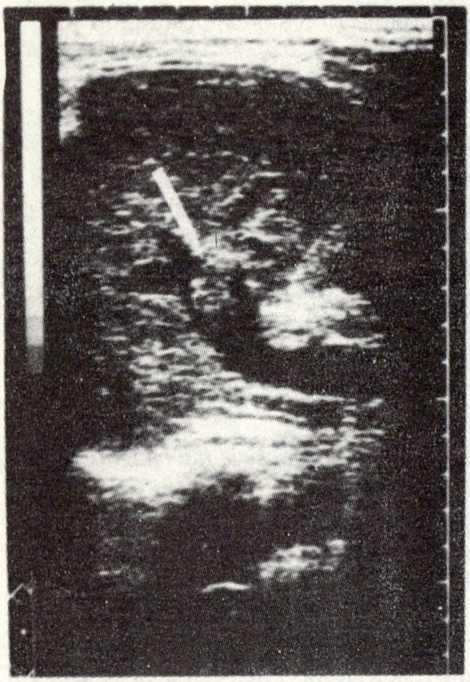

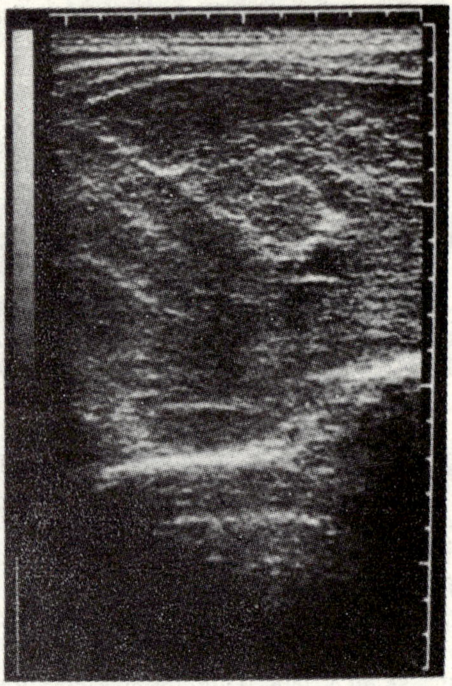

Fig. 15 *(left).* Portal vein invasion. The portal vein is clearly demonstrated in a case of HCC. An additional echogenic area with its irregular margin *(arrow)* is in the portal lumen near the bifurcation of right and left portal branches

Fig. 16 *(right).* Hepatosonogram of liver cirrhosis, showing an echo pattern of diffuse spots and mesh-like strips crossing

nothing abnormal was observed on echographic presentation in four cases of portal invasion confirmed surgically in this group. Portal vein invasion was a contraindication for hepatic resection.

V. Differential Diagnosis

Hepatocellular carcinoma may be confused with many diseases, and a careful differential diagnosis should be made (Green et al. 1977).

A. Liver Cirrhosis

Liver cirrhosis is common in patients with schistosomiasis japonica or chronic hepatitis. There are diffuse, coarse, crowded spots and mesh-like strips crossing on the hepatosonogram, with the spleen enlarged (Figs. 16, 17). Diffuse HCC also presents a diffuse echo in the entire liver with obvious hepatomegaly, but there are fewer mesh-like strips on the sonogram. A serum AFP examination is helpful for differentiation.

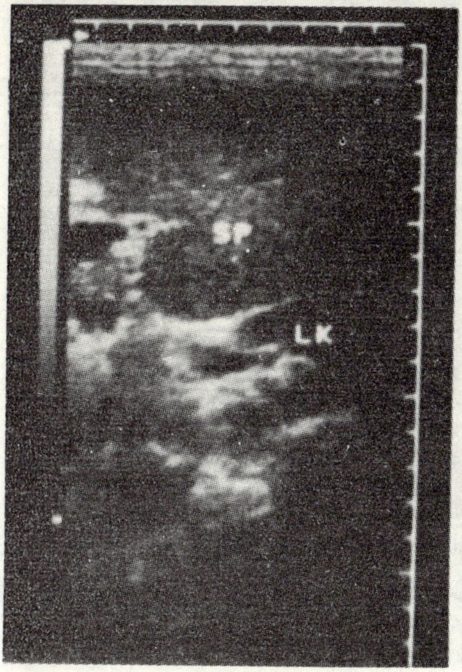

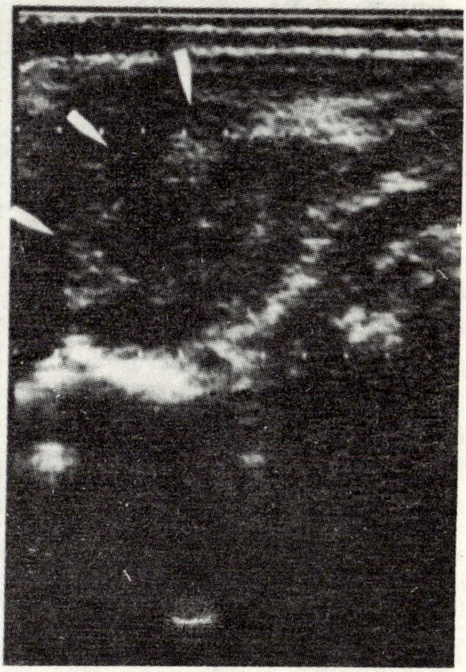

Fig. 17 *(left)*. Splenosonogram of liver cirrhosis. The enlarged spleen is displayed, with increased scattered echoes, in a case of schistosomiasis japonica. *SP*, spleen; *LK*, left kidney
Fig. 18 *(right)*. Capillary hemangioma. An echogenic mass is situated in the left lobe with ill-defined walls *(small arrows)*. The abdominal aorta is displaced by the compression of the tumor

B. Hemangioma

A hemangioma may have various echo reflections. Capillary hemangiomas often present echogenic patterns (Fig. 18), whereas cavernous hemangiomas display echo-free regions (Fig. 19). Multiple minute sonolucent areas in echogenic patterns favor the diagnosis of capillary hemangioma, while multiplicity of various echogenic and/or echo-poor patterns and rapid growth seem to be characteristic of HCC.

C. Hepatic Adenoma

A hepatic adenoma is a benign tumor and has an echogenic pattern which is difficult to differentiate from that of echogenic HCC (Fig. 20). However, hepatic adenomas are rare, being common in women with elevated blood estrogen levels and AFP within the normal range.

D. Hepatic Abscess

An amoebic hepatic abscess or a large, pyogenic hepatic abscess has thickened walls and liquid contents (Fig. 21). When necrosis occurs in HCC it is extremely dif-

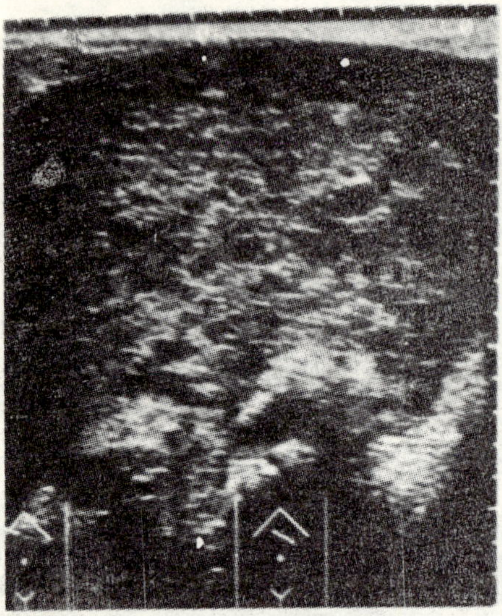

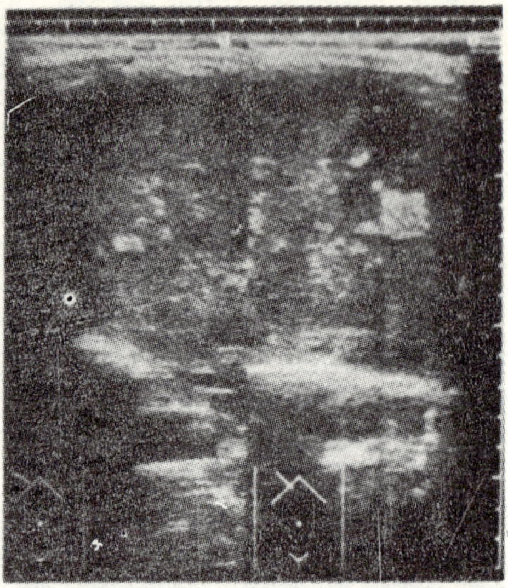

Fig. 19 *(left)*. Cavernous hemangioma. The right lobe is markedly enlarged and displays multiple echo-free (polycystic) lesions

Fig. 20 *(right)*. Hepatic adenoma demonstrates the swelling right lobe and diffused patterns. Some larger bright spots are caused by small foci of calcification

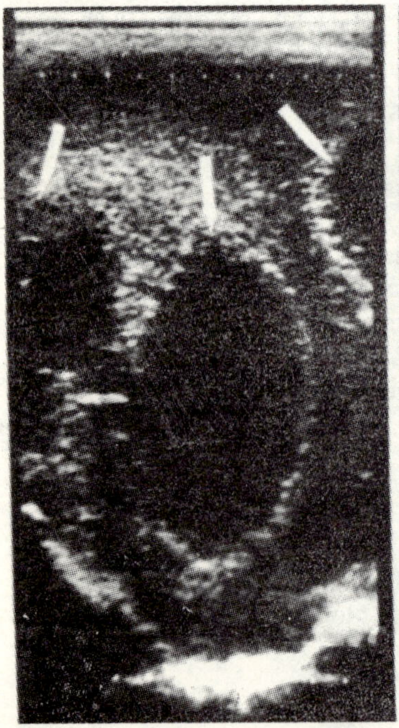

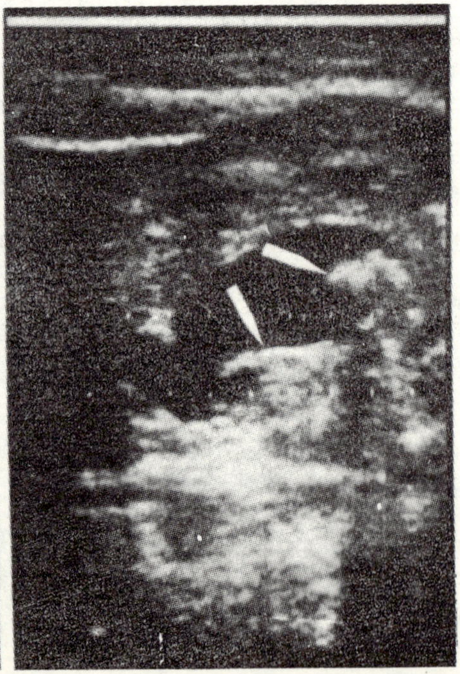

Fig. 21 *(left)*. Right hepatosonogram in a case of amoebic hepatic abscesses. These abscesses *(arrows)* have well-defined walls and liquid contents

Fig. 22 *(right)*. Carcinoma of gallbladder. The diseased gallbladder has thickened wall with the tumor tissue protruding to the bladder cavity *(arrows)*

ficult to distinguish (Fig. 13). Inflammatory leukocytosis and local tenderness are helpful in the diagnosis of liver abscess, which may be confirmed by liver biopsy.

E. Carcinoma of the Gallbladder

Carcinoma of the gallbladder may be confused with HCC in the portal region, the former having a locally thickened wall and tumor tissue possibly protruding into the cavity with an irregular surface (Fig. 22).

F. Right Adrenal Chromatocytic Tumor (Chromaffinoma)

This kind of tumor, originating from the upper pole of the right kidney, can generally be distinguished from the liver tissue. When enlarged, the tumor may press on the posterior margin of the right lobe; it can be differentiated during abdominal respiration. The movement of posterior liver surface has a different range and different manner from that of the anterior surface of the adrenal tumor. In addition, periodic hypertension often occurs in patients with chromatocytic tumors.

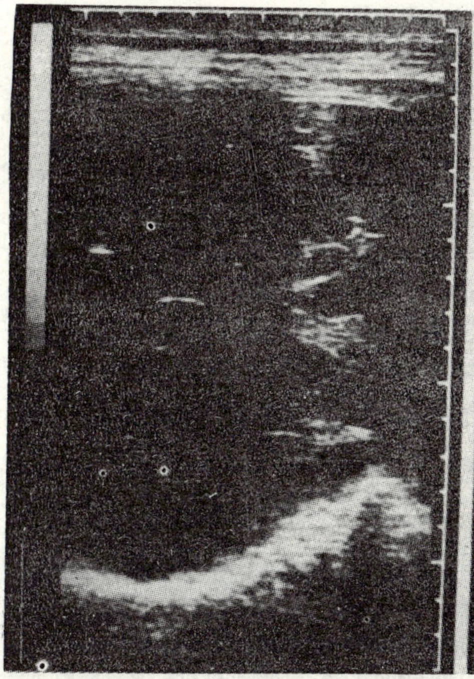

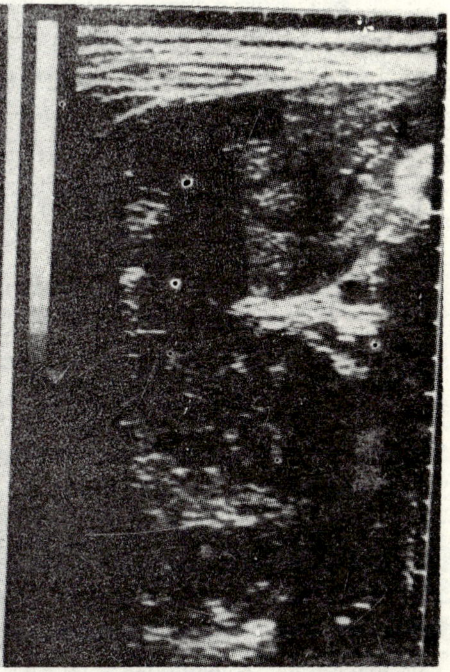

Fig. 23 *(left)*. Metastasis from lymphosarcoma. Multiple echo-poor infiltrations are shown in the right lobe of the liver

Fig. 24 *(right)*. Metastasis from renal carcinoma. Multiple metastases are displayed as echogenic nodules of similar manner and size

G. Metastatic Liver Tumors

As is the case with primary HCC, metastatic liver tumors have various echo patterns (Sumino et al. 1980). If single, the metastatic focus is rather difficult to differentiate from primary malignancy. When multiple metastatic nodules occur they often have the same manner and similar size. Some tumors of primary origin have certain metastatic echo appearances. Carcinoma originating from the breast (Smith et al. 1976) often displays multiple target configuration (Fig. 7); liver metastases from lymphoma, sarcoma, and Hodgkin's disease (Glees et al. 1977) always display homogeneous, echo-poor infiltration (Fig. 23); and metastatic adenocarcinomas originating from the ovary, kidney, pancreas, colon, and stomach have echogenic patterns in the majority of cases (Fig. 24). Calcification of the liver may often be seen in metastatic colonic carcinoma.

References

An S, Wang TH, An SY, et al (1962) The use of pulsed ultrasound in clinical diagnosis. Chin Med J [Engl] 81: 315–325

Carlsen EN, Filly RA (1976) Newer ultrasonographic anatomy in the upper abdomen: I. The portal and hepatic venous anatomy. J Clin Ultrasound 4: 85–96

Cosgrove DO (1978) Evaluation of liver tumors. In: Hill CR, Mc Cready VR, Cosgrove DO (eds) Ultrasound in tumor diagnosis. Pitman, Kent, pp 104–126

Cosgrove DO (1981) Liver. In: Goldberg BB (ed) Ultrasound in cancer. Churchill Livingstone, Edinburgh, pp 1–18

Glees JP, Taylor KJ, Gazet JC, et al (1977) Accuracy of gray-scale ultrasonography of liver and spleen in Hodgkin's disease and the other lymphomas compared with isotope scans. Clin Radiol 28: 233–238

Green B, Bree RL, Goldstein HM, et al (1977) Grey-scale ultrasound evaluation of hepatic neoplasms: patterns and correlations. Radiology 124: 203–208

Ito T, Ochiai Y, Shinagawa A, et al (1980) Comparison of ultrasonography and biochemical data in hepatic cell carcinoma. Japanese Society of Ultrasound in Medicine, Proceedings, Jpn J Med Ultrasonics (Monograph) pp 147–148

Kuwajima A, Aburano T, Tada K, et al (1980) Comparison of ultrasound and adionuclide liver imaging in the detection of focal hepatic lesions. Japanese Society of Ultrasound in Medicine, Proceedings, Jpn J Med Ultrasonics (Monograph) pp 149–150

Marks WM, Filly RA, Callen PW (1979) Ultrasonic anatomy of the liver: A review with new applications. J Clin Ultrasound 7: 137–146

Sakaguchi S, Ozaki T, Ichida F, et al (1979) Ultrasonic diagnosis of liver cancer. 2nd Meeting of WFUMB – 4th World Congress on Ultrasonics in Medicine. SCIMED, Tokyo, (abstract) p 267

Sample WF, Po JB, Gray RK, et al (1975) Gray-scale ultrasonography: techniques in pancreatic scanning. Applied Radiology 4: 63–67, 90–91

Shanghai Ultrasonic Medical Research Group (eds) (1961 a) Diagnostic ultrasound. Shanghai Sci and Technical Publisher, Shanghai, pp 106–110[1]

Shanghai Ultrasonic Medical Research Group (eds) (1961 b) Diagnostic ultrasound. Shanghai Sci and Technical Publisher, Shanghai, pp 233, 258–259[1]

Shen ZW, Xu ZZ, Yang MZ, et al (1983) Application of sectional anatomy of the liver in its echographic lobulation and segmentation. Natl Med J China 63: 602–605[1]

Smith IE, Taylor KJ, McCready VR (1976) A comparison of grey-scale ultrasound with other methods for the detection of liver metastasis from breast carcinoma. Clin Oncol 2: 47–53

Sumino Y, Hosaka H, Abei T, et al (1980) Diagnosis of intrahepatic tumor with real-time ultrasonic scanning. Japanese Society of Ultrasound in Medicine, Proceedings, Jpn J Med Ultrasonics (Monograph) pp 139–140

Tang ZY, Lu JZ, Zhou NQ, Yu YQ (1982) Small hepatocellular carcinoma-VI. Value of hepatoarteriography, B-scan ultrasonography and liver scintiscan in the localization of small HCC: a comparative study based on operative finding. Acta Acad Med Primae Shanghai 9: 101–105[1]

Taylor KJ, Hill CR (1975) Scanning techniques in grey-scale ultrasonography. Br J Radiol 48: 918–920

Taylor KJ, Carpenter DA, McCready VR (1973) Grey-scale echography in the diagnosis of intrahepatic disease. J Clin Ultrasound 1: 284–287

Taylor KJ, Carpenter DA, McCready VR (1974) Ultrasound and scintigraphy in the differential diagnosis of obstructive jaundice. J Clin Ultrasound 2: 105–116

Wells PNT (1977) Ultrasonics in clinical diagnosis, 2nd edn. Churchill Livingstone, Edinburgh, p 24

Xu ZZ, Tang ZY, Chen MH, et al (1982) Diagnostic value of ultrasound in liver cancer. Chin J Digest 2: 223–227[1]

Xu ZZ, Yang MZ (1983) B-mode real-time ultrasonography in the diagnosis of hepatic carcinoma. Chin J Radiol 17: 43–45[1]

1 Chinese

5 General Considerations on Treatment of Subclinical Hepatocelluar Carcinoma

Tang Zhao-you

Nearly a century has gone by since the establishment of the scientific basis for hepatocellular carcinoma. Endeavors have been made in both basic and clinical aspects; a substantial amount of knowledge, particularly of etiology and diagnosis, has been accumulated. Nevertheless, the therapeutic pattern as well as the prognosis for this malignancy has not altered remarkably. Thanks to the discovery of subclinical HCC by means of AFP serosurvey, however, dramatic alterations in therapeutic and prognostic patterns have recently been observed. A brief history of the treatment of HCC and the changing therapeutic pattern in recent years is delineated, and choices of therapeutic modality, as well as guidelines in the treatment of SCHCC, are also discussed.

I. Evolution in Treatment of HCC

The history of the treatment of HCC was thoroughly reviewed by Foster and Berman (1977), who traced it back to 1888. With advances in the fields of anesthesia, bacteriology, antiseptics, and abdominal surgery, a left lobe tumor with a pedicle had been removed by Langenbuch. In 1891 a malignant hepatic tumor was successfully resected by Lucke. Unfortunately, no substantial advance was observed in the ensuing years. Owing to a series of serious problems concerning the intrahepatic anatomy, the biochemistry of the liver, the disturbance of liver function after major hepatic resection, and particularly the close association with liver cirrhosis, only 16 cases of resected HCC were reported by Yeomans in 1915.

In the 1950s the anatomical basis of modern hepatic surgery was established (Healey et al 1953; Goldsmith and Woodburne 1957). Hepatic lobectomy by the hilium dissection technique was first reported by Lortat-Jacob and Robert in 1952; a similar report was made by Quattlebaum (1953), and a right hepatic lobectomy was presented by Pack the following year (Pack et al. 1953). The rapidly increasing recognition of pathophysiological disturbance after massive hepatic resection has resulted in a large number of hepatic resection reports, particularly from the Eastern world where the disease is prevalant (Wang and Lee 1963; Ong and Leong 1969; Lin 1970; Balasegaram 1972; Honjo and Mizumoto 1974). A total of 503 cases of hepatic resection for cancer worldwide were reported by Foster and Berman (1977).

The first clinical trial of liver transplantation for cancer was performed in 1963 (Starzl 1969). Bloodless hepatectomy by using organ isolation hypothermic perfusion (Fortner et al. 1971) or without hypothermia (Huguet et al. 1976) was also developed. These might provide more chances for patients with advanced HCC and increase the resectability rate.

Progress was also made in the surgical treatment of unresectable HCC. Intra-arterial infusion of chemotherapeutic agents (Bierman et al. 1951; Clarkson et al. 1962), hepatic artery ligation (Rienhoff and Woods 1953), cryosurgery (Zhou et al. 1979), and laser vaporization (Yu et al. 1981) have been employed and good palliation has been demonstrated.

Radiation therapy remains the conservative treatment of choice. Its history can be traced back to the 1950s. Acceptable results were reported by Ariel (1956) and Phillips (1960); however, the majority of reports from other authors were disappointing. Encouraging long-term survival was obtained in a major series in China (Yu 1981). Internal radiation with isotopes was also reported (Ariel 1965). A more sophisticated technique using isotopic immunoglobulin therapy for primary liver cancer (Ettinger et al. 1982) has aroused lively interest, and hepatic artery embolization with acceptable palliation has been reported in the past few years (Yamada et al. 1979; Chuang et al. 1982).

Systemic chemotherapy for HCC was also started in the 1950s, but the results were disappointing. The present status mimics that described by Eckhardt in 1979: of the drugs adequately tested, only methotrexate, adriamycin and 5-fluorouracil show activity against primary liver cancer.

Chinese medicinal herbs have been employed for decades in the treatment of clinically confirmed HCC, and palliative results have been observed in some cases. The mechanism, however, deserves to be investigated (Tang and Chen 1981).

A variety of immunotherapeutic agents, including modified tumor vaccine, anti-AFP serum, transfer factor, immune RNA, BCG, *Corynebacterium parvum,* and levamisole, have been tried to control residual tumor after surgery, radiation, and chemotherapy; a final evaluation remains to be made (Lin and Tang 1981). However, the rapid accumulation of knowledge in the fields of interferon, relative specific antibodies, and monoclonal antibodies has given new scope to the problem (Son et al. 1982; Ghose et al. 1980; Shouval et al. 1982).

II. Changing Therapeutic Pattern

A. Proportion of Hepatic Resection in the Overall Series

An extremely low overall 5-year survival rate is recorded in the literature: 3% in the United States – 913 cases of PLC from 1955 to 1964 (Axtell et al. 1972); 2.4% in Japan – 1424 cases of HCC from 1968 to 1977 (Okuda et al. 1980); 2.6% in China (Zhong Shan Hospital, Shanghai), 387 cases of PLC from 1961 to 1970 (Yang and Tang 1981). These dismal ultimate outcomes were accepted as a result of far advanced disease. It is universally acknowledged that hepatic resection remains the modality of choice which may provide long survival. Indeed, the close correlation between low 5-year survival and low proportion of hepatic resection in the overall series was found both in the East (China 5.3% – Shanghai Coordinating Group, Tang et al. 1974; Japan 9.0% – Okuda et al. 1980) and in the West (USA 7.0%–11.0% – Axtell et al. 1972) (Table 1). However, as a result of AFP serosurvey, a markedly increasing proportion of SCHCC accompanied by a markedly increasing resection rate was noted in our series (Table 2).

B. Alteration in Proportion of various Therapeutic Modalities

An unbelievably high proportion of untreated PLC has been reported in the past several decades, owing to far advanced disease. According to data from the United States, it was 95% in 1940–1949, 89% in 1950–1954, 74% in 1955–1964, and 62% in 1965–1969 (Axtell et al. 1972). However, a slow decrease in the no-treatment rate and an increase in the resection rate did occur with improvements in diagnosis and therapy. Most encouraging was the improvement in patterns of therapy (Table 3). Resection, hepatic artery ligation and/or catheterization, cryosurgery, and laser

Table 1. Proportion of hepatic resection in overall series

Reference	Country, period	Total no. of cases	Resection	
			No. of cases	%
Axtell et al. 1972	USA 1955–64 1965–69	913	64	7.0 11.0
Tang and Yang 1974	China 1967–72	3254	171	5.3
Okuda et al. 1980	Japan 1968–77	4031	361	9.0

Table 2. Correlation between increasing resection rate and increasing proportion of SCHCC (Zhong Shan Hospital, Shanghai, China)

Period	Total no. of cases	In the whole series	
		SCHCC (%)	Resection (%)
1961–1970	387	0 (0)	60 (15.5)
1971–1976	250	23 (9.2)	61 (24.4)
1977–1982	316	77 (24.4)	114 (36.1)

Table 3. Alteration in proportion of various therapeutic modalities

	U.S.A. (%)			Zhong Shan Hospital (%)	
	1940–49	1955–64	1965–69	1961–70	1971–82
Resection	2	7	11	15.5	31.0
Cryosurgery and/or laser					6.0
Hepatic artery ligation and/or perfusion				7.0	16.8
Radiation	3	5	5	10.3	3.7
Chemotherapy and/or herbs	0	11	20	45.5	33.4
No treatment	95	74	62	21.7	9.1

vaporization were feasible in only 22.5% of cases from 1961 to 1970 versus 53.8% in 1971–1982; on the other hand, the no-treatment rate decreased further from 21.7% to 9.1% in our series.

A more detailed comparison of therapeutic patterns was made between SCHCC and CHCC. Exciting results demonstrated that surgery, the modality which best provides radical cure or good palliation of HCC, was feasible in 85.0% of SCHCC cases as compared with 47.0% of CHCC cases. The dramatically high resection rate deserves special notice (60.0% versus 24.7%).

To sum up, in the early years the doctors could do nothing for patients in a relatively late stage of disease; with progress in the 1960s they could do something, and with AFP serosurvey in the 1970s a great deal could be done to rescue the dying. For CHCC patients a more effective conservative treatment must be sought, while for SCHCC patients attempts should be made to increase resectability, to decrease operative mortality, and to find other effective surgical approaches to eliminate or eradicate the tumor. The development of local treatment such as cryosurgery or high-power laser was of significance in the treatment of SCHCC but less useful in CHCC. In contrast, hepatic artery ligation and/or catheterization with chemotherapeutic perfusion seems more useful in CHCC with huge tumors (Table 4).

III. Selection of Therapeutic Modality in Management of SCHCC

There are two types of liver function: compensated and noncompensated. Patients with reversed albumin and globulin ratio and/or impairment of prothrombin time ($\leqslant 50\%$ of normal value), and/or bilirubin $\geqslant 2.0$ mg/dl are considered to have non compensated liver function.

A. SCHCC with Compensated Liver Function

Surgery is strongly indicated for SCHCC patients with compensated liver function. Segmentectomy or lobectomy is indicated for a left lobe tumor; however, local resection (wedge-shaped resection, partial hepatectomy, or even enucleation of the tumor nodule) is preferred for a right lobe small HCC with cirrhosis. Bloodless surgery with or without hypothermic perfusion is indicated for patients with a tumor

Table 4. Comparison of therapeutic patterns for SCHCC and CHCC

Therapeutic modality	SCHCC (%) (*n*=100)	CHCC (%) (*n*=466)
Resection	60.0	24.7
Cryosurgery and/or laser	11.0	4.9
Hepatic artery ligation and/or perfusion	14.0	17.4
Radiation	3.0	3.9
Chemotherapy and/or herbs	10.0	38.4
No treatment	2.0	10.7

located near the hepatic portal or the inferior vena cava. Cryosurgery or high-power laser vaporization is indicated in unresectable cases with a superficially located tumor; hepatic artery ligation and/or catheterization is preferred in unresectable cases with deeply located, multiple tumors. A combination of two or three modalities mentioned above may provide a better ultimate outcome.

Local radiation therapy can be employed for patients who have an accurately localized tumor but refuse surgery.

B. SCHCC with Noncompensated Liver Function

Conservative treatment is suggested for SCHCC patients with noncompensated liver function; this includes small or moderate doses of chemotherapy and intravenous injection or oral administration, combined with Chinese traditional medicinal herbs to strengthen the patient's general condition and to counteract the side effects of chemotherapy. If the patient does not tolerate chemotherapy, Chinese herbs are preferred, principally to strengthen the general condition, to improve the appetite and the circulation, and to reverse blood stasis.

However, the ultimate outcome of conservative treatment has been disappointing, no 5-year survivor having been encountered among the pathologically proven SCHCC cases in this series. Fortunately, conservative treatment was indicated for only a small proportion of SCHCC patients.

IV. Guidelines on Treatment of SCHCC

Both early detection and early effective treatment are necessary for a favorable ultimate outcome. Treatment of SCHCC can be early, radical, aggressive, or multimodal.

A. Early Treatment

Once the diagnosis of SCHCC is established, it is suggested that the patient be treated as a subemergency. As shown in Table 5, the smaller the tumor, the better the 5-year survival. It should be noted that the size of 5 cm seems to be the point at which a tumor spreads. A sudden decline in the 5-year survival rate was noted in

Table 5. Relation between tumor size and 5-year survival rate after resection of single nodule HCC

Tumor size (cm)	No. of cases	5-year survival[a]
≤3.0	18	87.5
3.1–5.0	24	65.8
>5.0	90	20.2

[a] Life table method

cases with tumors >5 cm, even after resection. As has been mentioned before, the median tumor size in our series of SCHCC cases was 4.5 cm; therefore, it is important to operate as early as possible. However, deterrents to the treatment of SCHCC include not only technical but also social factors. Generally, CHCC patients readily agree to treatment including surgery to relieve symptoms. However, SCHCC patients tend to refuse surgery because of the lack of symptoms and the impression of a high operative mortality and the dismal results of surgery. Many patients do not undergo surgery until symptoms occur several months later, and the opportunity for early resection is lost. Therefore, every effort should be made to persuade the SCHCC patient with compensated liver function to undergo surgery as early as possible. Superselective infusion hepatic arteriography detects small HCC in the majority of cases, thus helping the patient as well as the doctor to make the decision.

B. Radical Treatment

Pathological data reveal that the earlier the stage of disease, the higher the incidence of well-encapsulated single nodular tumor without tumor emboli (Table 6), which provides a good opportunity for radical cure of the disease. Therefore, radical extirpation of the tumor is of prime importance. Resection has been proven as the method of choice. The trouble is that in 68.9% (64/93) of SCHCC cases the tumor was located in the right lobe and portal area, that 85.7% (78/91) of SCHCC cases were associated with cirrhosis, and that the macronodular type was found in 75.6% (59/78) of the cirrhosis cases. It has long been documented that right hepatic lobectomy of small HCC leads to high operative mortality. The key is to remove the tumor completely but to preserve normal liver parenchyma as far as possible. It has been demonstrated that a revision of the surgical principle of hepatectomy for cancer is crucial. Local resection instead of lobectomy has proven to be of prime importance for this particular purpose.

C. Aggressive Treatment

Endeavors must also be made to prolong survival after resection. Long-term, periodic (every 2 months) AFP follow-up studies are important for early detection of subclinical recurrence. Contrary to the previous concept that further surgery is contraindicated for recurrent and metastatic cancer, reoperation has proven necessary for recurrence detected in the subclinical stage, and has resulted in a significant prolongation of survival after radical resection of SCHCC.

Table 6. Comparison of some pathological data on SCHCC and CHCC

Items	SCHCC	CHCC
Single nodule %	66.7 (60/90)	39.3 (118/300)[a]
Well encapsulated %	50.0 (42/84)	15.8 (46/291)[a]
No tumor emboli %	96.6 (57/59)	53.4 (78/146)[a]

[a] $P < 0.01$

D. Multimodality Treatment

Approaches other than surgical resection are needed to destroy (eradicate or eliminate) the tumor as much as possible in unresectable SCHCC. Various "local treatment" modalities are of importance. For example, adequate cryosurgery by repeated a "freeze-thaw" cycle covering the whole tumor area has led to an outcome in superficially located small HCC similar to that achieved with resection. The priority of an aggressive approach with a combination of two or three modalities has also been demonstrated. Figure 1 shows an SCHCC patient detected by AFP serosurvey who was operated on in March 1975, Palliative resection of a small tumor, measuring 2 cm in diameter (Fig. 2) and located in the caudal lobe, was performed. Cryo-

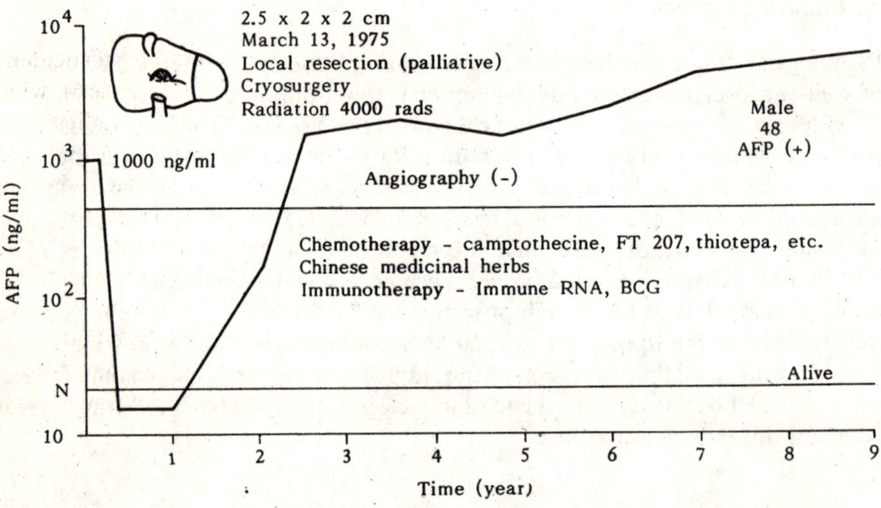

Fig. 1. Multimodal treatment of an SCHCC patient +, above normal; –, negative finding

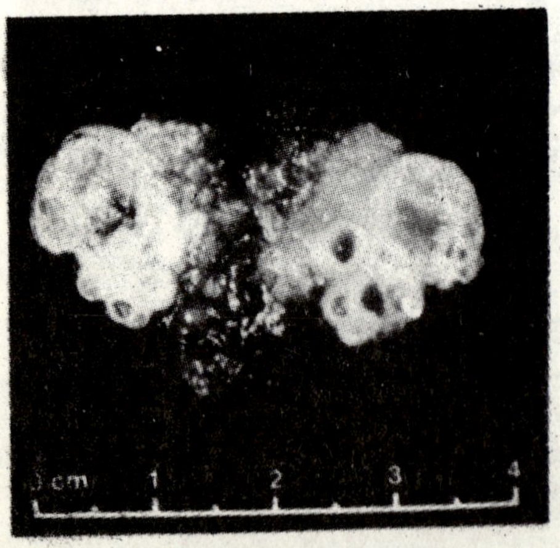

Fig. 2. Surgical specimen, showing a 2-cm tumor of the caudal lobe

surgery was also employed on the cut surface because of the resection was inadequate, and immediately after the operation external local radiation therapy was given, with a total dose of 6000 rads. AFP dropped to normal after the operation, increased somewhat by the end of the first postoperative year, and persisted at a low level. During the ensuing years, the patient received long-term conservative treatment consisting of chemotherapy, Chinese medicinal herbs, and immunotherapy. Despite slowly increasing AFP, selective hepatic arteriography did not reveal any space-occupying lesion. The patient is still in good health without any symptoms 100 months after the operation.

V. Unsolved Problems

Unsolved problems in the treatment of SCHCC include: (a) lack of an effective approach to the prevention of recurrence and distant metastasis after radical resection: (b) lack of effective modalities for local treatment of deeply located tumors in unresectable SCHCC; (c) lack of effective modalities for conservative treatment of SCHCC cases with noncompensated liver function. Studies on the biological characteristics of HCC and development of isotope-labeled and drug- or toxin-binding specific antibodies may be helpful.

References

Ariel IM (1956) The treatment of primary and metastatic cancer of the liver. Surgery 39: 70–91

Ariel IM (1960) Treatment of inoperable primary pancreatic and liver cancer by the intra-arterial administration of radioactive isotopes. Ann Surg 162: 267–278

Axtell IM, Cutler SJ, Myers HM (1972) End results in cancer – report No. 4. US Department of Health, Education and Welfare, Public Health Service, NIH, NCI, Bethesda, Maryland, pp 72–76

Balasegaram M (1972) Hepatic surgery – a review of a personal series of 95 major resections. Aust NZ J Surg 42: 1–10

Bierman HR, Miller ER, Byron RI Jr, et al. (1951) Intra-arterial catheterization of viscera in man. AJR 66: 555–568

Chuang VP, Wallace S, Soo CS, et al. (1982) Therapeutic Ivalon embolization of hepatic tumors. AJR 138: 289–294

Clarkson B, Young C, Dierick W, et al. (1962) Effects of continuous hepatic artery infusion of antimetabolites on primary and metastatic cancer of the liver. Cancer 15: 472–488

Eckhardt S (1979) Chemotherapy of primary liver cancer. J Toxicol Environ Health 5: 395–400

Ettinger D, Order SE, Wharam MD, et al. (1982) Phase I–II study of isotopic immunoglobulin therapy for primary liver cancer. Cancer Treat Rep 66: 289–298

Fortner JG, Shiu MH, Howland WS, et al. (1971) A new concept in hepatic lobectomy: experimental studies and clinical application. Arch Surg 102: 312–315

Foster JH, Berman MM (1977) Solid liver tumors. Saunders, Philadelphia, pp 9–27, 62–104

Ghose T, Tai J, Guclu A, et al. (1980) Use of cell surface localizing antihepatoma antibody for tumor imaging and therapy with drug-linked antibody. Transplant Proc 12: 192–194

Goldsmith NA, Woodburne RT (1957) The surgical anatomy pertaining to liver resection. Surg Gynecol Obstet 105: 310–318

Healey JE Jr, Schroy PC, Sorensen RJ (1953) The intrahepatic distribution of the hepatic artery in man. J Int Coll Surg 20: 133–148

Honjo I, Mizumoto R (1974) Primary carcinoma of the liver. Am J Surg 128: 31–36

Huguet C, Gallot D, Offenstadt G, et al. (1976) Total hepatic vascular exclusion and hemostatic glue for extensive resection of the liver. Nouv Presse Med 5: 1189–1192
Lin TY (1970) Primary cancer of the liver, quadrennial review. Scand J Gastroenterol 6: 223s
Lin ZY, Tang ZY (1981) Immunostatus and immunotherapy of primary liver cancer. In: Tang ZY (ed) Primary liver cancer. Shanghai Sci and Technical Publisher, Shanghai, pp 319–333[1]
Lortat-Jacob JL, Robert HG (1952) Hepatectomie droite reglec. Nouv Presse Med 60: 549–551
Okuda K, Kasai Y, Sugawara K, et al (1980) Primary liver cancer in Japan. Cancer 45: 2663–2669
Ong GB, Leong CH (1969) Surgical treatment of primary liver cancer. J R Coll Surg 14: 42–55
Pack GI, Baker HW (1953) Total right hepatic lobectomy – report of a case. Ann Surg 138: 253–258
Phillips R, Murikami K (1960) Primary neoplasm of the liver. Cancer 13: 714–720
Quattlebaum JK (1953) Massive resection of the liver. Ann Surg 137: 787–796
Rienhoff WF Jr, Woods AC (1953) Ligation of hepatic and splenic arteries in treatment of cirrhosis and ascites. JAMA 152: 687–690
Shouval D, Wands JR, Zurawski VR, et al. (1982) Selective binding and complement-mediated lysis of human hepatoma cells (PLC/PRF/5) in culture by monoclonal antibodies to hepatitis-B surface antigen. Proc Natl Acad Sci USA 79: 650–654
Son K, Kew M, Rabson AR (1982) Depressed natural killer cell activity in patients with hepatocellular carcinoma. In vitro effects of interferon and levamisole. Cancer 50: 2820–2825
Starzl TE (1969) Experience in hepatic transplantation. Saunders, Philadelphia
Tang CL, Chen BW (1981) Chinese traditional medicine and primary liver cancer. In: Tang ZY (ed) Primary liver cancer. Shanghai Sci and Technical Publisher, Shanghai pp 293–306[1]
Tang ZY, Yang BH (1974) Primary liver cancer – clinical analysis of 3254 cases (from 11 provinces, 21 hospitals in China). Tumor Prevent Treat Study 2: 207–215[1]
Wang CE, Lee GC (1963) Surgical treatment of primary carcinoma of liver. Chin Med J [Engl] 82: 65–78
Yamada R, Nakatsuka H, Nakamura K, et al. (1979) Transcatheter arterial embolization therapy in unresectable hepatoma – experience in 15 cases. Acta Hepatol Jpn 20: 595–603
Yang BH, Tang ZY (1981) Primary liver cancer, a clinical analysis of 1045 cases. in: Tang ZY (ed). Primary liver cancer. Shanghai Sci and Technical Publisher, Shanghai, pp 366–374[1]
Yeomans FC (1915) Primary carcinoma of the liver. JAMA 64: 1301
Yu EX (1981) Radiation therapy of liver cancer. In: Tang ZY (ed), Primary liver cancer. Shanghai Sci and Technical Publisher, Shanghai, pp 283–292[1]
Yu YQ, Tang ZY, Zhou XD, et al. (1981) Treatment of primary hepatic cancer by YAG laser: a preliminary report. Acta Acad Med Primae Shanghai 8: 29–31[1]
Zhou XD, Tang ZY, Yu YQ, et al. (1979) Cryosurgery for liver cancer – experimental and clinical study. Chin J Surg 17: 480–483[1]

1 Chinese

6 Surgical Treatment of Subclinical Hepatocellular Carcinoma

Tang Zhao-you

During the past decades, unquestionable progress has been made in the surgical management of HCC (Tang 1981). In the 1950s the anatomical basis was established; the 1960s brought the elucidation of pathophysiological alteration after massive hepatectomy. New concepts of surgical oncology began in the 1970s (Fisher 1977). As a result of great advances made in early detection and early treatment using AFP serosurvey in the 1970s, surgery has assumed a greater role. An increasing resectability rate (from 20% to 40%), a decreasing operative mortality (from 20–30% to 5–10%), and an improving 5-year survival rate after resection (from < 10% to around 20% in Asian patients) are noteworthy. Large series comprising 100 cases of PLC managed with hepatic resection have been common (Table 1). In light of the surgical management of early-stage HCC, some concepts may have to be changed and some principles revised.

I. Changing Role of Surgery in Treatment of SCHCC

It has long been universally accepted that surgery is the modality of choice in the treatment of HCC. Unfortunately, the role of surgery was limited owing to the extremely low series resection rate, the relatively high operative mortality and the dismal prospects for long-term survival. However, after more than 10 years of experience in the surgical management of SCHCC it was clear that the role of surgery had become greater. A comparison between SCHCC and CHCC revealed that resection was feasible for 60.0% of SCHCC patients versus 24.7% of CHCC patients, and that palliative surgical procedures, including hepatic artery ligation, cannulation, cryosurgery, and laser-beam vaporization, were feasible for 25.0% of SCHCC patients and 22.3% of CHCC patients. In other words, surgery (resection and palliative procedures) is indicated for the majority of SCHCC patients, while conservative procedures remain the major mode of treatment for CHCC patients (Table 2).

II. Indications for Surgery of SCHCC and Preoperative Care

A. Indications

Laparotomy is indicated as follows: (a) For SCHCC patients with accurate diagnosis – AFP level with positive CIEP (or AFP ⩾500 ng/ml) persisting for 3 weeks, or AFP ⩾200 ng/ml persisting for 8 weeks without coexistent active liver disease

Table 1. Selective data on resection of PLC

Reference	Cases resected	Resect-ability (%)	Operative mortality	Survival rate (%) 1-year	3-year	5-year
1963 Wang and Li	130	24.6	25.4	21.9	5.8	2.3
1970 Foster – World	296		24	42.3		14.0
Asian	236		24	23		6
Non-Asian	60		22	59		36
1970 Lin[a]	82	30.3	12.1	33.8		19.1
1971 El-Domeiri et al.	32	27.5	34			15.6
1972 Axtell (USA 1955–1964)	64			34	24	20
1974 Yu and Tang	258		14.7	34.1	15.5	
1974 Honjo and Mizumoto	23	32	9	43	22	13
1976 Lin[a]	118	44.3	11.8	35.0	20.0	19.0
1976 Ishikawa (Japan)	297	18.1	21.9	35.4	14.8	8.4
1977 Foster and Berman (USA 1960–1974)	127		21	80	53	30
1977 Tang and Qian (Qidong, China)[d]	91	45.0	3.3	60.8	33.3	
1979 Sorensen et al.	31		25.9			16
1979 Lin[a]	132	44.4	10.6	34.7	18.2	18.1
1980 Starzl et al.	30		3.3		49	49
1980 Wu et al.[b]	181	48.6	8.8	55.9	28.9	16.0
1980 Yan and Shen[c]	114	27.7	10.5	50.0	20.4	18.9
1980 Okuda et al. (Japan 1968–1977)	222		21.5	33.3	19.6	11.8
1981 Adson and Weiland	46		5.0		65	36
1981 Fortner et al.	35			85	50	37
1981 Tang et al.	153[e]	43.6	12.4	56.3	31.5	23.6
1982 Takasaki et al.	60			52	34	8
1982 Li et al.	114	21.3	11.4	58.6	32.7	20.5
1982 Huang and Zhang[d]	181[f]	52.3	2.8	55.6	29.4	27.6
1982 Wu et al.[b]	274		6.2	59.9	33.7	24.8
1983 Shen et al.[c]	195	34.0	8.2	60.2	28.7	22.9

[a, b, c, d] represent the same institution
[e] 20.3% of 153 cases were SCHCC
[f] 49.2% of 181 cases were SCHCC

(without abnormal serum ALT, etc.) and with pregnancy or teratoma of the gonads excluded. In AFP-negative HCC, positive findings by real-time ultrasonography and selective angiography are needed; (b) when there is a normal value of serum bilirubin (<2 mg/dl), prothrombin time >50% of normal value, and albumin/globulin ratio within normal; (c) when there is no obvious systemic disorder or diseases of the heart, lung, and kidney. Localization, particularly by ultrasonography

Table 2. Changing role of surgery in treatment of SCHCC

	SCHCC (n=100)	CHCC (n=466)
Series resection rate %	60.0	24.7
Operative mortality in resection %	1.7	6.1
Resection + other surgical procedures %	85.0	47.0
5-year survival rate %		
In whole series	43.9	4.2
In resection group	72.9	16.1

and/or angiography, is of importance in confirming the diagnosis, in predicting resectability, and in designing the operative procedure.

B. Preoperative Care

As in the case of large HCC, perfect preoperative care is required. Owing to the close association with liver cirrhosis (85.7% in this series) and to the fact that the smaller the tumor, the higher the risk of right lobectomy with cirrhosis, aggressive preoperative care is needed. Since most SCHCC patients appear "healthy," it is necessary to resect the tumor both radically and safely. Preoperative care includes: (a) intravenous administration of glucose, vitamin K, and vitamin C, (b) administration of plasma or albumin if necessary, (c) oral administration of kanamycin, neomycin, or streptomycin 2 days before operation, and (d) Chinese herbs to strengthen the patient's general condition.

III. Anesthesia, Transfusion, and Surgical Incision

A. Anesthesia

Epidural anesthesia is routinely used. General anesthesia is needed in a transthoracic and abdominal approach for right lobe surgery. Sufficient oxygen supply is necessary to minimize liver function damage.

B. Transfusion

Transfusion through an upper extremity is recommended. Fresh blood proves to be superior to bank blood.

C. Incision

An upper abdominal rectus incision was routinely employed in our series. Generally, an extension to the xiphoid process was sufficient for surgery of left lobe cancer; a transverse abdominal extension was needed for partial hepatectomy of right lobe cancer in the lower pole; a transthoracic and abdominal approach was routinely employed for right hemihepatectomy or partial hepatectomy of right lobe cancer in the upper pole. Good exposure was necessary, both to shorten operative time and to minimize blood loss.

IV. Localization of Small HCC During Surgery

Data from a high-risk area (Qidong County) reveal that the surgeon failed to locate the small tumor in 14.6% (13/89) of the survey patients and in 27.1% (13/48) of SCHCC patients who underwent surgery but whose tumor eventually proved to be HCC (Tang and Qian 1977); in the Shanghai series this was so for 7.5% (4/53) of SCHCC patients (Tang et al. 1979). Of the 90 cases of SCHCC operated on in this series, the tumor failed to be located in only two cases. Our experience in the localization of small HCC during surgery showed that the identification limit was 1 cm for selective angiography and 2 cm for real-time ultrasonography (Tang et al. 1982). A systematic survey of the whole liver by meticulous palpation with both hands, one in front of and the other behind the liver, is required to minimize the rate of tumors missed (Yu et al. 1980a). Generally, small HCC situated in a surface area or along the margin of the liver can easily be found, but a deep small HCC is often difficult to locate in macronodular cirrhosis. It should be noted that 16.7% of SCHCC patients had two nodules and another 16.7% had three or more. Patients who have AFP $\geqslant$ 500 ng/ml persisting for over 6 months will probably have multiple nodules.

In this series, the tumor was on the left lobe in 16.1% of cases, on the right lobe in 45.2%, and on the hepatic hilum in 23.7%. Particular attention should be paid to the bare area of the right lobe, the caudal lobe, the area under the triangular and coronary ligaments, and the area just behind and beneath the gallbladder. Usually the falciform, coronary, triangular, hepatorenal, and gastrohepatic ligaments should be divided to facilitate the exposure of the liver.

In some individual cases with deep tumors, an aspiration biopsy for frozen section is necessary. Inasmuch as the accuracy rate of AFP diagnostic criteria (Chap. 3) was reported to be as high as 98%, every effort should be made to locate the small HCC. Recently, intraoperative ultrasonography has been claimed to be of value in locating small HCC during surgery (Ryu et al. 1982).

V. Experience in Surgical Resection of SCHCC

Of the 100 patients with SCHCC in this series, 90 underwent surgery, and successful resection of cancer was achieved for 60 of them (66.7%). A long-term follow-up study revealed that resection of SCHCC provided a much higher 5-year survival as compared with resection of CHCC and nonresectional treatment of either SCHCC or CHCC (72.9% versus 16.1%, 0%, and 0%). Therefore, every effort should be directed toward increasing the resectability rate, decreasing operative mortality, and further prolonging survival.

A. Approach to Increasing Resectability Rate

Although relatively high series resection rates (resection in the whole series of PLC) were reported at individual centers (23.4%, EL-Domeiri et al. 1971; 30%, Lin 1979), the majority of other series with large numbers of cases remained disappointing, being only 5.3% of 3254 cases (1967–1972) in China (Tang et al. 1974), 9.0% of 4031 cases (1968–1977) in Japan (Okuda et al. 1980), 7% (1955–1964) and 11% (1965–1969) in the United States (Axtell et al. 1972), and 4.5% of 511 cases (1960–1970) in Thailand (Plengvanit et al. 1974). The ratio of resectable PLC to the number of cases explored was similar to that mentioned above. It was around 40% at a few centers but only 20%–30% at the majority (Table 1). The relatively low resection rate for series and for PLC in general was mainly the result of relatively late-stage disease with dissemination of cancer and of coexisting liver cirrhosis and the involvement of the hepatic portal. According to our experience, early detection remains the key to the dramatic increase in the resection rate (60% of SCHCC versus 24.7% of CHCC in this series). A marked increase in the risk of dissemination and a decrease in the resection rate might occur when the tumor reaches 5 cm (see Chap. 14).

Local resection or partial hepatectomy instead of a typical right lobectomy for small HCC in the presence of cirrhosis helps to increase the resection rate and provides a similar survival. Regular lobectomy has been the accepted approach to hepatic resection for cancer since the 1950s. Curutchet et al. (1971) reviewed the litera-

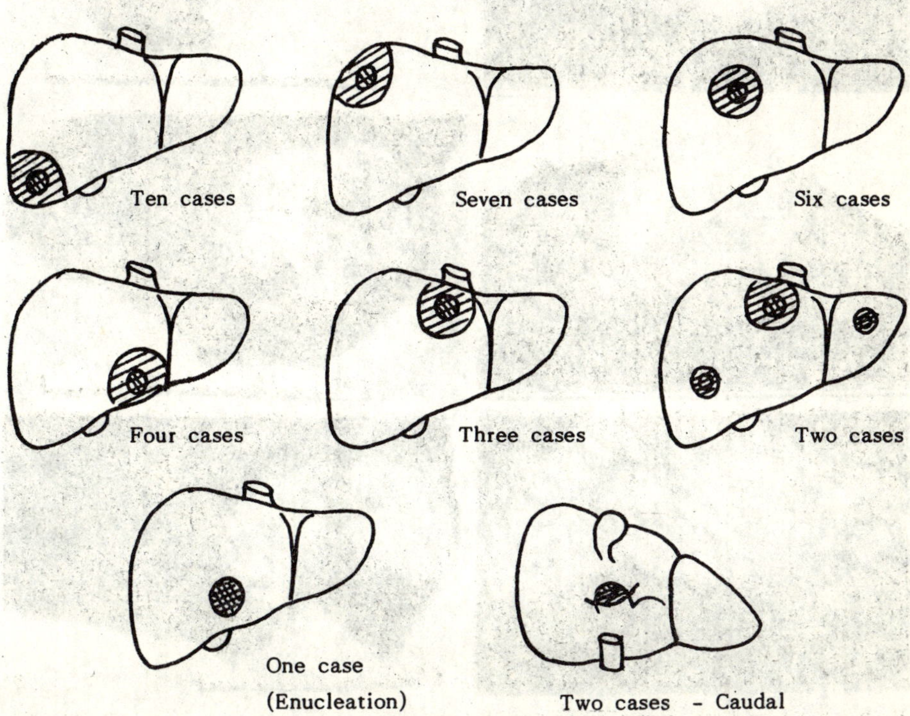

Fig. 1. Various modes of local resection of 35 SCHCC cases

ture worldwide, and found that in all of the eight cases of PLC with 3-year survival prior to 1950 local resection had been performed, but that of the 53 patients achieving 3-year survival during the 1950–1970 period, only 16 had undergone local resection. It has long been emphasized that right lobectomy cannot be tolerated in the presence of liver cirrhosis (Lin 1979). This is not a great problem in the West because of the relatively low rate of coexistent cirrhosis, which was 20.5% (26/127) in the United States during the period 1960–1974 (Foster and Berman 1977). However,

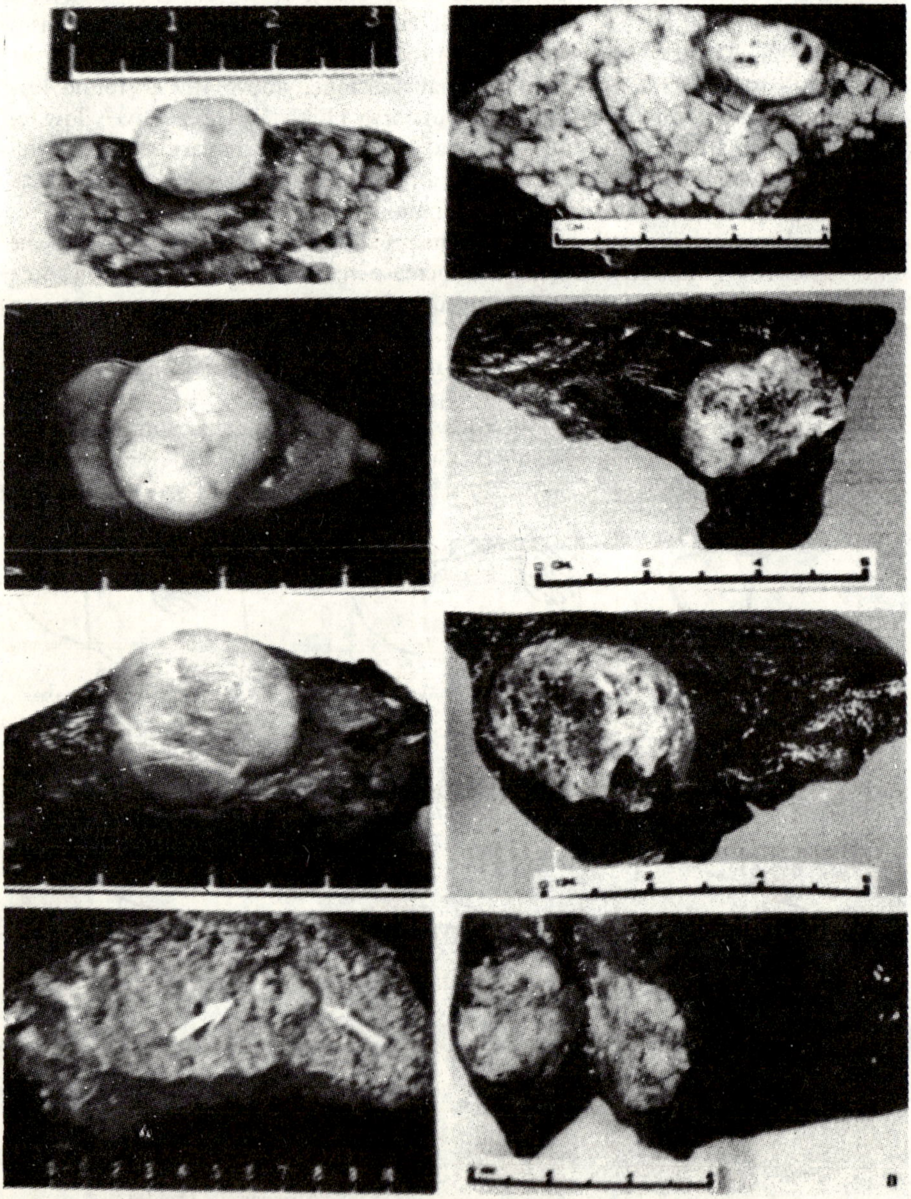

Fig. 2 a, b Surgical specimens from SCHCC patients

it is a great trouble to Asian patients. The rate of coexistent cirrhosis was 85.7% for SCHCC patients in this series, 45.2% of tumors being located in the right lobe and another 23.7% of tumors in the hepatic portal area. Thus, the resection rate is severely limited. The dramatically high series resection rate (60.0%) of SCHCC in this series was indeed a result of revision of the principles of hepatic surgery of cancer (Table 2). The types of resection performed in SCHCC and CHCC cases are listed in Table 3. For CHCC, regular lobectomy remained the principal type of resection (71.3%); however, local resection (including wedge-shape resection, partial hepatectomy, and enucleation of the tumor nodule in a few individual cases) became the main resection type for SCHCC (Figs. 1 and 2). A long-term follow-up

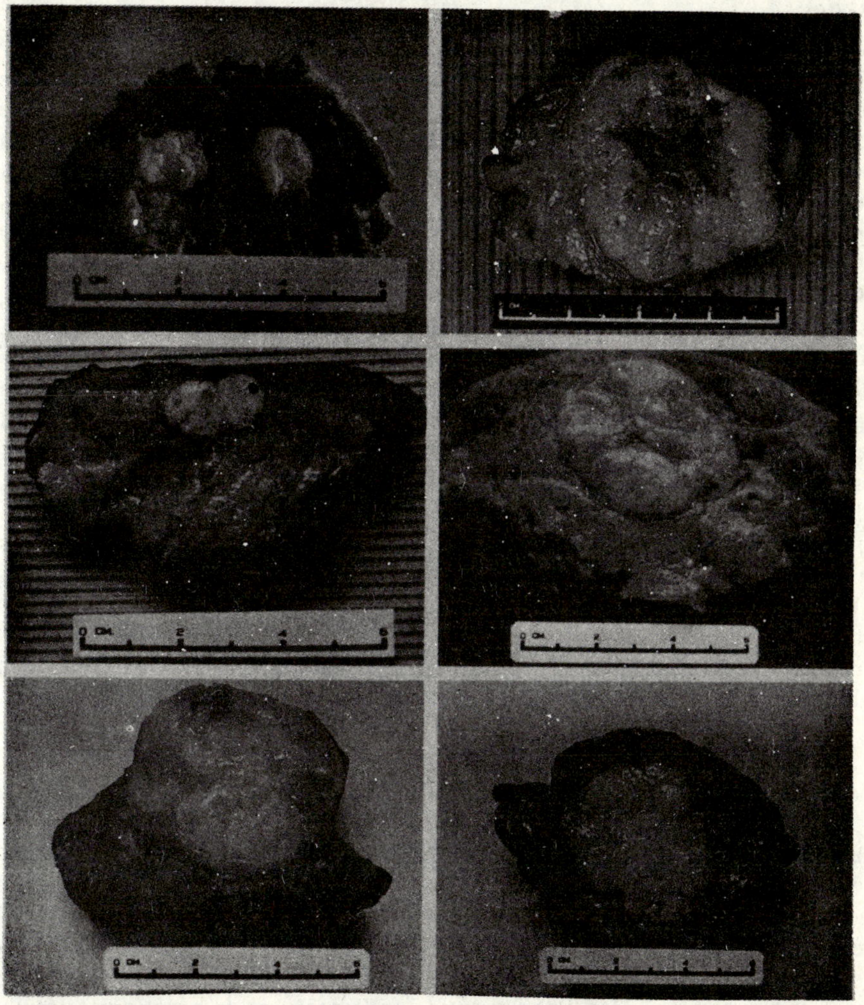

Fig. 2b

Table 3. Types of resection in SCHCC and CHCC

	SCHCC	CHCC
Local resection	35 (58.3%)	33 (28.7%)[a]
Left lateral segmentectomy	8 (13.3%)	22 (19.1%)
Left hemihepatectomy	4 (6.7%)	36 (31.3%)[a]
Extended left hemihepatectomy	2 (3.4%)	3 (2.6%)
Right posterior lobectomy	5 (8.3%)	0 (0)/za
Right hemihepatectomy	3 (5.0%)	18 (15.7%)[b]
Extended right hemihepatectomy	0 (0)	1 (0.9%)
Middle lobectomy	3 (5.0%)	2 (1.7%)
Total	60 (100.0%)	115 (100.0%)

[a] $P<0.01$
[b] $P<0.05$

study revealed that local resection and lobectomy yielded similar survival rates (Chap. 7). It is therefore justified to remove the small HCC with an area wide enough to eradicate the lesion but to save the noncancerous hepatic parenchyma as much as possible. According to pathological findings, removal of an area of 2 cm from the capsule of the tumor is usually sufficient to eradicate the small HCC lesion.

"Bloodless operation" by vascular isolation, with (Fortner et al. 1974; Yu et al. 1980b) or without hypothermic perfusion (Offenstadt et al. 1978; Wu et al. 1981), has further increased the resection rate and was successful in five cases of SCHCC. However, it is indicated only for patients with tumors located near the porta hepatis and the inferior vena cava and without severe cirrhosis. Treatment of large PLC in stages (two-step resection) is another approach to increasing the resection rate (Yu et al. 1983). As mentioned before, not all SCHCC cases are small HCC; a few of them have large tumors. Patients with huge encapsulated but unresectable tumors, with or without micronodular cirrhosis are good candidates for two-step resection. Combined hepatic artery ligation and cannulation for perfusion is presently ideal as the first-step procedure, and leads to 50% tumor regression in about 25% of cases within 3–6 months. Second-step resection was successfully carried out in three cases of the SCHCC group and three cases of the CHCC group. The ultimate outcomes were encouraging (Fig. 3). Similar results are reported in the literature dealing with regionally confined hepatic metastases (Tilchen et al. 1981).

B. Approach to Decreasing Operative Mortality

The high operative mortality has been one of the major deterrents to PLC surgery; however, it has decreased from around 20% to around 10%, or even less than 5% in recent years (Table 1). Hemorrhage and hepatic failure are the two major causes of operative mortality. In our series the hepatic clamp (Zhou et al. 1980) or the cross-interrupted mattress suture was employed for cancer located in the periphery of the liver to minimize blood loss. Temporary occlusion of the porta hepatis was usually performed for tumors located deep in the liver or near the portal area to control bleeding.

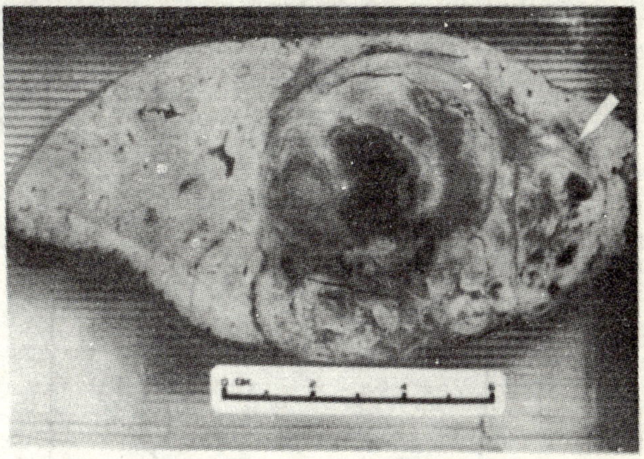

Fig. 3. Treatment of large PLC in stages – 52-year-old man. Four month after hepatic artery ligation plus perfusion, tumor size decreased from 15 × 10 × 9 cm to 9.5 × 9 × 7.5 cm; surgical specimen showed massive necrosis with only 3 × 2 × 2 cm residual tumor

The key, however, is to carefully judge the extent of hepatic resection reguired in right lobe carcinoma with cirrhosis. Therefore, local resection instead of lobectomy has also proved to be an important approach to decreasing operative mortality in Asian patients (Wu et al. 1980; Takasaki et al. 1982). Aggressive postoperative care is needed in right-side resection with a cirrhotic background. A dramatically low operative mortality was observed in this series, being 1.7% in SCHCC and 6.1% in CHCC.

C. Approach to Further Prolonging Survival After Resection

The dismal outcome of PLC resection, with a 5-year survival rate seldom exceeding 10% for Asian patients (Table 1) was considered to be the result of a high incidence of recurrence and metastases. The larger the tumor, the higher the risk of spreading. Another factor is coexistent cirrhosis. An analysis of factors influencing the PLC resection survival rate demonstrated that patients with (a) normalization of AFP after resection, (b) radical resection, (c) tumors ⩽5 cm, (d) single nodules, (e) SCHCC, and (f) negative findings in nuclide imaging, and survey patients have a better prognosis. Therefore, early detection and early radical resection are essential to improving the prognosis (Tang et al. 1981). Every effort should be made to perform the resection as early as possible and as radically as possible. SCHCC patients should be managed as subemergencies. Long-term periodic follow-ups using AFP and ultrasonography are of prime importance to the discovery of subclinical recurrence or subclinical metastasis.

Reoperation for subclinical recurrence in liver and solitary lung metastasis is of proven value for the further prolongation of survival after an initial radical resection (Yu et al. 1980c). The 5-year survival rate of SCHCC patients after resection has increased from 60.5% (1972–1980, Tang et al. 1983) to a present 72.9%. Of 60 patients with resection of SCHCC, nine subsequently underwent reoperation (with seven resections) owing to subclinical recurrence (Fig. 4) or solitary lung metastasis (Fig. 5), the longest record for recurrence being 5 years after initial resection.

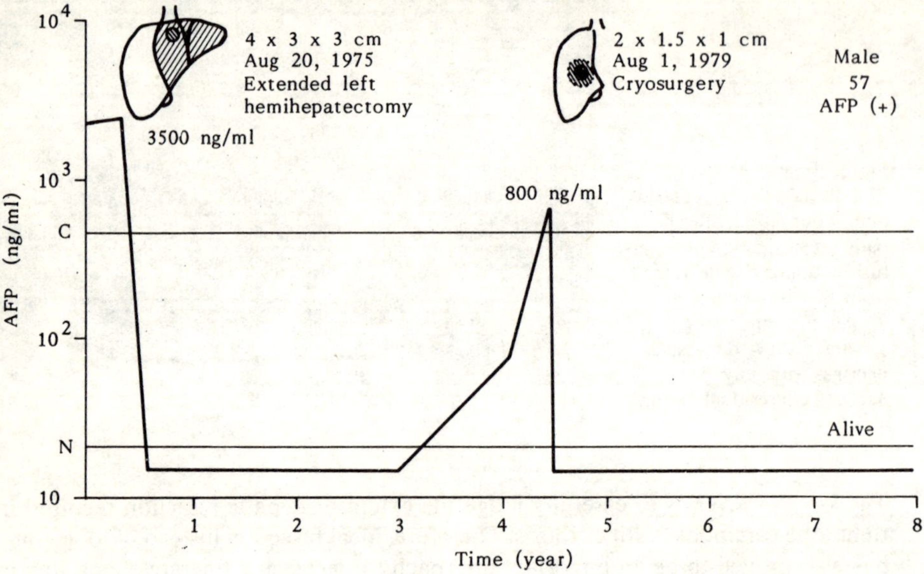

Fig. 4. Reoperation of subclinical recurrence in the liver

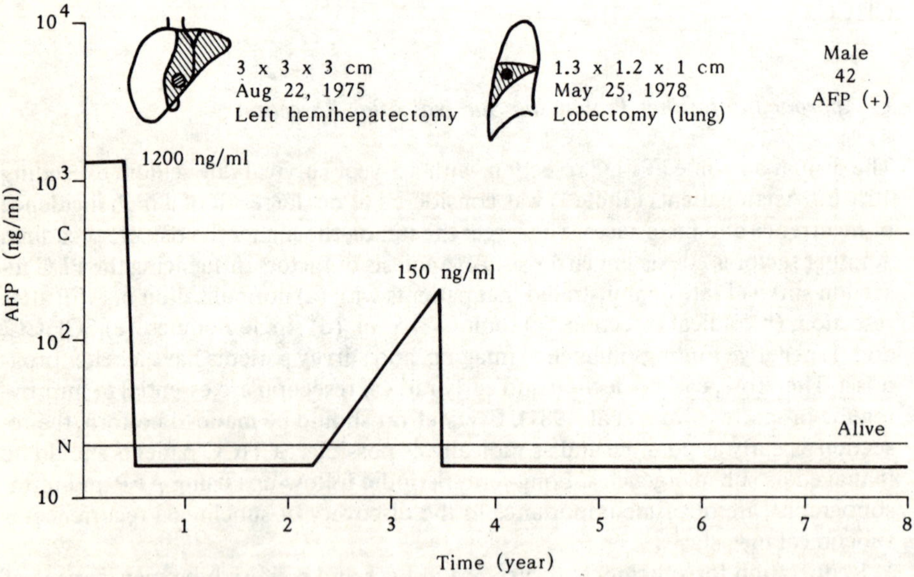

Fig. 5. Reoperation of solitary lung metastasis

Multimodality postoperative treatment is recommended for patients after palliative resection of SCHCC; a dramatic prolongation of survival can be observed in some cases.

VI. Surgical Management of Nonresectable SCHCC

According to new concepts in surgical oncology (Fisher 1977), the immunostatus as well as the host resistance to cancer might well be changed after complete or partial removal of tumor bulk, thus facilitating other procedures to control the residual tumor. Therefore, an aggressive approach with multimodality treatment seems to be justified.

A. Cryosurgery and Laser Beam Vaporization

Cryosurgery (Zhou et al. 1979) and high-power YAG laser beam vaporization (Yu et al. 1981) have been demonstrated as effective measures for eradicating superficially confined PLC. These were the principal therapeutic measures in 11 cases of SCHCC with tumor located near the porta hepatis and coexisting macronodular cirrhosis. Sixty percent of 1-year survivals, 20% of 2-year, and 10% of 3-year survivals were observed in the cryosurgery group.

B. Hepatic Artery Ligation or Embolization

Hepatic artery ligation or embolization is of proven merit in the palliation of nonresectable PLC (Yamada et al. 1979; Chuang et al. 1982; Lin et al. 1983). They have been less frequently employed in SCHCC cases with small tumors, with only two cases treated to date.

C. Hepatic Artery Cannulation and Perfusion

Hepatic artery cannulation and chemotherapeutic perfusion were employed in nine cases of nonresectable SCHCC; 1-year survival amounted to 44.4% but there were no 2-year survivors. Acceptable palliation is also reported in the literature (Reed et al 1981).

D. Multimodality Treatment

Multimodality treatment with hepatic arterial infusion plus occlusion (Berjian et al. 1980; Chuang et al. 1981) or arterial infusion plus irradiation (Friedman et al. 1979) seems to be the latest trend in the treatment of nonresectable liver cancer. Three SCHCC patients and 18 with nonresectable CHCC were treated by means of hepatic artery ligation plus perfusion. Better long-term results were obtained as compared with those using each procedure alone (Table 4). Jaundice, ascites, emboli in the portal trunk, and noncompensated liver function are contraindications for these procedures.

Table 4. Comparison of long-term results with different palliative surgical procedures for CHCC

Modality	No. of cases	Survival	
		1-year (%)	2-year (%)
Hepatic artery ligation + perfusion	18	40.5	21.6
Cryosurgery	21	35.4	8.8
Hepatic artery perfusion alone	49	22.5	3.4
Hepatic artery ligation alone	14	9.4	0

VII. Postoperative Care and Follow-up AFP Monitoring

A. Postoperative Care

Technically, surgery of small HCC is a relatively minor procedure as compared with surgery of large HCC; however, the same degree of attention is required as is given after major hepatectomy. The operative risk of right lobectomy for small HCC is even higher than that for large HCC. Careful monitoring of serum bilirubin, prothrombin time, and A/G ratio is necessary. Aggressive supportive treatment, particularly with plasma or albumin, vitamin K, and sufficient oxygen, is important with right lobe surgery. Chest fluid appears not infrequently after the transthoracic abdominal approach has been used for resection of a right lobe tumor with a cirrhosis background. Local injection of *Corynebacterium parvum* into the chest cavity is usually helpful in controlling chest fluid.

B. Follow-up Studies

Long-term follow-up AFP monitoring after resection provides valuable information. Serial AFP monitoring can objectively represent the priority of resection in SCHCC. The normalization rate (to $\leqslant$20 ng/ml) of AFP after treatment was 84.2% in resections of SCHCC, 38.5% in resections of CHCC, 14.8% in a nonresection group of SCHCC patients, and only 4.2% in a nonresection group of CHCC patients. Normalization of AFP after resection proved to be the leading factor influencing prognosis, occurring in 95.8% of SCHCC patients within 60 days postoperatively. The median time for normalization was 35.5 days (8–152 days). Thus, it is possible to predict the survival of the patient 2 months after surgery by using a microcomputer with high accuracy (Tang et al. 1981).

Generally, serum AFP will be eliminated according to its half-life (3.5–4 days). Therefore, the normalization time usually depends on the original AFP level. The median times for AFP to return to normal after resection of SCHCC with relation to original AFP levels are listed in Table 5. The failure of AFP to decline according to

Table 5. AFP normalization after resection of SCHCC, with relation to original AFP level

Original AFP (ng/ml)	AFP return to normal (median days)
⩽500	23.5
501– 5000	35.5
5001–50000	50.0
>50000	100.5

half-life, and to return to normal, always reveals a palliative resection, and early adjunctive treatment is indicated. Long-term follow-up monitoring of AFP at 2-month intervals is of prime importance for early detection of subclinical recurrence or subclinical metastasis. Reappearance of abnormal AFP without associated evidence of active liver disease always represents recurrence. Regeneration of liver after human hepatic resection is almost never accompanied by elevation of serum AFP. If reappearance of AFP meets the AFP diagnostic criteria, with or without positive imaging findings, reoperation is recommended.

The postoperative follow-up studies for AFP-negative SCHCC after resection include periodic examination by means of real-time ultrasonography, serum γ-GTP, ALP, and skin delayed hypersensitivity reaction to old tuberculin.

VIII. Problems to Be Solved

Problems to be solved in the surgical treatment of SCHCC include multinodular cancer and coexistent macronodular cirrhosis with noncompensated liver function, in which surgery cannot be tolerated, even in the subclinical stage.

References

Adson MA, Weiland LH (1981) Resection of primary solid hepatic tumors. Am J Surg 141: 18–21

Axtell IM, Cutler SJ, Myers MH (1972) End results in cancer – report no. 4. US Department of Health, Education and Welfare, Public Health Service, NIH, NCI, Bethesda, pp 72–76

Berjian RA, Douglass HO, Nava HR, Karakousis C (1980) The role of hepatic artery ligation and dearterialization with infusion chemotherapy in advanced malignancies. J Surg Oncol 14: 379–387

Chuang VP, Wallace S, et al. (1981) The palliative role of hepatic arterial infusion and arterial occlusion in colorectal carcinoma metastatic to the liver. Lancet 1: 349–351

Chuang VP, Wallace S, Soo CS, et al. (1982) Therapeutic Ivalon embolization of hepatic tumors. AJR 138: 289–294

Curutchet HP, Terz JJ, Kay S, Lawrence W Jr (1971) Primary liver cancer. Surgery 70: 467–479

El-Domeiri AA, Huvos AG, Goldsmith HS, et al. (1971) Primary malignant tumors of the liver. Cancer 27: 7–11

Fisher B (1977) The changing role of surgery in the treatment of cancer. In: Becker FF (ed) Cancer-6 – A comprehensive treatise. Plenum, New York, pp 401–421

Fortner JG, Shiu MH, Kinne DW, et al. (1974) Major hepatic resection using vascular isolation and hypothermia perfusion. Ann Surg 180: 644–652

Fortner JG, Maclean BJ, Kim DK, et al. (1981) The seventies evolution in liver surgery for cancer. Cancer 47: 2162–2166

Foster JH (1970) Survival after liver resection for cancer. Cancer 26: 493–502
Foster JH, Berman MM (1977) Solid liver tumors. Saunders, Philadelphia, pp 62–104
Friedman MA, Volberding PA, Cassidy MJ, et al. (1979) Therapy for hepatocellular carcinoma with intrahepatic arterial adriamycin and 5-fluorouracil combined with whole liver irradiation – a Northern California Oncology Group Study. Cancer Treat Rep 63: 1885–1888
Honjo I, Mizumoto R (1974) Primary carcinoma of the liver. Am J Surg 128: 31–36
Huang XY, Zhang QM (1982) Results of surgical treatment of carcinoma of the liver – report of 181 cases. Chin J Surg 20: 68–70[1]
Ishikawa K (1976) Follow-up study of patients with primary liver cancer. Report 3. Acta Hepatol Jpn 17: 460–465
Li GC, Wang CE, Zhu SL, et al. (1982) Surgical treatment of 563 cases of primary liver cancer. Cancer (Chin) 1: 9–18[1]
Lin TY (1970) Primary cancer of the liver, quadrennial review. Scand J Gastroenterol 6: 223s
Lin TY (1976) Recent advance in technique of hepatic lobectomy and results of surgical treatment for primary carcinoma of the liver. In: Popper H, Schaffner F (eds) Progress in liver diseases, vol V. Grune and Stratton, New York, pp 668–682
Lin TY (1979) Resectional therapy for primary malignant hepatic tumors. Int Adv Surg Oncol 2: 25–54
Lin ZY, Lu JZ, Cao YZ, et al. (1983) Therapeutic embolization for primary liver cancer. Chin J Oncol 5: 197–201[1]
Offenstadt G, Huguet C, Gallot D, Bloch P (1978) Hemodynamic monitoring during complete vascular exclusion for extensive hepatectomy. Surg Gynecol Obstet 146: 709–713
Okuda K, Kasai Y, Sugawara K, et al. (1980) Primary liver cancer in Japan. Cancer 45: 2663–2669
Plengvanit U, Viranuvatti V, Chearanai O (1974) Treatment of primary liver carcinoma. Med Chir Digest 3: 301–306
Reed ML, Vaitkevicius VK, Al-Sarraf M, et al. (1981) The practicality of chronic hepatic artery infusion therapy of primary and metastatic hepatic malignancies – ten-year results of 124 patients in a prospective protocol. Cancer 47: 402–409
Ryu M, Uematsu S, Watanabe Y, et al. (1982) The significance of intraoperative ultrasonography for hepatic surgery. APASL Meeting, Hong Kong, (abstract no. 4)
Shen KN, Yan ZB, Qin WX, et al. (1983) Results of surgical treatment of primary liver cancer – an analysis of 195 cases. Cancer (Chin) 2: 81–83[1]
Sorensen TI, Aronsen KF, Aune S, et al. (1979) Results of hepatic lobectomy for primary epithelial cancer in 31 adults. Am J Surg 138: 407–410
Starzl TE, Koep LJ, Weil R III, et al. (1980) Right trisegmentectomy for hepatic neoplasms. Surg Gynecol Obstet 150: 208–214
Takasaki K, Muto H, Harada M, et al. (1982) Experience with hepatic resection of 60 cases of hepatocellular carcinoma. Acta Hepatol Jpn 23: 159–164
Tang ZY (1981) Surgical resection of primary liver cancer. In: Tang ZY (ed) Primary liver cancer. Shanghai Sci and Technical Publisher, Shanghai, pp 238–258[1]
Tang ZY, Qian SG (1977) Surgical treatment of primary liver cancer. Jiangsu Med 3: 501–505[1]
Tang ZY, Li JH (1981) Prediction of survival time by means of microcomputer after resection of primary hepatic cancer. Shanghai Med J 4: 470–473[1]
Tang ZY, Yang BH (1974) Primary liver cancer – clinical analysis of 3254 cases (from 11 provinces, 21 hospitals in China). Tumor Prevent Treat Study 2: 207–215[1]
Tang ZY, Yu YQ, Zhou XD, Chen QM (1981) Factors influencing primary liver cancer resection rate. Chin Med J [Engl] 94: 749–754
Tang ZY, Yu EX, Wu CE, Gu XY (1979) Diagnosis and treatment of primary hepatocellular carcinoma in early stage – report of 134 cases. Chin Med J [Engl] 92: 801–806
Tang ZY, Lu JZ, Zhou NQ, et al. (1982) Small hepatocellular carcinoma. VI. value of hepatoarteriography, B-scan ultrasonography, and liver scintiscan in the localization of small HCC – a comparative study based on operative findings. Acta Acad Med Primae Shanghai 9: 101–105[1]
Tang ZY, Yu YQ, Lin ZY, et al. (1983) Subclinical hepatocellular carcinoma. Chin J Oncol 5: 226–228[1]
Tilchen E, Patt YZ, McBride CM et al. (1981) Sequence of regional chemotherapy and surgery – management of colorectal adenocarcinoma confined to the liver. Arch Surg 116: 959–960
Wang CE, Li GC (1963) Surgical treatment of primary carcinoma of liver. Chin Med J [Engl] 82: 65–78

Wu MC, Chen H, Zhang XH et al. (1980) Primary hepatic carcinoma – resection over 18 years. Chin Med J [Engl] 93: 723–728

Wu MC, Zhong JP, Zhang XH, et al. (1981) Normothermic hepatic vascular exclusion for hepatectomy. Chin J Surg 19: 36–40[1]

Wu MC, Zhang XH, Chen H, Wu BW (1982) Experiences with hepatectomy in 467 cases. Chin J Digest 2: 190–193[1]

Yamada R, Nakatsuka H, Nakamura K, et al. (1979) Transcatheter arterial embolization therapy in unresectable hepatoma – experience in 15 cases. Acta Hepatol Jpn 20: 595–603

Yan ZB, Shen KN (1980) Camptothecin as adjunctive treatment of primary liver cancer. Cnin J Surg 18: 361–362[1]

Yu YQ, Tang ZY (1974) Surgical resection of primary liver cancer – analysis of 258 cases. Tumor Prevent Treat Study 2: 215–218[1]

Yu YQ, Tang ZY, Zhou XD (1980a) Experience in resection of small hepatocellular carcinoma. Chin Med J [Engl] 93: 491–494

Yu YQ, Tang ZY, Zhou XD et al. (1980b) Bloodless hepatectomy. Chin J Surg 18: 146–147[1]

Yu YQ, Tang ZY, Zhou XD, et al. (1980c) Evaluation of reoperation of primary liver cancer. Jiangsu Med 6 (11): 4–6[1]

Yu YQ, Tang ZY, Zhou XD, et al. (1981) Treatment of primary hepatic cancer by YAG laser, a preliminary report. Acta Acad Med Primáe Shanghai 8: 29–31[1]

Yu YQ, Tang ZY, Zhou XD, et al (1983): Treatment of large primary liver cancer in stages. Chin J Surg 21: 92–93[1]

Zhou XD, Tang ZY, Yu YQ, et al. (1979) Cryosurgery for liver cancer – experimental and clinical study. Chin J Surg 17: 480–483[1]

Zhou XD, Tang ZY, Yu YQ, Yu TT (1980) Hepatectomy using hepatic clamp. Jiangsu Med 6 (12): 9–11[1]

1 Chinese

7 Factors Influencing Resectability and Resection Survival Rates of Subclinical Hepatocellular Carcinoma

Zhou Xin-da, Tang Zhao-you

Surgical resection is accepted as the treatment of choice for SCHCC. One of the major problems is how to provide a simple and objective approach to preoperative prediction of the resectability rate (RR) and a postresection prediction of the survival rate (SR). This chapter analyzes factors that influenced RR in 90 cases of SCHCC explored and SR in 60 cases of SCHCC resected and treated at Zhong Shan Hospital, Shanghai First Medical College, from January 1971 to January 1983.

I. Clinical Data

Over the past 12 years, exploratory laparotomy has been performed in 90 cases of SCHCC. Of these, 70 cases (77.8%) were discovered in a mass survey, and 20 cases (22.2%) on follow-up monitoring of chronic hepatitis and cirrhosis or on physical examination. Pathologically 65.6% were associated with macronodular cirrhosis and 34.4% without, or with micronodular cirrhosis. Small HCC ($\leqslant 5$ cm) was found in 70.0%. Surgical resection was performed in 60 of the 90 patients, the RR being 66.7%. The resection method was right hepatectomy in 18.3%, and local and left hepatectomy in 81.7%. The operative mortality was 1.7%. Survival rates calculated by the life table method were 1-year, 85.0%; 3-year, 72.9%; and 5-year, 72.9%.

II. Factors Influencing Resectability Rate

A. Single-Factor Analysis of SCHCC

The RR of $\leqslant 30$-year-old patients was higher than those of >30- to <50-year and $\geqslant 50$-year-old patients, being 88.9% versus 68.6% and 56.7% respectively. The RR of cases with or without micronodular cirrhosis was higher than that of cases with macronodular or severe macronodular cirrhosis, i.e., 80.6% versus 59.3% (Table 1).

Of 90 SCHCC cases explored, 97.8% were AFP-positive before operation. Of these, the patients with AFP <500 ng/ml had a slightly higher RR (85.7% versus 76.1%). Similar results were observed in our previous report, the RR being 62.5% among patients with AFP <500 ng/ml and 33.6% among patients with AFP $\geqslant 5000$ ng/ml ($P<0.05$) (Zhou et al. 1982).

The RR of cases with γ-GTP (Orlowski's method, normal level <6 units) $\leqslant 20$ units was higher than that of cases with γ-GTP >20 units, the RR being 67.1% versus 44.4%. Similar results were observed in our previous report, the RR being 47.0% versus 21.5% ($P<0.001$) (Zhou et al. 1982).

In this series, the localization of SCHCC was done by liver scan, selective celiac or hepatic arteriography, or ultrasonography. The position of the SCHCC was determined before operation in 88 patients (97.8%). The RR of patients with a single tumor in the left lobe was higher than that of patients with a single tumor in the right lobe or the porta hepatis, and with bilateral multiple tumors, the RR being 93.3%, 83.8%, 54.5%, and 21.4% respectively. Unfortunately, only 15 patients (16.7%) had the tumor in the left lobe. It is similar to our previous report, in which the RR for these four groups were 68.4%, 53.3%, 8.3%, and 4.5% respectively ($P < 0.01$) (Zhou et al. 1982).

The RR of patients with negative A-mode ultrasound findings was slightly higher than that of patients with positive findings (66.2% versus 57.1%). No significant difference was observed from our previous report, where the RR were 45.7% versus 38.5% ($P > 0.05$) (Zhou et al. 1982).

The RR of patients with normal right diaphragm roentgenography was slightly higher than that of patients with abnormal right diaphragm roentgenography (66.2% versus 57.1%). However, in our previous report, a statistically significant difference ($P < 0.001$) was found between the RR of patients with normal right diaphragm roentgenography and that of patients with abnormal right diaphragm roentgenography (56.9% versus 23.9%, $P < 0.001$) (Zhou et al. 1982). The reason may

Table 1. Factors influencing resectability rate before SCHCC exploration (90 cases)

Item	No. of cases	No. of resections	Resectability rate (%)
Age ⩽ 30 years	9	8	88.9
> 30 years – < 50 years	51	35	68.6
⩾ 50 years	30	17	56.7
None or micronodular cirrhosis	31	25	80.6
Macronodular cirrhosis	59	35	59.3
AFP < 500 ng/ml	21	18	85.7
⩾ 500 ng/ml	67	51	76.1
γ-GTP < 20 unit	70	47	67.1
⩾ 20 unit	9	4	44.4
Tumor site – left	15	14	93.3
right	37	31	83.8
hepatic portal	22	12	54.5
bilateral	14	3	21.4
A-mode ultrasound (–)	68	45	66.2
(+)	7	4	57.1
Right-diaphragm X-ray (–)	66	46	69.7
(+)	6	3	50.0
Tongue substance – normal	35	27	77.1
abnormal	51	27	52.9
History of hepatitis or cirrhosis (–)	33	24	72.9
(+)	57	36	63.2

be that 70% of cases in this series had small HCC of ⩽5 cm, which usually appeared on normal right diaphragm roentgenography. In this series, tongue substance observed before operation was recorded in 86 cases (95.6%). Thirty-five cases (40.7%) had a normal tongue appearance and 51 cases (59.3%) a red or reddish-purple tongue appearance. The normal tongue substance group had a higher RR (77.1% versus 52.9%). Similar results were observed in our previous report (55.0% versus 39.6%) (Zhou et al. 1982).

There was a slight difference between patients with and those without a history of chronic hepatitis or cirrhosis, the RR being 63.3% versus 72.7%, similar to our previous report (49.2% versus 63.3%) (Zhou et al. 1982).

B. Multivariate Analysis of HCC

Single-factor analysis leads to a false conclusion owing to the interference of other factors; multivariate analysis may have a more reliable conclusion. However, in this series the number of SCHCC cases with complete data was too small for multivariate analysis. Our previous data from a multivariate analysis of 83 HCC cases including SCHCC and clinical HCC were as given in Table 2 (Zhou et al. 1982).

Subjects. Eighty-three cases with complete data on 17 variables probably related to the RR were subjected to multivariate analysis, 39 were resected and 44 were not.

Method. It is appropriate to apply "The Theory of Quantification 1" (Dong et al. 1979) to perform multivariate analysis and discrimination. The 17 indices, four quantitative and 13 qualitative, can be analyzed to decide whether or not a cancer can be resected. The frequency distribution curves of the scores for the 83 cases are shown in Fig. 1, from which one can see that discrimination according to these indices was rather satisfactory. The curves between resectable and nonresectable groups are far apart and the misclassification rate is very low.

Results. Multivariate analysis indicated a higher RR in patients with the following factors: mass screening, subclinical (stage 1), AFP < 500 ng/ml, left-side cancer, normal X-ray of right diaphragm, γ-GTP < 20 units, and normal tongue substance. The partial correlation coefficients of the items range from 0.0881 to 0.6617 (Department of Health Statistics, Shanghai First Medical College, 1979).

The mean accuracy of predicted RR with computer indices was 92.8% (77/83), being 92.3% (36/39) in the resected group and 93.4% (41/44) in the nonresected group.

In predicting the RR using the 17 indices from Table 2, i.e., all quantitative and qualitative markers, a total score <0 indicates a resectable cancer, >0 a nonresectable cancer. For example, the scores of cases 25 and 59 were as follows (Table 2):

$$25 = 32 \times 0.1 + 450 \times 0.0001 + 0.05 \times 3 + 10 \times 0.05 + 0 + 0 + 0 + 0 + 0 + 0 + 0 + 0 + 0 + 0 + 0.53 + 0 + 0 - 15.65 = -11.22$$

Total score <0; it was a resectable cancer.

$$59 = 42 \times 0.1 + 16000 \times 0.0001 - 0.05 \times 13 + 0.05 \times 6 - 0.64 + 0 + 5.83 + 0 + 0 + 0 + 1.78 + 1.82 + 0 + 11.35 + 0.53 + 0.16 + 0 - 15.65 = 10.15$$

Total score >0; it was a nonresectable cancer.

Table 2. Multivariate analysis of factors influencing resectability rate before exploration (83 cases of SCHCC and CHCC)

Item	Resected cases (%)	Scores	Case 25	Case 59
Age ⩽ 30 years				
> 30– < 50 years	0.47	0.1 × yr	32	42
⩾ 50 years				
Stage I (SCHCC)	0.31	0	×	
II (moderate)	0.16	−0.64		×
Without cirrhosis	0.45	0	×	×
With cirrhosis	0.02	−4.13		
Mass-survey patients	0.36	0	×	
Clinical patients	0.11	1.82		×
Symptoms (−)	0.33	0	×	×
(+)	0.14	1.59		
Signs (−)	0.29	0	×	×
(+)	0.18	−1.78		
AFP ⩽ 20 ng/ml				
< 500 ng/ml				
< 5000 ng/ml	0.47	0.0001 × AFP	450	16000
⩾ 5000 ng/ml				
γ-GTP ⩽ 20 units	0.47	−0.05 × γ-GTP	3	13
and/or ALP > 20 units		0.05 × ALP	10	6
Tumor site – left	0.13	0.22	×	
right	0.10	3.95		
hepatic portal	0	5.83		×
bilateral	0	9.96		
A-mode ultrasound (−)	0.35	0	×	×
(+)	0.12	2.06		
Right-diaphragm X-ray (−)	0.43	0	×	×
(+)	0.04	1.89		
ALT ⩽ 40 units	0.43	0	×	×
> 40 units	0.04	0.15		
OT test (−)	0.01	5.25		
(+)	0.46	0	×	×
Tongue substance normal	0.39	0	×	
Tongue substance abnormal	0.08	11.35		×
History of hepatitis (−)	0.22	0		
(+)	0.53	0.35	×	×
History of cirrhosis (−)	0.46	0	×	
(+)	0.01	0.16		×
	Constant	−15.65		
	Total		−11.22	10.15

OT, old tuberculin

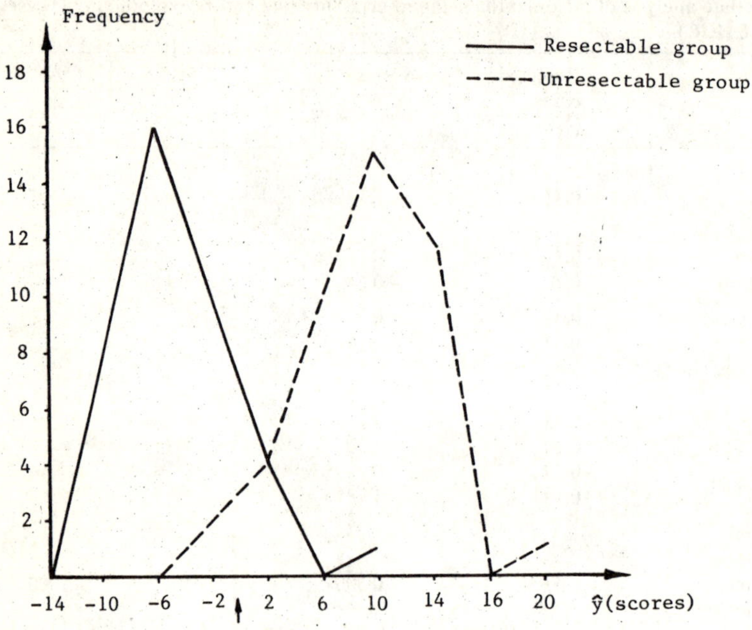

Fig. 1. Frequency distribution curves of scores of the 83 cases

C. Discussion

According to our data, all the factors that significantly influence the RR can be grouped into three categories:

Size of the tumor. Smaller tumors are often detected in mass screening, AFP <500 ng/ml, subclinical stage, normal X-ray of right diaphragm and γ-GTP <20 units. This is not only logical, as the AFP level is correlated with the size of the tumor as well as with the stage of the disease, but it can also explain the higher RR in SCHCC.

Site of the tumor. Patients with tumors located in the left lobe had a significantly higher RR (93.3%). However, tumors located in the hepatic portal or very close to the inferior vena cava were formerly considered "off limits" by surgeons. Recently, the technique of organ isolation with hypothermic perfusion has been employed with some success in resection of HCC near that region in five patients in this series.

Number of tumors. Multiple cancers also limit resection, the RR being only 21.4%. Therefore, bilateral partial hepatectomy has been performed instead of typical lobectomy for some individual patients. It is our conclusion that early detection of SCHCC and employment of new techniques for radical tumor extirpation remain the principal means of increasing the RR and prolonging survival. Mass screening of populations in areas with a high incidence of HCC, and of patients with a long history of cirrhosis or hepatitis, was the main approach to early identification as well as to achieving a higher proportion of resectable cases and a higher percentage of radical resections. According to our previous results, a comparative study showed that resection and radical resection in mass surveys and clinical patients were statistically different ($P < 0.001$) (Zhou et al. 1982).

It is generally accepted that the RR is also limited by concomitant severe macronodular cirrhosis. According to our data, the RR of patients with or without micronodular cirrhosis was higher than that of patients with macronodular or severe macronodular cirrhosis (80.6%) versus 59.3%). In patients who also had severe macronodular cirrhosis, partial hepatectomy was done instead of hemihepatectomy, and in our experience most patients with cirrhosis were able to tolerate partial resection. In any case, we believe that coexistent severe macronodular cirrhosis limits the RR to a certain extent.

The tongue substance may provide valuable information for preoperative prediction of the RR. Our previous study of the relation between tongue substance and HCC demonstrated (Tang et al. 1978) that in most patients with normal tongue substance the tumor was in a subclinical stage and of a simple type clinically, with single nodules, and accompanied by mild or no cirrhosis; moreover, a high RR and longer survival were observed. This series also showed that the patients with normal tongue substance had a higher RR than those with cardinal red tongue appearance (77.1% versus 52.9%). According to our previous data, a statistically significant difference was also found in those two groups, using multivariate analysis (Zhou et al. 1982).

III. Factors Influencing Resection Survival Rate of SCHCC

Patients with AFP returning to ≤20 ng/ml after resection of SCHCC had a much better prognosis, the 5-year SR being 82.0% however, no patients in the group with abnormal AFP after resection survived 5 years (Table 3). This is similar to our form-

Table 3. Factors influencing survival rate after resection of SCHCC (60 cases)

Item	No. of cases	Survival rate (%) (Life table method)		
		1-year	3-year	5-year
Postoperative AFP ≤20 ng/ml	48	93.2	82.0	82.0
>20 ng/ml	8	42.9	–	–
Tumor ≤5 cm	42	86.2	78.3	78.3
>5 cm	18	76.5	61.8	–
Single nodule	45	92.3	83.7	83.7
Multiple nodules	15	62.2	40.0	–
Local and left hepatectomy	49	86.4	76.4	76.4
Right hepatectomy	11	67.5	56.3	56.3
Age ≤30 years	9	88.9	88.9	88.9
>30 years–<50 years	34	87.2	74.0	74.0
≥50 years	17	69.6	60.9	60.9
None, or micronodular cirrhosis	25	87.0	82.1	82.1
Macronodular cirrhosis	35	80.3	64.5	64.5

er report, where the 5-year SR were 64.9% and 0% respectively ($P<0.01$) (Tang et al. 1981).

Patients with small HCC ≤5 cm had a better prognosis than those with tumors >5 cm. Our previous studies demonstrated that the 5-year SR was 56.2% for the former and 17.0% for the latter, and a statistically significant difference was found in these two groups, using multivariate analysis. (Tang et al. 1981).

The long-term survival of patients with single tumors (single small HCC or massive tumor without infiltrating nodules) was much better than that of patients with multinodular tumors (multinodular small HCC, multinodular or massive HCC with infiltration). Similar results were observed in our former series where the 5-year SR was ten times higher with single nodular tumors than with multiple nodular tumors (45.0% versus 4.8%, $P<0.01$) (Tang et al. 1981).

It seems that the prognosis of local and left hepatectomy was slightly better than that of right hepatectomy, although our previous reports showed that there was no statistical significance ($P>0.05$) (Tang et al. 1981).

It also seems that the SR was slightly higher in patients ≤30 years of age. Foster reviewed the world literature in 1970 and found that the 5-year SR was 14% in adults, but 33.3% in infants and children (Foster 1970). Ishikawa (1976) reported that the 3-year SR in patients <15 years of age was 24.9% while it was only 14.8% in adults.

The prognosis was likely to be better in patients with or without coexisting micronodular cirrhosis than in those with macronodular cirrhosis, concurring with the results of our previous reports (Tang et al. 1981).

In conclusion, early and radical resections are recognized as the most important factors influencing prognosis after resection of SCHCC; biological characteristics and coexisting cirrhosis also deserve to be noted.

References

Department of Health Statistics, Shanghai First Medical College, China (1979) Multiple linear regression and curvilinear regression. In: Department of Health Statistics, Shanghai First Medical College (ed). Methods of medical statistics. Shanghai Scientific and Technical Publishers, Shanghai, pp 87–98[1]

Dong WQ, Zhou GY, Xia LX (1979) The theory of quantification 1. In: Dong WQ, Zhou GY, Xia LX (eds) The theory of quantification and its application. Jilin People Publishers, Jilin, pp 1–32[1]

Foster JH (1970) Survival after liver resection for cancer. Cancer 26: 495–502

Ishikawa K (1976) Follow-up study of patients with primary liver cancer. Report 3. Acta Hepatol Jpn 17: 460–465

Tang CL, Tang ZY (1978) Clinical relationship between tongue substance and primary liver cancer. New Med J 7: 33–35[1]

Tang ZY, Yu YQ, Zhou XD, et al. (1981) Factors influencing primary liver cancer resection survival rate. Chin Med J [Engl] 94: 749–754

Zhou XD, Tang ZY, Yu YQ, et al. (1982) Factors influencing resectability rate of primary liver cancer. Chin J Surg 20: 595–597[1]

1 Chinese

8 Bloodless Hepatectomy and Hepatic Clamp in Resection of Small Hepatocellular Carcinoma

Zhou Xin-da, Tang Zhao-you

I. Bloodless Hepatectomy

Surgical resection is still considered to be the most effective modality for treatment of HCC. Not uncommonly, however, the tumor is very close to, or directly invades the inferior vena cava, hepatic vein, or portal vein. Such a tumor, even small, has often been declared unresectable, as its removal may lead to alarming iatrogenic morbidity and mortality (Wang et al. 1963; Foster 1970; Brasfield et al. 1972; Shiu et al. 1975). In most instances death is due to uncontrollable hemorrhage during operation. To permit safer resection of hepatic neoplasms located in such areas, Fortner and his associates (1971, 1974a) devised a new method of organ isolation hypothermic perfusion – bloodless hepatectomy with hypothermic perfusion. Based on their previous experience in total hepatectomy and orthotopic liver transplantation (Fortner et al. 1970), they believed that the liver could be temporarily isolated from the general circulation and preserved by hypothermic perfusion for several hours, and that the liver function after isolation perfusion would be satisfactory, even after 80% had been resected. Forty-one hepatic lobectomies, in cases where the tumors were previously considered nonresectable, have been performed by this method with encouraging results, 30-day operative mortality being 17% (Fortner et al. 1981). In addition to enabling lobectomy to be carried out in a controlled bloodless field, the technique also allows the surgeons to extract the tumor emboli and to cut and repair the involved vascular walls without the risk of massive hemorrhage.

Based upon canine experiments in our laboratory, bloodless hepatectomy with the hypothermic perfusion technique has been successfully performed by the authors in five patients since August 1978, for resection of HCC which was close to, or invaded the inferior vena cava, and was previously deemed nonresectable (Yu et al. 1980). The technique details, intraoperative physiological monitoring and management, and postoperative metabolic changes are described in this chapter.

A. Technique

If abdominal exploration reveals the tumor to be resectable, the incision is extended through a convenient right intercostal space, usually the sixth or seventh. The diaphragm is incised radially toward the inferior vena cava. The round ligament is divided and the falciform ligament incised to the inferior vena cava. The bilateral coronary, triangular, hepatorenal and hepatogastric ligaments should be divided, in that order. The right adrenal vein is then divided and ligated, and the dissection is continued behind the vena cava until the vena cava is completely free posteriorly, from the diaphragm to just above the right renal vein. The hepatic artery, common bile ducts, and gastroduodenal artery must be isolated individually. At this time, the entire liver is completely separated from all of its attachments except the major blood vessels and the extrahepatic bile ducts.

The gastroduodenal artery is then cannulated to the proper hepatic artery by means of a polyethylene catheter with a 2-mm internal diameter. The portal vein is cannulated with a 3-mm internal diameter catheter via a venotomy or its collateral vein. The hepatic artery and portal vein are temporarily occluded proximal to the cannula using noninvasive clamps. The common bile duct is also temporarily occluded. The vena cava above and below the liver is also separately occluded temporarily by means of vascular clamps and a cavotomy is performed immediately between the lower border of the liver and the lower occluding clamp to drain the perfusion fluid (Fig. 1). Ringer's lactate solution, which is cooled to 4 °C with 10 mg heparin, 10 mg procaine, and 1000 mg chloramphenicol per 1000 ml cold fluid, is then perfused at 100–120 ml per minute through the catheters of the hepatic artery and portal vein. This cooled solution passes through the liver parenchyma via the hepatic artery and portal vein, out the hepatic veins, into the vena cava, and out through the cavotomy. A few minutes later, when the liver parenchyma is adequately chilled, the liver becomes pale and is ready for the resection of the tumor. The affected lobe is removed using digital fracture or the scalpel handle, as described for hepatic lobectomy.

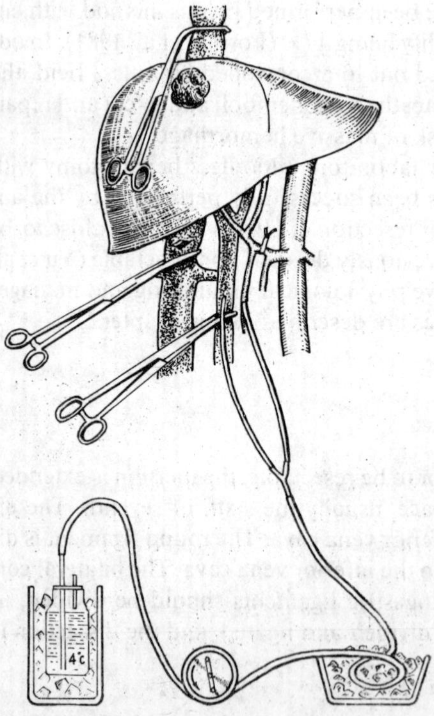

Fig. 1. Bloodless hepatectomy with hypothermic perfusion

Major intrahepatic vascular structures and bile ducts should be sutured. The involved wall of the vena cava can be included with the specimen and the defect is then repaired. The tumor emboli can also be extracted from the vessel. After removal of the tumor, the resection edge and remaining liver should be checked for leakage of perfusate, which would lead to bleeding or bile leakage when hepatic circulation is reestablished. Generally, the raw surface is covered by a free graft of omentum or covered with anterior and posterior flaps of the liver tissue. After that, the cavotomy is closed and hypothermic perfusion stopped. First the clamp on the suprahepatic inferior vena cava is removed, then those on the infrahepatic vena cava, the hepatic artery, portal vein, and common bile duct. The catheters are removed from the portal vein and hepatic artery, the venotomy is then closed and the gastroduodenal artery is ligated. After hepatic circulation is reestablished, the liver regains its color and warms rapidly. Free drainage of the subdiaphragmatic space should be maintained to prevent the formation of a subphrenic abscess. A chest drainage tube is provided. The thoracic and abdominal incisions are closed.

According to the authors' experience, the key points in using this technique may be as follows: (a) The liver must be completely detached from all but the major vascular attachments and the extrahenatic bile ducts at the first hepatic portal. Sometimes one or two vertebral veins must also be dealt with, as they enter the posterior aspect of the vena cava. The hepatic parenchyma can thus be isolated from the systemic circulation after the portal vein, hepatic artery, and infra- and suprahepatic inferior vena cava have been clamped so as to ensure that there is no bleeding when the hepatic parenchyma is transected. Fortner et al. (1971) reported unexpected complications with this technique in their first case. Although the surgical procedure seemed uneventful, perfusate from the cavotomy was pink, indicating some leakage of blood into the isolated system. The liver had been isolated from the circulation for approximately 1 h, and there was a gradual leakage of blood during the entire time, until cardiac arrest suddenly occurred. Therefore, it is of prime importance for this technique that the liver be completely isolated from the systemic circulation. (b) In order to keep the liver cells alive, it is necessary to ensure the effective and continuous hypothermic perfusion of the liver parenchyma through both the hepatic artery and portal vein, using Ringer's lactate solution at 4 °C. (c) After removal of the tumor, the cut surface should be checked carefully to make sure that there is no leakage of perfusion fluid, which would indicate bleeding sites when hepatic circulation is reestablished.

B. Case Reports

Case 1 (Table 1). A 22-year-old man, picked up by AFP mass screening with no symptoms or signs, was admitted to our hospital on January 13, 1978. His liver scintiscan was normal, but a selective hepatic arteriogram showed two small tumors on the right lobe, the right lower tumor measuring 1.7 cm in diameter and the right upper tumor 4 cm in diameter, very close to the inferior vena cava. The first operation was performed on February 1 of the same year – the right lower was tumor resected. Pathological examination showed that the tumor was HCC associated with micronodular cirrhosis. As the right upper tumor could not be resected by means of routine hepatectomy, hepatic artery catheterization was performed and postoperative perfusion chemotherapy with 5-fluorouracil carried out. After the first operation, however, the patient's AFP level failed to drop and the right upper tumor failed to regress. The second operation, using bloodless hepatectomy with hypothermic perfusion, was carried out 6 months later, on August 31 of the same year, the right upper tumor with a 1.5 × 0.2 cm wall of the inferior vena cava being resected and the defect of the inferior vena cava repaired under a bloodless field. The liver was isolated from the systemic circulation for 76 min. On the 8th day after surgery the patient was up and about. Both hepatic and renal functions returned to normal within 11 days postoperatively. AFP also declined to normal 1 month following the operation. Five years after surgery the patient is still alive, with negative AFP, and has returned to work.

Case 2 (Table 1). A 51-year-old man discovered by AFP mass screening, entered the hospital on October 10, 1978. An operation was performed on November 28 of the same year, and a 7 × 6 × 5 cm tumor was found at the bare area near the inferior vena cava, associated with severe macronodular cirrhosis. Using bloodless hepatectomy with hypothermic perfusion, the tumor and two pieces of the inferior vena cava wall – 0.8 cm and 0.6 cm in diameter – were resected, and the defects of the inferior vena cava were repaired. The liver was isolated from the systemic circulation for 96 min. Pathological examination showed the tumor to be HCC associated with severe macronodular cirrhosis. Both the AFP level and liver function returned to normal within 14 days, AFP remaining normal for 8 months. Unfortunately, the patient died 9 months after surgery noncompensated liver function because of severe macronodular cirrhosis.

Case 3 (Table 1). A 38-year-old man, discovered by AFP mass screening, was hospitalized on February 1, 1979. His liver scintiscan was normal, but the chest X-ray showed localized elevation of the right diaphragm. An operation was performed on February 21 of the same year and confirmed that the main tumor of 4 × 3.5 × 3.5 cm was located at the second hepatic portal, close to the middle hepatic vein entering the inferior vena cava, and that there was a satellite nodule of 0.5 × 0.5 × 0.4 cm surrounding the main tumor, associated with severe macronodular cirrhosis. Both tumors were successfully resected and the 0.7 × 0.3 cm defect of the middle hepatic vein was repaired, using bloodless hepatectomy with hypothermic perfusion. The liver was isolated from the systemic circulation for 86 min. Pathological examination showed that the tumors were HCC, associated with severe macronodular cirrhosis. Twenty-four hours after surgery the patient's general condition was good and the changes in hepatic and renal function were similar to those observed after a routine hepatectomy. Thirty-three hours after surgery chill, high fever, and a drop in blood pressure appeared suddenly during transfusion. Although a great deal of broad-spectrum antibiotic and cortisone was used, the patient died of irreversible shock on the 3rd day after operation. A blood bacteria culture demonstrated *Escherichia coli* in the blood, so the death may have resulted from sepsis.

Case 4 (Table 1). A 40-year-old woman entered the hospital on January 17, 1980, because of a vague pain in the right upper quadrant and a low elevation of AFP for

Table 1. Position, size of tumor, type of resection, and circulatory changes during bloodless hepatectomy in five patients

Sex, age Operation date	Illustration of operation		Hepatic ischemia (min)	Gold perfusate (ml)	Blood transfusion (ml)	Transfusion prior to ischemia (ml)	Systolic BP (mmHg)		Ventral venous pressure (cm H_2O)	
							Before ischemia	During ischemia	Before ischemia	During ischemia
Male, 22 years Aug. 31, 1978	4x4x4 cm HCC 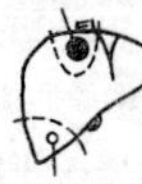 1.7x1.7x1.7 cm HCC resected on Feb. 1, 1978	Micronodular cirrhosis 1.5x0.2 cm inferior vena cava wall resected and repaired	76	8000	2600	1550 (including blood 800)	110	38	11	11 - 14
Male, 51 years Nov. 28, 1978	7x6x5 cm HCC 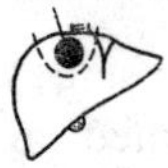	Severe macronodular cirrhosis Two pieces of inferior vena cava (0.8 cm and 0.6 cm diameter) resected and repaired	96	11 500	2800	4050 (including blood 2200)	88 - 100	44	12 - 15	9 - 14
Male, 38 years Feb. 21, 1979	4x3.5x3.5 cm HCC 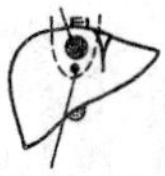 0.5x0.5x0.4 cm satellite HCC	Severe macronodular cirrhosis Middle hepatic vein repaired	86	11 500	1900	3700 (including blood 1200)	111 - 130	60	/	/
Female, 40 years Feb. 27, 1980	5x5x4.5 cm HCC 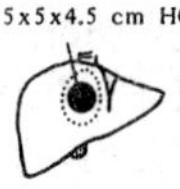	Micronodular cirrhosis Small left lobe, extended rigth lobectomy cannot be toleranted	39	5500	2400	2650 (including blood 1400)	80	60	11	6 - 7
Male, 37 years Jan. 12, 1981	5.5x3x3 cm HCC 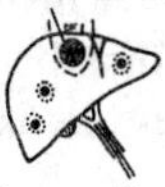 Three satellite nodules resected	Macronodular cirrhosis 0.3 cm inferior vena cava wall resected and repaired Hepatic arterial catheter consered	86	11 500	2700	2400 (including blood 1400)	110	32	11	9 - 9.5
	Mean		77.6	9600	2480	2870 (blood 1400)	102.8	46.8	11.8	9.9

6 months. A liver scan showed nothing, but B-scan sonography revealed space-occupying lesions in the right lobe. An operation was performed on February 27 of the same year, and a 5 × 5 × 4.5 cm tumor was found in the right lobe, very close to the inferior vena cava and associated with micronodular cirrhosis. The tumor was successfully resected using bloodless hepatectomy with hypothermic perfusion. The liver was isolated from the systemic circulation for 39 min. Pathological examination revealed a moderately differentiated HCC associated with micronodular cirrhosis. The postoperative course was uneventful, both hepatic and renal function returning to normal within 10 days postoperatively and AFP also declining to normal on the 12th day following the operation. It is now more than 3 years after the operation and the patient is still in good health with negative AFP.

Case 5 (Table 1). A 37-year-old man, discovered by AFP mass screening, entered the hospital on December 13, 1980. An operation was performed on January 12, 1981, revealing a main tumor of 5.5 × 3 × 3 cm located near the inferior vena cava, two small satellite nodules in the right lobe, and another small spread nodule in the left lobe, associated with macronodular cirrhosis. All tumors were successfully resected by using bloodless hepatectomy with hypothermic perfusion. Pathologically, the tumor was HCC associated with macronodular cirrhosis. The liver was isolated from the systemic circulation for 86 min. During the operation, 1000 mg 5-fluorouracil and 10 mg mitomycin C were administered through the hepatic catheter, which was then preserved for continuous perfusion of the chemotherapeutic drugs postoperatively. AFP declined to normal within 10 days and both liver and renal functions also returned to normal within 21 days postoperatively; however, 3 months following the operation the patient had mild jaundice, most probably due to obstruction of the bile duct. Reoperation was planned to relieve his jaundice, but the patient unfortunately refused. He was then discharged from the hospital, his condition rapidly deteriorated, and he died of liver function failure 6 months later.

C. Physiological Monitoring, Biochemical Changes, and Their Management During Surgery

Major hemodynamic and other acute physiological changes are encountered with this technique as a result of abrupt occlusion of the vena cava and portal vein and cold ischemia followed by resection of normal hepatic tissue (Howland et al. 1975).

1. Circulatory Changes and Transfusion

The changes in circulation that occurred in the five patients are shown in Table 1. The first patient, who had an inadequate expansion of circulatory volume prior to liver isolation, suffered severe hypotension for a long time after occlusion of the inferior vena cava. An ECG showed a remarkable decrease in the ST segment and reversal of the T wave until the second day after operation; this may have been due to lower blood pressure for an extended period, resulting in inadequate perfusion of the coronary artery. This complication was avoided in the four subsequent cases through deliberate overexpansion of the circulatory volume with blood and glucose solution prior to the isolation of the liver.

2. Changes in Serum Electrolytes and Acid-Base Balance, and Their Management

Arterial and central venous blood samples were drawn during the six different periods of the operation: (a) Following induction of anesthesia, (b) at the onset of isolation perfusion, (c) 30 min after isolation perfusion, (d) 60 min after isolation perfusion, (e) at the end of isolation perfusion, and (f) at the end of the operation. The blood samples were analyzed immediately for partial pressure of CO_2, excess base, pH, calcium, potassium and sodium. The changes in serum electrolytes and acid-base balance are shown in Fig. 2. The only significant changes were a decrease in the levels of pH and potassium immediately after perfusion, especially in the first patient, in whom the lowest level of pH was 7.22, excess base −6 to −14, and serum potassium 12 mg %. Since appropriate amounts of sodium bicarbonate were administered prior to isolation perfusion in subsequent cases, the changes in pH did not produce clinically significant acidosis. At the same time, respiratory compensation maintained the pH at the normal level or produced only slight alkalosis. The reason for the lower level of potassium was not clear, but an important cause of hypokalemia during the period after isolation perfusion might be the recovery of active uptake of potassium by the ischemic liver. Both metabolic acidosis and hypokalemia gradually improved following the restoration of hepatic circulation.

3. Changes in Hepatorenal Function and Serum Enzymes, and Their Management

During isolation perfusion of the liver, serum bilirubin and ALT increased remarkably, the average being 2.6 mg % total bilirubin with 0.7 mg % conjugated (direct) fraction bilirubin and 160 units of ALT (Fig. 2). The longer the occlusion of liver circulation, the more severe the disturbance of liver function. Serum albumin and globulin were maintained at relatively stable levels by the administration of large volumes of fresh blood and plasma. In case 2, damage to liver function with a slight elevation of serum bilirubin and ALT prior to the occlusion of liver circulation was the result of severe macronodular cirrhosis and oozing owing to the dissection procedure. When ALT, LDH, ALP, and creatine phosphokinase were monitored a significant increase in LDH at over 800 units and a slight elevation of ALT at 45–84 units were observed. There was no demonstrable change in ALP during isolation perfusion. These disturbances of liver function and enzymes were directly related to the damage to liver cells. It is emphasized, therefore, that the period of occlusion of liver circulation in patients with severe macronodular cirrhosis should be shortened as far as possible, and that effective cold perfusion must be ensured. The volume of urine decreased significantly to between 10 and 70 ml during isolation of the liver, probably owing to increased back pressure on the renal veins. The urine output gradually improved after restoration of hepatic circulation. A diuretic and mannitol were administered when necessary. Although there were some red cells, grannular casts, and protein in urine after occlusion of the liver circulation, the renal function was essentially normal.

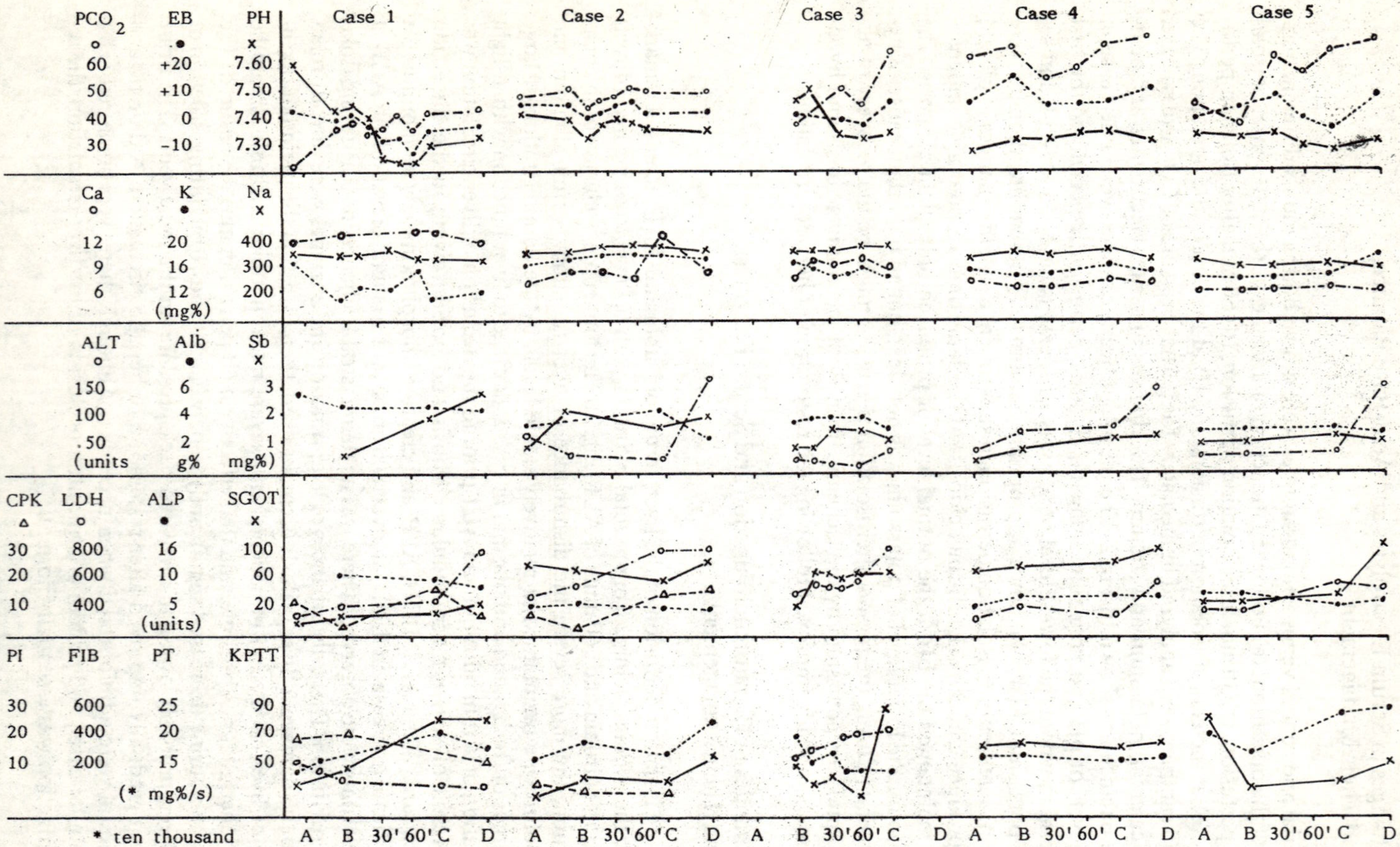

Fig. 2. Biochemical changes in five patients. A, following induction of anesthesia; B, onset of isolation perfusion; C, end of isolation perfusion; D, end of operation; PCO_2, Partial pressure of carbon dioxide; EB, excess base; Ca, calcium; K, potassium; Na, sodium; ALT, alanine tine phosphokinase; LDH, lactate dehydrogenase; ALP, alkaline phosphatase; SGOT, serum glutamic-oxaloacetic transaminase; PI, prothrombin index; FIB, fibrinogen; PT, prothrombin time; KPTT, kaolin partial thromboplastin time

4. Changes in Coagulation, and Their Management

Samples of blood for prothrombin indes (PI), fibrinogen (FIB), prothrombin time (PT) and kaolin partial thromboplastin time (KPTT) were obtained at five different stages of the operation: following induction of anesthesia, before, during, and after isolation of the liver, and at the end of the operation (Fig. 2). Major coagulation changes occurred in prolongation of KPTT, PT, and PI, but FIB and platelet levels showed no significant changes. These coagulation changes were probably due to the transfusion of large volumes of bank blood, deficiency of clotting factors, and perfusion of heparin contained in cold fluid, as well as to the disturbance of the liver function, because many coagulation factors are manufactured in the liver. Routine administration of fresh blood, vitamin K_1, and calcium during surgery, therefore, might help to decrease hemorrhage during and after the operation.

These disturbances of coagulation gradually returned to normal several days after operation. Disseminated intravascular coagulation (DIC) using this technique was reported in the literature (Fortner et al. 1974), but no case in our series showed evidence of DIC.

D. Changes in Liver Function and AFP After Bloodless Hepatectomy, and Their Management

The changes in liver function and AFP after employment of this technique were slightly more severe than, or similar to, those following a routine hepatectomy (McDermott et al. 1963; Lin et al. 1965; Zhou et al. 1980a, 1981). The ALT level rose strikingly immediately after bloodless hepatectomy and fell to normal rapidly, within a week. The changes in serum bilirubin after surgery were mainly in the conjugated (direct) fraction, increasing gradually within 3–5 days and returning to normal in 10 days. Serum AFP assessed by RIA became negative ($\leqslant 20$ ng/ml) in 1 month in all four surviving patients. The postoperative course was even more uneventful in case 4, with micronodular cirrhosis: ALT rose to 266 units and gradually returned to normal in 10 days; serum total bilirubin increased to 2.2 mg % and fell to normal rapidly within 6 days; AFP also gradually decreased to normal within 12 days after resection and remained normal for 3 years (Fig. 3). The postoperative disturbances of liver function were closely related to the duration of occlusion of the liver circulation, to the absence or presence of associated cirrhosis of the liver, to the amount of normal hepatic tissue resected, and to preoperative liver function. For example, in case 2, with severe macronodular cirrhosis and 96 min occlusion of liver circulation, as well as bile leakage with inadequate drainage, the patient's liver function did not return to normal for over 1 month following the operation.

More aggressive supportive treatment, especially 7–10 days after bloodless hepatectomy, is of great importance for an uneventful recovery. It was therefore necessary to take the following measures after operation: transfusion of plasma, fresh whole blood, or albumin every day or every other day; administration of vitamin K_1 and other coagulants; periodic examinations of liver function, prothrombin time, and electrolytes. Oxygen inhalation was used routinely for 4–5 days. Antibiotics that cause no damage to the liver should be used. Hypertension glucose, insulin,

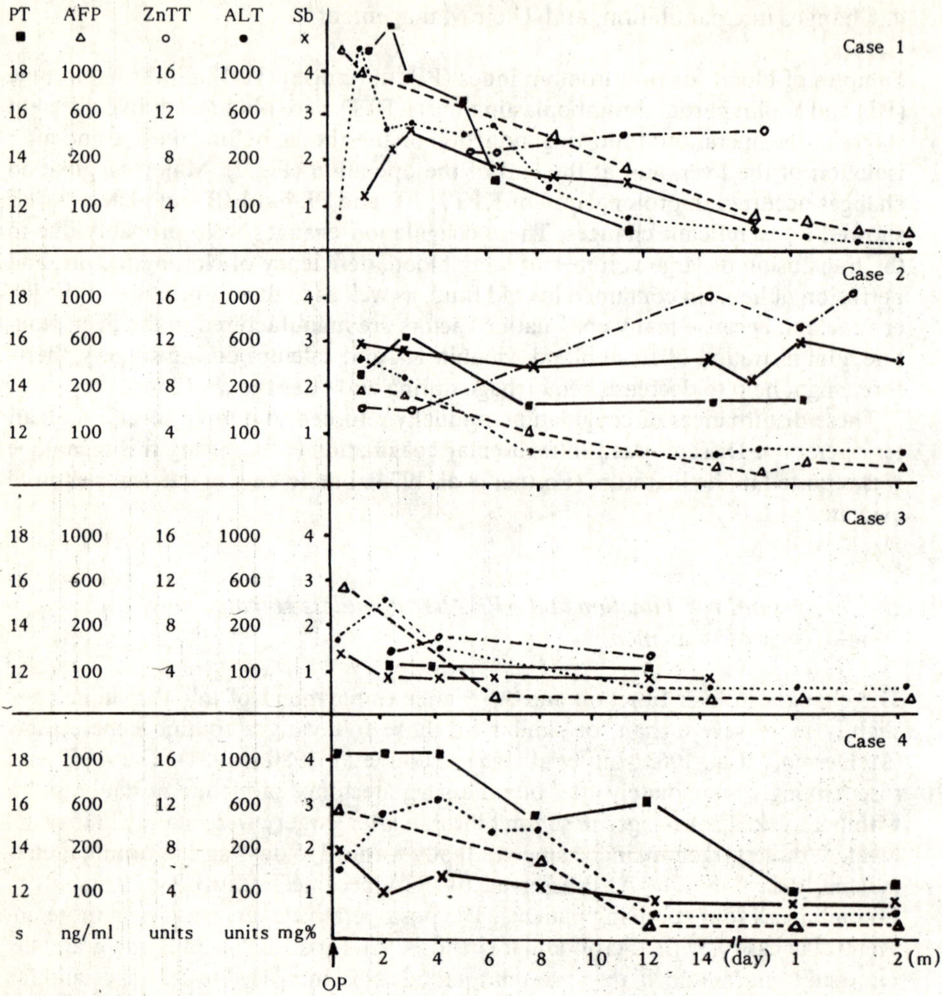

Fig. 3. Changes in liver function, AFP, and prothrombin time postoperatively in four patients. ZnTT, zinc sulfate turbidity test

ATP, and coenzyme A were given to patients whose liver function was severely impaired. When necessary, small doses of cortisone were also used for 2–4 days after the operation.

E. Evaluation

At present, hepatic resection is the only effective measure available for treating HCC; however, hemorrhage is an extensive operative risk during resection of a tumor close to the hepatic portal or inferior vena cava. Total clamping of the hepatic hilum is useless in the prevention of major venous bleeding, gaseous embolism, or both. On the other hand, complete hepatic vascular isolation with or without cold perfusion may theoretically reduce blood loss considerably during hepatic resection and decrease the hazard of lobectomy, as well as the resectability rate of liver tumors.

The technique of hepatic lobectomy by complete hepatic vascular isolation without the use of refrigeration, i.e., normothermic hepatic vascular exclusion, was first described by Heaney and associates (1966). A few instances of its use have been reported (Huguet et al. 1976, 1978; Offienstadt et al. 1978; Wu et al. 1981). With this technique, occlusion of the aorta above the celiac axis, cross-clamping of the portal triads, and occlusion of the inferior vena cava below and above the liver are done to avert the risk of uncontrollable caval hemorrhage. It is generally accepted, however, that the liver is one of the organs most sensitive to warm ischemia and that vascular exclusion at room temperature is tolerated only 15–20 minutes (Almersjö et al. 1968; Draz et al. 1971; Hirasawa et al. 1978; We et al. 1980). Such a short period is usually not enough for the performing of rather difficult hepatic resection or for the cutting and repairing of involved vessel walls. Moreover, dissection of the upper abdominal aorta above the celiac axis may be extremely difficult technically and even impossible when the left lobe of the liver is large, the large tumor is located on the left lobe of the liver, or both (Huguet et al. 1978). Furthermore, there is some risk related to hemodynamic alteration, as well as to ischemia of the intestine, kidney, and lower half of the body (Offienstadt et al. 1978; Adson et al. 1977). Thus, such a technique is usually indicated only in the emergency management of trauma to major hepatic veins or the vena cava, associated with liver injuries, and sometimes in resection of liver cancer which is located near to, but does not frankly invade the vena cava, and is without severe macronodular cirrhosis.

The adjunct measure of chilled perfusion of the liver, as first performed by Fortner et al. (1971), may thus be necessary to prevent hepatocellular damage during the anoxic period and to facilitate precise repair of veins. Hepatic tolerance to prolonged cold ischemia up to 87.6 $\pm$ 33.5 min is surprisingly good in the absence of severe cirrhosis and preoperative extensive hepatic dysfunction (Fortner et al. 1974a). Major hemodynamic and other acute physiological changes are encountered with this technique as a result of abrupt occlusion of the vena cava and portal vein and cold ischemia. However, with keen observation and prompt corrective measures when indicated, these changes can be minimized to ensure a safe and smooth resection. Finally, it must be emphasized that hepatic resection using the isolation–perfusion technique is only potentially useful in particular instances where cancer involvement of the vena cava or a tumor thrombus in the hepatic vessels requires management in a bloodless field (Fortner et al. 1974b, 1977). Routine employment of such a technique does not seem justified because it necessitates a prolonged operative procedure and postoperative hospitalization. For more favorably located lesions, the standard technique including the use of the hepatic clamp usually ensures good results and makes the procedure less sophisticated. The value of isolation and high-dose chemotherapy perfusion needs further evaluation (Fortner et al. 1975, 1981).

II. Hepatic Clamp in Resection of Small Hepatocellular Carcinoma

Because of the nature of the liver, hepatic resection is a complicated operative procedure, even for a skilled surgeon, which often involves massive blood loss, lengthy operating time, and difficulty in manipulating and controlling the cut surface of the liver. To lessen these complications and to improve the efficiency of the surgeon, some authors have reported that several hepatic clamps can be used for right, left, and partial hepatectomies (Doty et al. 1970; Storm et al. 1971; Lin 1973, 1974; Zhou et al. 1980b; Sha et al. 1980). A hepatic crush clamp has also been used in hepatic resection to crush the liver parenchyma and expose the intrahepatic vascular and ductal structures to direct vision (Lin 1974).

In China, a number of cases of small HCC have been reported since the application of AFP examination in a mass survey in 1971. In view of the fact that in 83.3% of patients with HCC there was coexistent liver cirrhosis (Tang et al. 1979), local resection rather than hemihepatectomy in surgical treatment of small HCC has yielded higher resectability, lower operative mortality, and similar ultimate outcome, especially in small HCC located at the right lobe with obvious cirrhosis (Tang et al. 1982). Since 1974, the authors have used a "two-jaw hepatic clamp" for various hepatectomies in HCC cases with cirrhosis and have found it to be quite satisfactory.

A. Instrument

The instrument is made of stainless steal; it consists of two clamping jaws and one handle (Fig. 4) and is similar to Storm's clamp (Storm and Longmire 1971). Each clamping jaw is 0.1 cm thick and 1 cm in breadth. Clamping jaws are of three different lengths, 21, 16, and 12.5 cm, to be used according to the size of the liver resected. The upper jaw has two fulcrum suspensions, while the lower one is fixed, with one point suspension. The flexible clamping jaws can be used to grip the liver parenchyma evenly, with minimal damage to liver tissue and more efficient control of bleed-

Fig. 4. Side view of the hepatic clamp with jaws 16 cm in length

ing from the cut surface of the liver because of three point suspensions and three troughs of the long axis of the jaws. The handle of the clamp is 33.5 cm in length.

The design of this clamp provides greater versatility of approach in the technique of hepatic resection. The surgeon may exert many pounds of uniform pressure on the liver and may release the clamp partially or completely.

B. Operative Technique

After complete detachment of all the ligaments of involved liver lobe, the hepatic clamp is placed on the healthy part of the affected liver lobe or on the liver at the anatomic boundary of the hepatic lobes. A resection line is made about 1 cm from the side of the clamp and Glisson's capsule is incised by means of electrocautery for the insertion of fingers or scalpel. Both intrahepatic vessels and ducts can be isolated, divided, and ligated under direct vision, at which time the assistant who holds the clamp should exert mild force on the clamp toward the remaining lobe so that the jaws may not slip down from the remaining liver as hepatic resection continues. After resection, the hepatic clamp is loosened slightly to check for bleeders; if there are any, they are sutured. The hepatic clamp is then totally removed. Usually, the affected lobe can be removed completely and almost bloodlessly in about 10 min (Fig. 5).

C. Results

Since 1974 the authors have used the hepatic clamp for resection of HCC in our department as well as in areas with a high-incidence of HCC and have reported 19 cases with complete clinical data. We found the technique to be feasible, simple, and safe (Zhou et al. 1980a). Of the 19 cases, nine were small HCC with cirrhosis.

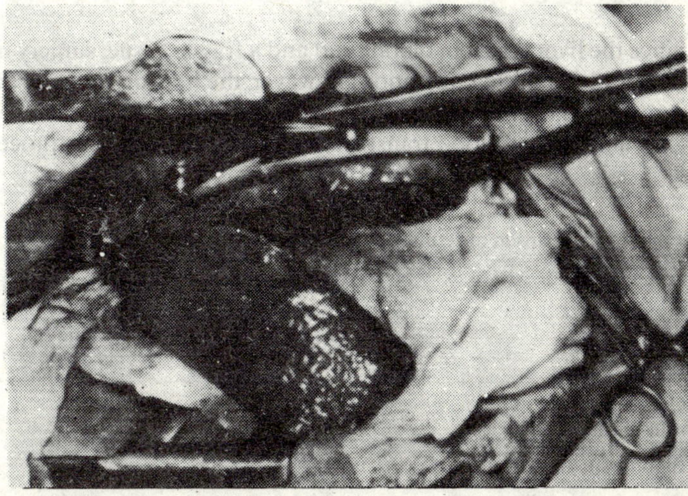

Fig. 5. Right hemihepatectomy with the hepatic clamp, showing almost bloodless field

Right hemihepatectomy was carried out in one case, right posterior hepatectomy in one case, right partial hepatectomy in six cases, and left partial hepatectomy in one case. Thoracolaparotomy was performed in five cases and abdominal incision in four. Liver function and AFP were checked periodically pre- and postoperatively. Pre- and postoperative management was the same as that mentioned in our previous reports (Zhou et al. 1980a).

The postoperative course in all patients was uneventful, even after right hemihepatectomy. There was no operative mortality, and no evidence of secondary bleeding, bile leakage, or liver function failure following surgery.

D. Evaluation

According to the data mentioned above and in comparison with an other 19 patients in whom the size and position of tumor, the degree of cirrhosis, and the type of resection were all similar to those of this series, it appears that hepatectomy using the hepatic clamp can reduce the operation time, decrease blood transfusion during the operation, and reduce operative mortality (Table 2).

1. Simplifying Transection of the Liver and Reducing Operation Time

Detachment of the falciform, coronary, and triangular ligaments of the affected lobe is all that is required before proceeding to actual resection of the liver. Since the extrahepatic vascular and ductal structures do not require individual isolation with scrupulous precaution, the operation time is significantly reduced. Average operative time (skin to skin) was 2.89 h in this series, but 4.63 h in the control group ($P < 0.01$). Using this technique, hepatectomy becomes simple, even in inexperienced hands.

2. Decreasing Blood Loss During Transection of the Liver

Since the liver is rich in blood fluid and a fragile tissue, surgery may result in a great loss of blood during operation; however, the hepatic clamp provides uniform pressure on hepatic tissue and almost absolute hemostasis in the cut surface of the liver. Less amounts of blood transfusion are required with this procedure than with the

Table 2. Comparison of results of hepatic resection in hepatic clamp group and control group

	Hepatic clamp group (19 cases)	Control group (conventional technique) (19 cases)	*P* value
Operation time, skin-to-skin (h)	2.89	4.63	<0.01
Blood transfusion (ml)	510	1468	<0.01
Operative mortality	0/19	2/19	>0.05

conventional technique because there is less damage to the hepatic artery, portal vein, and hepatic vein during the operation. Mean blood transfusion during the operation was 510 ml in this series as opposed to 1468 ml in the control group ($P < 0.01$). Complications resulting from large amounts of bank blood transfusion can thus be decreased.

3. Increasing Operative Safety

Since the first and second hepatic hila do not require extrahepatic isolation, unnecessary major vascular injuries, hemorrhage, air embolization, or iatrogenic tumor cell dissemination resulting from this isolation can be avoided. Moreover, according to our previous experience with changes in liver function after conventional hepatectomy, ALT rose to the mean level of 272.5 units and fell to normal 3 weeks later, serum bilirubin elevated to the average level of 3.15 mg % and returned to normal in 1 month, and serum albumin and prothrombin time decreased in most patients. However, liver function disturbances following the resection of the liver using this technique are only very slight, especially as regards serum bilirubin, which is only slightly elevated to the average level of 1.3 mg %, and returns to normal within 5 days after the operation. There was no operative mortality in our series, but it was 11% in the control group.

Nevertheless, the hepatic clamp is by no means suitable for every kind of liver resection. The only shortcoming is that when the tumor extensively involves the inferior vena cava, an entire hepatic lobe, or more, there may be no room to apply the hepatic clamp. In such instances, the technique of complete hepatic vascular isolation and cold perfusion, mentioned in the foregoing section, or transient occlusion of hepatic inflows at the first hilum may be resorted to for hepatic resection.

References

Adson MA, Beart RW Jr (1977) Elective hepatic resections. Surg Clin North Am 57: 339–360

Almersjö O, Bengmark S, Engevik L, et al. (1968) Serum enzyme changes after hepatic dearterialization in man. Ann Surg 167: 9–17

Brasfield RD, Bowden L, McPeak CJ (1972) Major hepatic resection for malignant neoplasm of the liver. Ann Surg 176: 171–177

Doty DB, Kugler HW, Moseley RV (1970) Control of the hepatic parenchyma by direct compression: A new instrument. Surgery 67: 720–724

Draz S, Minami R, Byfield J, et al. (1971) Biochemical evaluation of hepatic preservation techniques in the isolated rat liver. Surgery 70: 446–451

Fortner JG, Beattie EJ Jr, Shui MH, et al. (1970) Orthotopic and heterotopic liver homografts in man. Ann Surg 172: 23–32

Fortner JG, Shiu MH, Howland WS (1971) A new concept for hepatic lobectomy. Arch Surg 102: 312–315

Fortner JG, Shiu MH, Kinne DW, et al. (1974a) Major hepatic resection using vascular isolation and hypothermic perfusion. Ann Surg 180: 644–652

Fortner JG, Kinne DW, Kim DK, et al. (1974b) Vascular problems in upper abdominal cancer surgery. Arch Surg 109: 148–153

Fortner JG, Penneman R, Krakoff IH (1975) Actinomycin-D perfusion of the isolated liver for cancer. Bull Soc Int Chir 5: 399–403

Fortner JG, Kallum BO, Kim DK (1977) Surgical management of hepatic vein occlusion by tumor. Arch Surg 112: 727–728

Fortner JG, Maclean BJ, Kim DK, et al. (1981) The seventies evolution in liver surgery for cancer. Cancer 47: 2162–2166
Foster JH (1970) Survival after resection for cancer. Cancer 26: 493–502
Heaney JP, Stauton WK, Halbert DS, et al. (1966) An improved technique for vascular isolation of liver: Experimental study and case reports. Ann Surg 163: 237–241
Hirasawa H, Chaudry IH, Baue A (1978) Improved hepatic function and survival with adenosine triphosphate magnesium chloride after hepatic ischemia. Surgery 83: 655–662
Howland WS, Schweizer O, Fortner JG, et al. (1975) Intraoperative physiologic monitoring and management during hepatic lobectomy using the liver isolation-perfusion technique. Am J Surg 129: 608–615
Huguet C, Gallot D, Offenstadt G (1976) Normothermic complete hepatic vascular exclusion for extensive resection of the liver. N Engl J Med 294: 51–52
Huguet C, Nordlinger B, Calopin JJ, et al. (1978) Normothermic hepatic vascular exclusion for extensive hepatectomy. Surg Gynecol Obstet 147: 689–693
Lin TY, Chen CC (1965) Metabolic function and regeneration of cirrhotic and non-cirrhotic liver after hepatic lobectomy in man. Ann Surg 162: 959–972
Lin TY (1973) Results in 107 hepatic lobectomies with a preliminary report on the use of a clamp to reduce blood loss. Ann Surg 177: 413–421
Lin TY (1974) Most simplified technique for hepatic resection – crush method. Ann Surg 180: 285–290
McDermott WV Jr, Greenborger NJ, Isselbacher KJ, et al. (1963) Major hepatic resection: Diagnostic techniques and metabolic problems. Surgery 54: 56–66
Offienstadt G, Huguet C, Callot D, et al. (1978) Hemodynamic monitoring during complete vascular exclusion for extensive hepatectomy. Surg Gynecol Obstet 146: 709–713
Sha YW, Wang LM, Huang XY, et al. (1980) Right hemihepatectomy using hepatic clamp. Tianjin Med J Suppl 7: 37–37[1]
Shiu MH, Fortner JG (1975) Current management of hepatic tumors (collective review). Surg Gynecol Obstet 140: 781–787
Storm FK, Longmire WP (1971) A simplified clamp for hepatic resection. Surg Gynecol Obstet 133: 103–104
Tang ZY, Yu YQ, Lin ZY, et al. (1979) Small hepatocellular carcinoma – clinical analysis of 30 cases. Chin Med J [Engl] 92: 455–462
Tang ZY, Ying YY, Gu TJ (1982) Hepatocellular carcinoma – changing concepts in recent years. In: Popper H, Schaffner F (eds) Progress in liver disease, vol VII. Grune and Stratton, New York, pp 637–647
Wang CE, Li KT (1963) Surgical treatment of primary carcinoma of liver. Chin Med J [Engl] 82: 65–78
Wu MC, Chen H, Zhang XH, et al. (1980) Primary hepatic carcinoma resection over 18 years. Chin Med J [Engl] 93: 723–728
Wu MC, Zhong JP, Zhang XH, et al. (1981) Normorthermic total hepatic vascular exclusion for hepatectomy. Chin J Surg 19: 36–40[1]
Yu YQ, Tang ZY, Zhou XD, et al. (1980) Bloodless hepatectomy. Chin J Surg 18: 146–147[1]
Zhou XD, Yu YQ (1981) Changes in hepatic metabolism and their management after resection of primary liver cancer. In: Tang ZY (ed) Primary liver cancer. Shanghai Scientific and Technical Publishers, Shanghai, pp 258–270[1]
Zhou XD, Tang ZY, Yu YQ (1980a) Changes in liver function and their management after resection of primary liver cancer. Natl Med J China 60: 606–611[1]
Zhou XD, Tang ZY, Yu YQ, et al. (1980b) Hepatectomy using hepatic clamp. Jiangsu Med J 11: 9–11[1]

1 Chinese

9 Subclinical Recurrent Hepatocellular Carcinoma: Detection and Reoperation

Yu Ye-qin

Recurrence after resection for HCC is common, but reoperation has been reported only sporadically. As early as 1915, Yeomans reported on a patient operated on for recurrence 7 years after resection for primary carcinoma of the liver. In 1953, Quattlebaum suggested that second-look procedures be done on patients with liver cancer. Brunschwig, in 1957, reported on two patients who survived 5 years after right lobectomy for malignant hepatoma, one of these having a reoperation for recurrence 2½ years after the primary procedure. In 1965, Bradham and his colleagues mentioned a 21-month-old child who survived 4 years after a right lobe resection for malignant hepatoma and subsequent operations, including right pneumonectomy and resection of part of the chest wall, for recurrences. In 1967, Friesen et al. also delineated a case of hepatocarcinoma with seven reoperations in 4 years for recurrences; the patient remained well. Yu et al. (1980a, 1980b) and Chen et al. (1979) also stated that reoperation for recurrent liver cancer should be performed.

Although progress in resection for recurrent HCC has been made in the past few decades, the ultimate result is not satisfactory in the majority of cases. Faced with a highly malignant recurrent cancer, many surgeons find reoperation a decision most difficult to make and some might even adopt a defeatist attitude.

Since the advent of AFP determination in the 1970s, ultrasonography and selective hepatic angiography have also been widely employed and great advances achieved in the early diagnosis of HCC as well as subclinical or asymptomatic recurrent HCC. With aggressive management, including reoperation, survival could be prolonged.

In recent years some recurrent HCC cases in the subclinical stage have been treated by Yu et al. (1980b) with satisfactory results.

I. Subclinical Recurrence Can Be Detected in Time

Regular follow-ups at 1- to 2-month intervals should be routine for every postoperative patient. In addition to physical examination, chest roentgenography and others, AFP is the test of choice. When an AFP test turns from negative to positive or displays a low titer – for example, when AFP > 200 ng/ml persists for over 8 weeks while ALT is normal, recurrence and/or metastases should be highly suspected, calling for further examination of the liver and chest. Early recurrences can thus be detected.

II. Determining the Site of Recurrence and Reoperability

In addition to physical examination, a nuclide liver scan, mode-B ultrasonography, hepatoangiography, chest roentgenography, etc. are helpful in detecting the sites of recurrence and/or metastases. A second laparotomy for resection should be carried out in cases with unilateral or small, centrally located recurrent lesions within the remaining liver. A large palpable tumor often indicates nonoperability with intrahepatic dissemination. Pulmonary lobectomy should be performed in cases with unilateral solitary pulmonary metastatic lesions, provided there is no recurrence in the liver. The prognosis is fairly good in such cases.

III. Criteria for Reoperation

The general condition of the patient should be good; recurrent foci must be small; liver function and coagulation mechanisms should be adequate, without jaundice or ascites; and a serious complicating illness should not present.

IV. Selection of Surgical Procedures

Pulmonary lobectomy is sufficient for solitary or confluent metastatic HCC nodules in the lung. Partial resection should supersede regular resection in order to preserve as much functional liver tissue as possible. Otherwise, compromised liver reserve would lead to liver failure or even death. A central, superficially located small recurrent lesion in the right side of the liver could be resected locally or managed by cryosurgery (liquid nitrogen). In case of dense, inseparable adhesions precluding exposure of the recurrent mass, a polyethylene catheter can be inserted into the hepatic artery for postoperative infusion of chemotherapeutic agents. To put it in a nutshell, the surgical procedure selected should be optimal for the situation involved.

V. Clinical Material

From September 1977 to February 1983, 14 patients with recurrent HCC underwent reoperation in our hospital. Although asymptomatic, all these cases were detected by close follow-up and periodic monitoring of AFP levels. Ten of the 14 recurrences were in the remaining liver and four were in a lung. According to the site and size of the recurrences, various operative procedures were performed, including local resection, partial hepatectomy, cryosurgery, pulmonary lobectomy, and hepatic artery catheterization combined with postoperative chemotherapeutic drug infusion and exploration (Table 1, Fig. 1). The longest survival is 8 years after primary operation and reoperation, and the patient has resumed his original work.

Table 1. Data on reoperation in 14 cases of hepatocellular carcinoma

Case no.	Age	Primary operation			Reoperation						Result of reoperation
		Date	Cancer site	Operation	Date	Cancer site and size (cm)	Operation	Pathological diagnosis	AFP (ng/ml) Pre-operative	AFP (ng/ml) Post-operative	
1	36	Aug. 14, 75	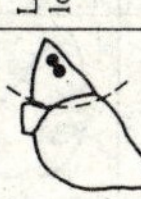	Left lateral lobectomy	Nov. 28, 77	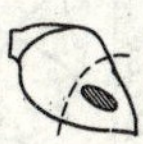 9x6x4	Partial hepatectomy	HCC	> 1000	100	Died at 8 months (total survival: 36 months)
2	51	April 24, 75	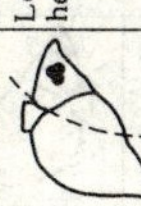	Left hemi-hepatectomy	April 25, 78	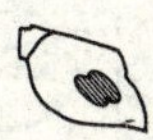	Exploration	Not biopsied	> 1000	> 1000	Died at 2 months (total survival: 38 months)
3	21	Dec. 16, 76	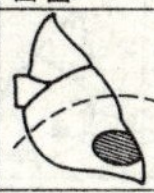	Right hemi-hepatectomy	Aug. 8, 78	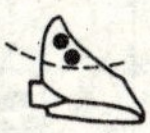 2.8x2x2 0.5x1x1	Partial hepatectomy	HCC	No determined	20	Died at 34 months (total survival: 54 months)
4	38	April 11, 78	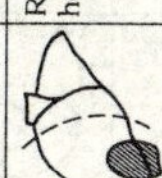	Right hemi-hepatectomy	Feb. 16, 79	Cancer could not be visualized due to dense adhesions	Hepatic artery catheterization	Not biopsied	1000	> 1000	Died at 16 months (total survival: 26 months)
5	57	Aug. 20, 75	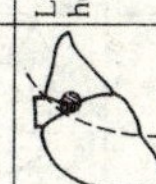	Left hemi-hepatectomy	Aug. 1, 79	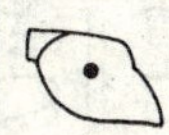 2x2	Cryo-surgery	HCC (needle biopsy)	1000	10	Well at 44 months (total survival: 92 months)
6	42	Aug. 22, 75	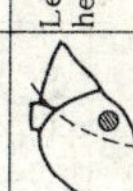	Left hemi-hepatectomy	May 24, 78	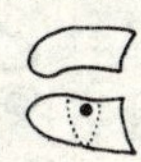 1.3x1.2x1	Right middle lobectomy	Metastatic HCC	280	<10	Well at 59 months (total survival: 92 months)
7	36	Jan. 20, 76	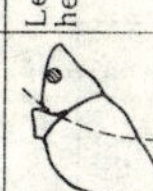	Left hemi-hepatectomy	Dec. 8, 79	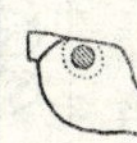 3.5x3.7x4.5	Local excision	HCC	310	20	Died at 27 months (total survival: 74 months)

VI. Critique on Reresection

Reoperation on recurrent or metastatic malignant tumors in selected patients has now become a trend in tumor surgery; it has been accepted because of successes with resection of pulmonary metastases from osteogenic sarcoma and of solitary hepatic metastases from colorectal carcinoma (Minton 1979; Beattie 1979; Ren and Shi 1979). Although some authors (Chen et al. 1979) state that results of reresection of the recurrent HCC were poor, we cannot concur. Of our 14 cases, nine patients survived, while five died 2 months to 3 years after reresection. The four patients with

Table 1. (continued)

Case no.	Age	Primary operation: Date	Primary operation: Cancer site	Primary operation: Operation	Reoperation: Date	Reoperation: Cancer site and size (cm)	Reoperation: Operation	Reoperation: Pathological diagnosis	Reoperation: AFP (ng/ml) Pre-operative	Reoperation: AFP (ng/ml) Post-operative	Result of reoperation
8	39	Nov. 6, 75	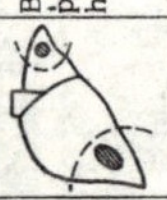	Bilateral partial hepatectomy	June 13, 78	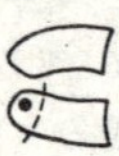 1.3x1.2x1	Right upper lobectomy	Metastatic HCC	30	20	Well at 58 months (total survival: 89 months)
9	45	April 22, 75	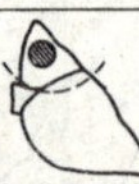	Left lateral lobectomy	Dec. 4, 78	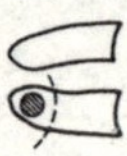 6x3x3	Right upper lobectomy	Metastatic HCC	> 1000	< 10	Well at 52 months (total survival: 96 months)
10	60	Sept. 2, 75	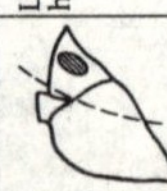	Left hemihepatectomy	Oct. 22, 79	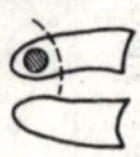 5x4x4	Left upper lobectomy	Metastatic HCC	30	< 10	Well at 42 months (total survival: 91 months)
11	48	July 26, 78	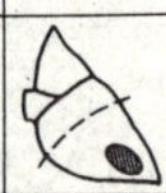	Right hemihepatectomy	July 8, 80	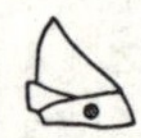 2.3x2.5	Cryosurgery	HCC (needle biopsy)	500	25	Well at 33 months (total survival: 57 months)
12	55	Dec. 2, 76	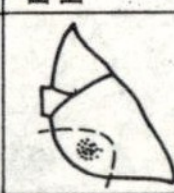	Partial hepatectomy	July 12, 82	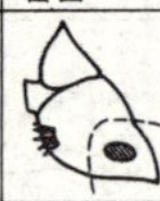 5x4x5	Partial hepatectomy	HCC	1000	< 20	Well at 9 months (total survival: 76 months)
13	50	Nov. 17, 80	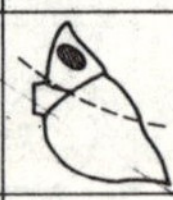	Left hemihepatectomy	July 2, 82	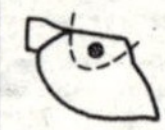 2x1.8x1.8	Partial hepatectomy	HCC	380	42	Well at 6 months (total survival: 26 months)
14	43	May 24, 82	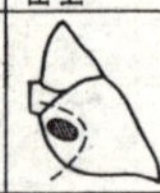	Partial hepatectomy	Feb. 9, 83	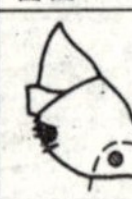 1.5x1.4x1.2	Partial hepatectomy	HCC	250	20	Well at 2 months (total survival: 11 months)

lung metastases remained well for 4–5 years. It should be noted that case 5 was subjected to cryosurgery only. After freezing of the recurrent tumor, AFP titers rapidly declined to normal within 2 weeks, and the patient is still alive. It can therefore be seen that cryosurgery is of value in the treatment of small recurrent HCC.

Our limited clinical material shows that the result of reoperation for highly malignant HCC in selected cases is reasonably good. Patients subjected to pulmonary lobectomy for solitary pulmonary metastases also seem to do better than those who undergo further resection for recurrence in the liver. Additional further studies will be made to substantiate this.

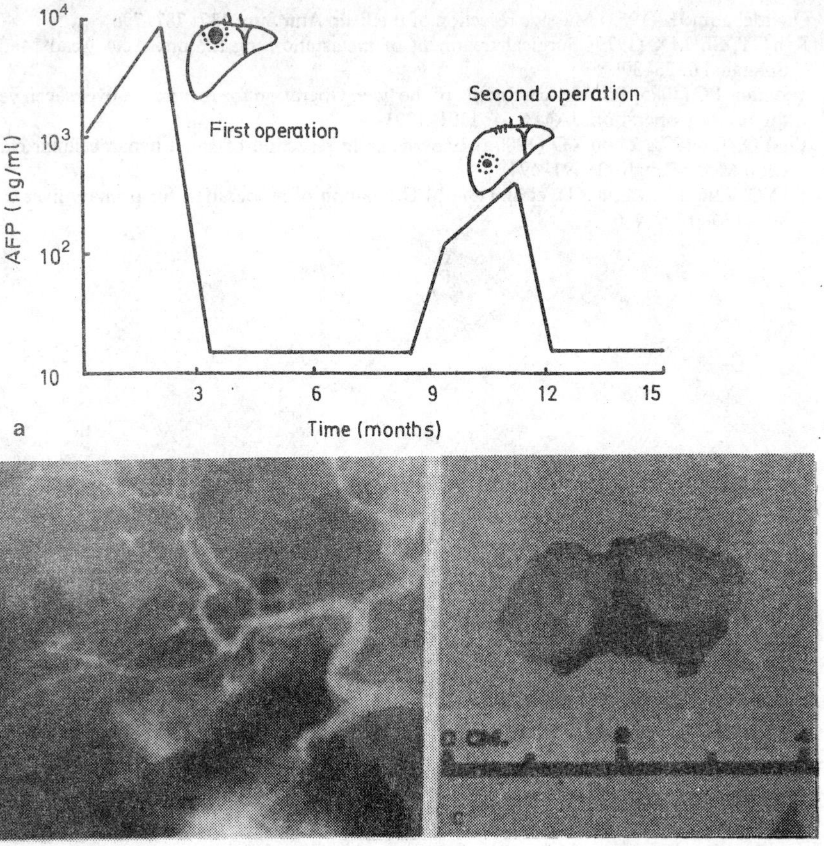

Fig. 1a–c. Reoperation of case No. 14, showing **a** AFP serial change, **b** angiographic finding *(bracket),* and **c** surgical specimen

References

Brunschwig A (1957) Long-term survival following right hepatic lobectomy. Am J Surg 94: 2–8

Bradham RR, Paul JR, Thrower WB, et al. (1965) Malignant hepatoma in a child: Survival following right hepatectomy, right pneumonectomy, and resection of diaphragmatic and parietal recurrence. Surgery 57: 767–773

Beattie EJ Jr (1979) Bone tumors – management of lung metastases of osteosarcoma. In: Canonico A, Estevez O, Chacon R, et al. (eds) Advances in medical oncology, research and education, vol XII. (Proc 12th Int Cancer Congr). Pergamon, Oxford, p 114

Chen H, Wu MC, Zhang SH (1979) Research on reoperation for primary liver cancer. Shanghai Med J 2: 794–796[1]

Friesen SR, Hardin CA, Kittle CF (1967) Prolonged survivals after partial hepatectomies and second-look procedures for primary and secondary carcinoma of the liver. Surgery 61: 203–209

Minton JP (1979) The use of serial carcinoembryonic antigen (CEA) determinations to predict recurrence of colon cancer and when to do a second-look operation. In: Canonico A, Estevez O, Chacon R, et al. (eds) Advances in medical oncology, research and education, vol XII. (Proc 12th Int Cancer Congr). Pergamon, Oxford, p 103

Quattlebaum JK (1953) Massive resection of the liver. Ann Surg 137: 787–796
Ren CY, Shi MX (1979) Surgical treatment of metastatic lung tumors. Acta Acad Med Primae Shanghai 6: 25–30[1]
Yeomans FC (1915) Primary carcinoma of the liver. Operation for recurrence over seven years after the primary operation. JAMA 64: 1301–1303
Yu YQ, Tang ZY, Zhou XD (1980a) Experience in resection of small hepatocellular carcinoma. Chin Med J [Engl] 93: 491–494
Yu YQ, Tang ZY, Zhou XD, et al. (1980b) Evaluation of reoperation for primary liver cancer. Jiangsu Med J 6: 4–6[1]

1 Chinese

10 Cryosurgery for Hepatocellular Carcinoma – Experimental and Clinical Study

Zhou Xin-da, Tang Zhao-you, Yu Ye-qin

Modern cryosurgery for the treatment of malignant neoplasms has been applied for more than two decades; however, it was mostly limited to surface or skin, rectal, prostatic, gynecological, head, and neck cancers (Holden and McKelvie 1972; Rand et al. 1968; von Leden et al. 1971). With visceral tumors, apart from the need to expose the tumor by laparotomy, the major problem is that destruction of large tumors by freezing is difficult. There were only a few reports on experimental studies (Cooper and Hirose 1966; Grady et al. 1973; Healey et al. 1971; Neel et al. 1971a, b; Serra and Brunschwig 1955; Zhou et al. 1979b). However, cryosurgery with liquid nitrogen had not yet been used for human HCC. The authors had used the method for treatment in 1979 (Zhou et al. 1979a).

This chapter presents the results of cryosurgery for HCC, including experimental and clinical studies, from June 1973 to December 1982. Devices for cryosurgery with liquid nitrogen (−196 °C), made by the Shanghai Institute of Technical Physics of the Academica Sinica, were employed (Fig. 1).

I. Experimental Study

A. Animals and Tumor Models

Group I consisted of 30 rabbits, four dogs and five head of young cattle, they were used in studies of cryosurgery of normal liver in order to observe the pathological changes, safety, and physical conditions during the operation. Group II was composed of 53 Kunming mice with hepatoma-22 solid ascitic tumors or S180 (pleomorphic cell) sarcomas; they were used to study the immunological effects of cryosurgery.

B. Experimental Methods

Animals in group I were anesthetized with intraperitoneal injections of sodium pentobarbital (4 mg per 100 g body wt.), and the liver was exposed through an upper midline incision. Cryosurgery of liver was applied in three ways (Cahan 1972; Dutta et al. 1977): direct contact freezing using a probe 3–5 cm in diameter, penetration freezing via a needle probe 0.3–0.4 cm in diameter, and spraying liquid nitrogen directly on the surface of liver. The duration of freezing was from 5 to 40 min. Needle thermocouples were placed on the liver surface and inserted 1 cm deep near the

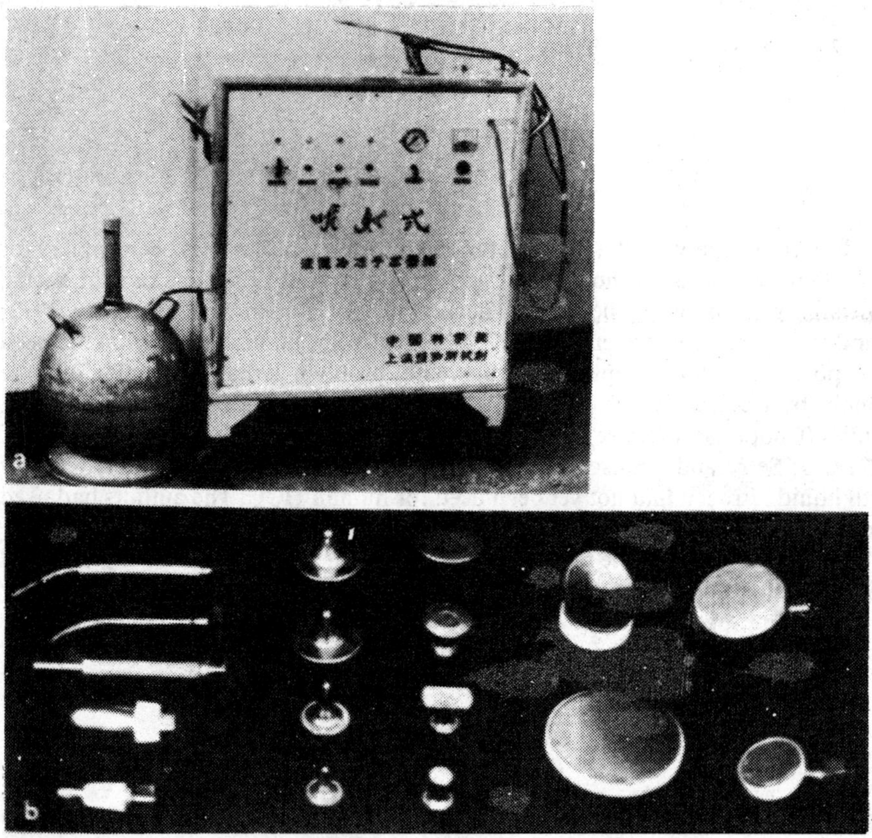

Fig. 1. **a** Cryosurgery unit with liquid nitrogen. **b** Various cryosurgery probes

center of the area of liver to be frozen; temperature records were traced on a recorder. Probe temperature was maintained at a constant −180 °C. The probe was applied to the same site twice. After each freezing, thawing was allowed to proceed spontaneously, and then the abdominal incision was closed without drainage. Laboratory data including serum ALT, total and conjugated (direct) bilirubin, and zinc sulfate turbidity test (ZnTT) were collected before cryosurgery, and on the 1st, 9th, and 16th day after cryosurgery. Animals were killed at 2 and 6 h and on the 1st, 3rd, and 7th day and every 2 weeks after cryosurgery. The liver was retained for detailed gross and microscopic examination. In group II animals, a 1-cm-diameter probe was in contact with the tumor for 1–2 min so that the temperature of the tumor base could be cooled to −20 °C. The tumor volume was measured periodically before and after cryosurgery; at the end, the growth rate of another implanted tumor was recorded.

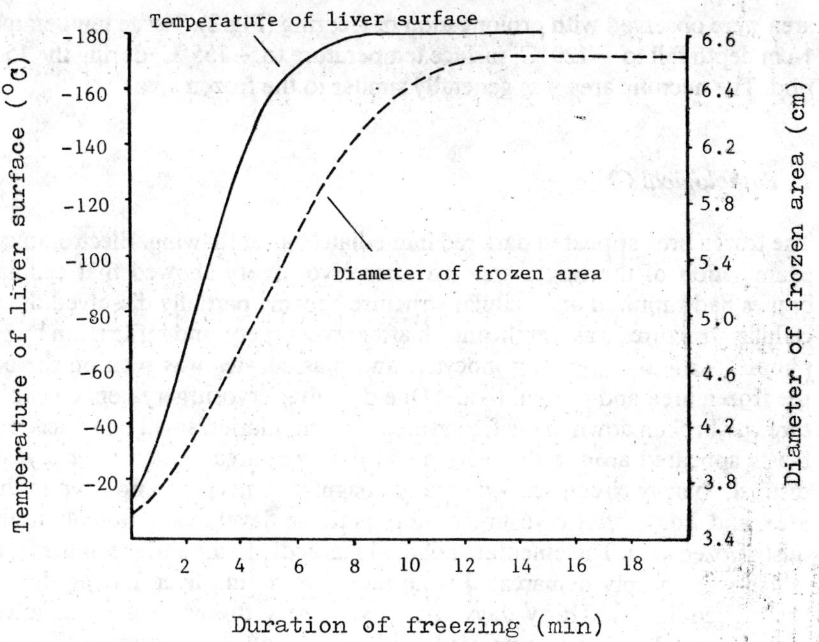

Fig. 2. Relation between drop in temperature and extension of frozen area (freezing liver of young cattle using 3-cm cryoprobe)

C. Safety of Hepatic Cryosurgery

Two rabbits died of hypothermia during cryosurgery. ALT rose to varying degrees in surviving animals immediately following cryosurgery and then returned to normal within 2 weeks. There were no significant changes in serum total and conjugated (direct) bilirubin and ZnTT before and after cryosurgery. During the operation, rupture of the hepatic capsule was observed with liquid nitrogen sprayed directly on the surface of liver, so that hemostasis was required. There was no evidence of rupture, delayed bleeding, or bile leakage after cryosurgery in any of the long-term survivors that were killed. If the gallbladder was frozen directly, there was no evidence of bile leakage either.

D. Physical Conditions

The volue of frozen tissue was directly related to probe size, duration of freezing, time of freeze-thaw, and blood supply of the tissue. For example, the largest surface diameter of frozen area was 8–9 cm, using 5-cm-diameter probe; however, the frozen area was about 6 cm in diameter with a 3-cm-diameter probe. Freezing with a cryoprobe produced a roughly hemispherical lesion. The freezing depth relative to the surface diameter was 1:2.0–2.8. The optimum effect was obtained after 12–14 min of freezing; only minor changes in temperature as well as in the frozen area were observed with prolongation of freezing (Fig. 2). Tissue temperature at the 1-cm depth fell to −120 °C, surface temperature to −155 °C, during the 15-min period. The necrotic area was generally similar to the frozen area.

E. Pathological Changes

The frozen area appeared dark red immediately after thawing. Electronmicroscopic examination of the target area 2 h after cryosurgery showed that cellular membranes had ruptured and cellular structure became partially dissolved. Necrosis of cellular structures was significant 6 h after cryosurgery, and infiltration by polymorphonuclear leukocytes, lymphocytes, and plasmacytes was seen on the border of the frozen area and normal tissue. One day after cryosurgery hepatocellular structure was broken down in the frozen area, and capillaries, small bile ducts, and fibroblasts appeared around the margin of the frozen area; 3 days after cryosurgery a distinct, sharply circumscribed area of coagulative necrosis appeared in the frozen area, and 7 days after cryosurgery fibrous tissue developed gradually in the previously frozen area. The omentum adhered markedly to the surface of the frozen area, which was sharply demarcated from the surrounding liver, having developed fibrous membranes. Thirty days after cryosurgery the area of coagulative necrosis was found to have contracted, and 45 days after cryosurgery there was only thin white, scar tissue left in the previously frozen area, with normal surrounding liver.

F. Immunological Findings

After we froze hepatoma-22 solid tumors, the growth of the original tumors, as well as that of the reimplanted tumors, was inhibited; this was considered to be a result of tumor-specific transplantation immunity induced by cryosurgery. Immunity was more significant 10 days after cryosurgery (Table 1). The more completely the tumor had been frozen, the stronger was the inhibition. There was no cross-immunity between hepatoma-22 solid tumors and S180 sarcomas.

Table 1. Comparison of the effects of cryosurgery on original and replanted solid hepatoma-22 tumors

Type of tumor	Group	No. of mice	Weight of tumor (g) (10th day)	Rate of tumor inhibition (%)	p value
Original tumor	Cryosurgery	17	5.07 ± 3.91	60	<0.01
	control[a]	12	12.64 ± 3.23		
Replanted tumor	Cryosurgery	17	0.68 ± 0.80	65	<0.01
	Control[a]	12	1.97 ± 1.48		

[a] Controls were sham operated (laparotomy)

II. Clinical Application

A. Indication

Cryosurgery for HCC was indicated for (a) relatively small and superficially located tumors, close to the first or second hepatic hilum or the inferior vena cava, which were unsuited for the conventional resection procedure; (b) tumors located at the right lobe in cases where the patient could not tolerate a right hemihepatectomy owing to coexisting severe cirrhosis with noncompensated liver function; (c) residual tumor at the cut surface or in the rest of liver after resection of the main tumor; (d) nonresectable recurrent HCC.

B. Patients

Zhou et al. (1979 a) reported on 35 HCC patients who had undergone cryosurgery with liquid nitrogen. Nine cases were at the early stage with no definite HCC symptoms or signs, 21 cases were at the moderate stage, between early and late stages, and five cases were at the late stage, with jaundice, ascites, or distant metastasis. Of the 35 cases, 11 had tumors ≤ 5 cm in diameter. All cases were confirmed histologically.

C. Operative Procedure

Epidural anesthesia was employed and the tumor was exposed through a right upper abdominal incision. Cryosurgery was performed with a 3–5 cm in diameter hollow, plate-like probe, which was in direct contact with the HCC. The probe and its handle met at the right or the bevel angle according to the site of the tumor. The probe was put on the tumor surface with minimal pressure, and the temperature began to drop. Neighboring organs and tissue should be protected with isolating materials; the temperature between the freezing and surrounding areas should also be determined by means of thermocouple needles in order to prevent damage. If the hepatic hilum was clear, it proved best to temporarily occlude the blood supply to the liver during cryosurgery in order to enhance freezing effects. Generally, the time for each freezing was from 15 to 20 min. Repetitive freeze-thaw cycles might augment the probability of necrosis, while hasty withdrawal of the probe before it was detachable, an insufficient number of freeze-thaw cycles, and hastening the thawing process could interfere with ultimate results. With larger tumors repeated freezing of separate areas comprising the whole tumor mass was employed. The vapor caused by the freezing process was removed with an aspirator. In cases with relatively large frozen area it was necessary to put a hot-water bag on the thoracic wall under the axilla to prevent general whole-body hypothermia. After cryosurgery the frozen area was covered by a graft of omentum to prevent bleeding. No drainage was necessary.

D. Pre- and Postoperative Management

Routine preoperative medication, including hypertonic glucose, vitamin K_1, and oral administration of streptomycin or Chinese medicinal herbs, was given for 2 days and an enema was administered before surgery. An uneventful postoperative course was observed in cases with a relatively small frozen area and a noncirrhotic liver; however, intensive care with albumin or plasma, fresh blood, and coagulants was necessary in cases with a large frozen area in cirrhotic liver. Oxygen inhalation was routinely given for 4–5 days. Chinese medicinal herbs, immunotherapy, and chemotherapy were needed for palliative cryosurgery. Liver function and serum AFP levels were also measured pre- and postoperatively.

E. Postoperative Reactions

Postoperative fever was slightly higher as compared with simple laparotomy, but it rarely exceeded 39 °C. A temporal elevation of ALT after cryosurgery was observed; however, it was not higher than that after routine hepatectomy, and returned to normal within 2 weeks. Elevation of ALT was closely related to the duration of freezing, the frozen area, and liver function before operation. There were usually no changes in the levels of total serum bilirubin and conjugated bilirubin, the ZnTT, and prothrombin time. Of the 35 cases, 24 cases were AFP positive, and in 17 of these 24 cases the AFP level dropped gradually after cryosurgery (70.8%). In one case, AFP returned to normal after cryosurgery, and remained AFP negative for 3.7 years; in another three cases, AFP remained negative for 2.5, 2.4, and 1.1 years after cryosurgery.

The postoperative course was uneventful in all of the 35 patients. There was no operative mortality, and there were no complications such as rupture of tumor, secondary bleeding, bile leakage, or abdominal infection.

F. Survival Rates

The longest survival was 7 years and 8 months after cryosurgery for treatment of residual tumor at cut surface, closing the inferior vena cava after resection of the main tumor. Chinese medicinal herbs, chemotherapy, and radiotherapy were used after the operation. Although AFP positive, the patient is still in good health. The 1-, 2-, and 3-year survival rates (calculated by the direct method) were 55.5% (19/34), 24.3% (8/33), and 10.0% (3/30) for the whole series (Zhou et al. 1979a). This rate was much higher than those for other conservative treatments with Chinese medicinal herbs and for chemotherapy (1- and 2-year survival rates were 13% and 0% respectively; Shanghai Coordinating Group for Liver Cancer Research, China 1974). Among the 11 patients with tumor nodules ⩽5 cm in diameter, 1-, 2-, 3-, and 5-years survival rates were 90.9% (10/11), 63.6% (7/11), 30.0% (3/10), and 12.5% (1/8) respectively.

G. Pathological Findings

Well-demarcated coagulative necrosis was observed in the frozen area, including both tumor and normal tissue, in autopsies. Collagen fibril hyperplasia could be seen in the marginal zone between the frozen area and normal tissue, and sometimes there was plasmocyte infiltration. A fibrous connective tissue capsule surrounding the frozen area was noticed in long-term observation (Fig. 3). There was only thin white, scar tissue left in the previously frozen tumor area (Fig. 4). The pathological changes mentioned above coincided with the experimental findings.

H. Case Reports

Case 1. A 62-year-old man entered the hospital on February 13, 1974 because of a pain in the upper right quadrant with positive AFP (both CIEP and AGD were positive) for 2 months. A liver scintiscan revealed a large filling defect on the right lobe. An operation was performed on February 28, and a tumor of 11 × 10 × 5 cm was found in the right lobe of the liver, associated with macronodular cirrhosis. Aspiration biopsy demonstrated HCC. The patient could not tolerate an extensive right hemihepatectomy owing to the coexisting cirrhosis and his age. Cryosurgery was carried out with a 3.5-cm probe which was in direct contact with the tumor for 20 min, with two freez-thaw cycles. AFP returned to normal 1 month after cryosurgery and remained negative for 3 years and 8 months. The size of the filling defect on the liver scintiscan had decreased remarkably 6 months after cryosurgery (Fig. 5).

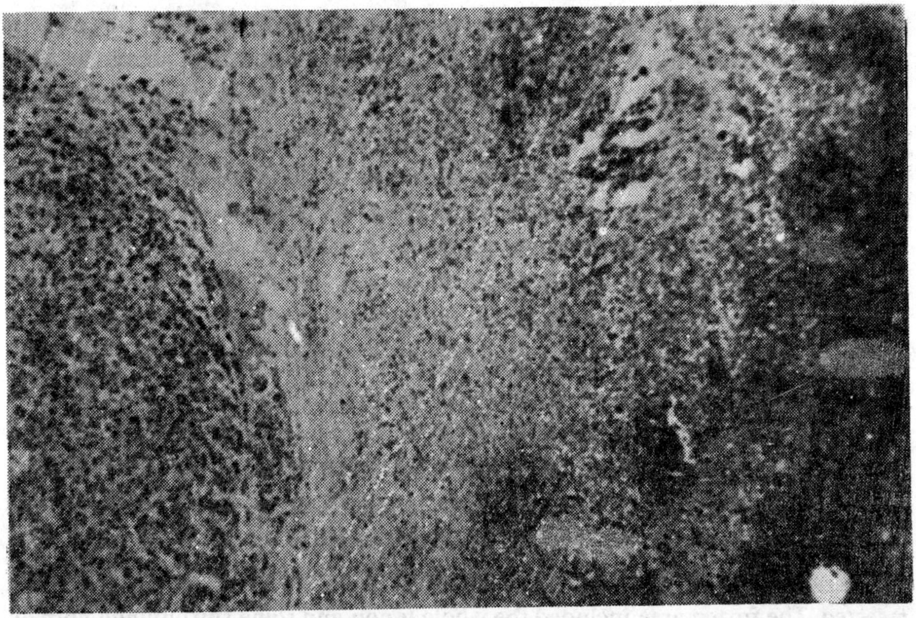

Fig. 3. Histology of marginal area of frozen necrosis. Coagulative necrosis with liquification and hemorrhage *(right),* surrounded by a thick fibrous capsule. H and E, × 100. (Reproduction by 25%)

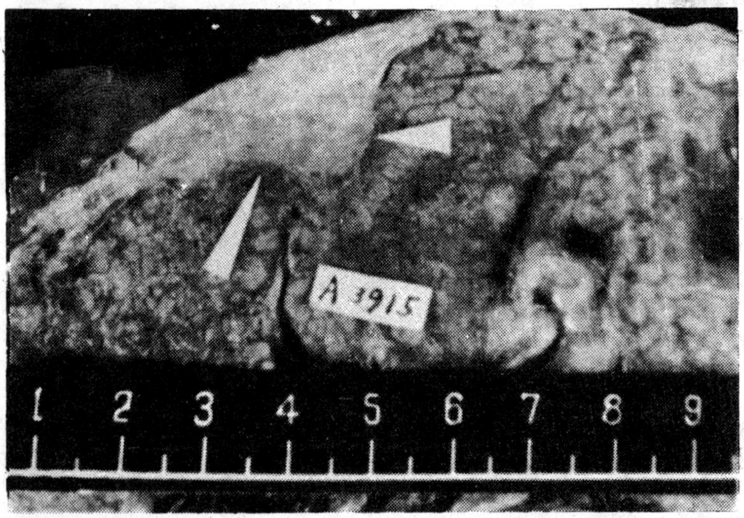

Fig. 4. Autopsy findings. Only thin, white scar tissue was left in previously frozen area of the tumor

Unfortunately, the patient died of pneumonia 4 years and 1 month following this operation. There was no tumor nodule in the original frozen area; only thick scar tissue was found on autopsy (Fig. 4).

Case 2. A 48-year-old man was picked up by AFP mass screening (RIA, > 1000 ng/ml). He underwent surgery on June 20, 1979 and two small tumors 1.5 and 0.8 cm in diameter were found, 1.0 cm deep in the middle hepatic lobe and associated with severe macronodular cirrhosis. Aspiration biopsy revealed HCC. Cryosurgery was carried out with a 3.5-cm probe which was in direct contact with each tumor for 20 min, with two freeze-thaw cycles. The frozen area involved all the nodules of the two tumors and some surrounding normal liver tissue. AFP returned to normal 2 weeks after cryosurgery and has remained negative. The patient is still alive and has been well for over 2 years and 6 months.

Case 3. A 57-year-old man was discovered by AFP mass screening. The first operation on August 20, 1975 revealed a well-encapsulated 3- × 3- × 4-cm tumor in the quadrate lobe near the second hepatic portal. An extensive left hemihepatectomy was performed. Pathologically, the tumor was HCC associated with micronodular cirrhosis. AFP declined to normal following resection, but reappeared at a level > 1000 ng/ml 3 years later. Subclinical recurrence of HCC was considered, despite the excellent condition of the patient; another operation was performed on August 1, 1979 and a tumor of 1 × 1.5 × 2 cm was found in the right lobe. Aspiration study confirmed HCC. Cryosurgery was carried out because no more liver could be resected. The frozen area included the whole lesion and some surrounding normal liver. The AFP level declined to normal again 2 weeks after cryosurgery. The patient has been in good condition for over 2 years and 4 months, with negative AFP.

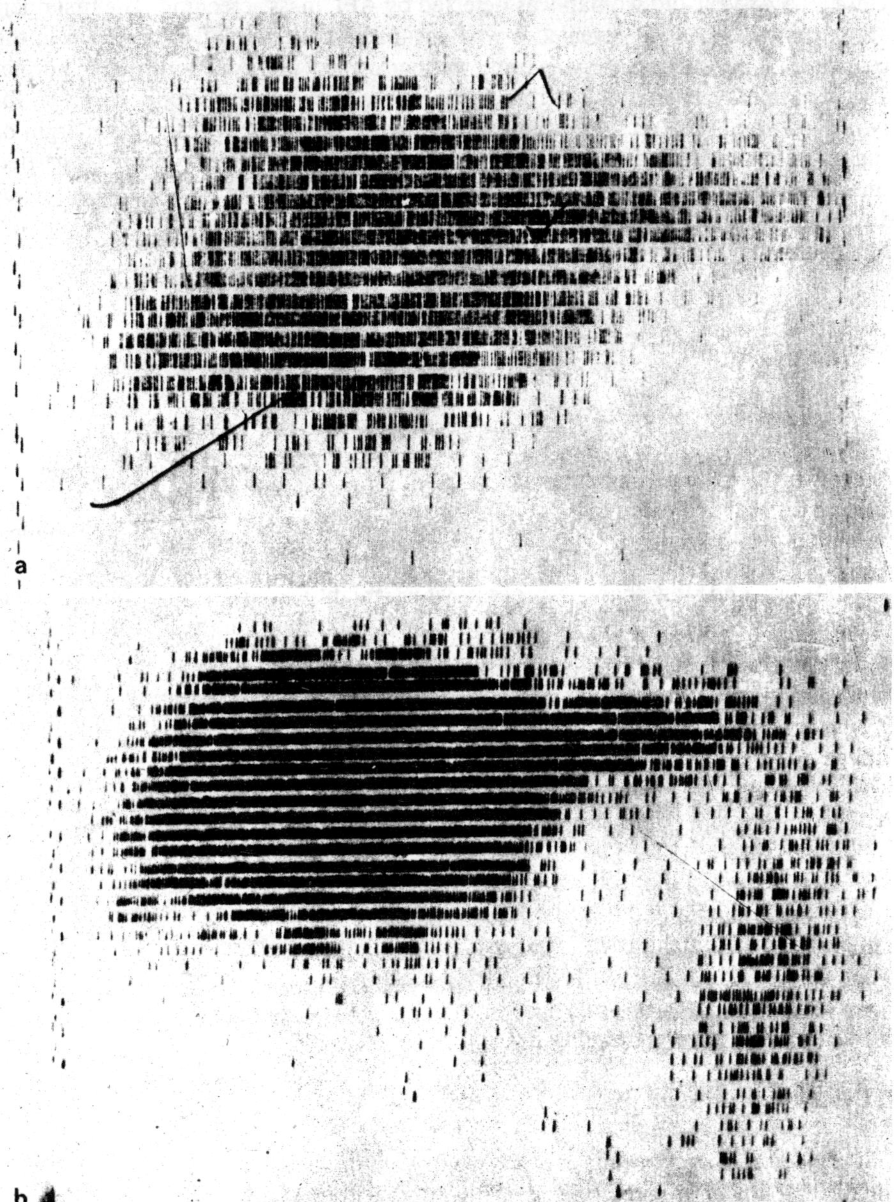

Fig. 5. a Before cryosurgery, liver scintiscan revealed a large filling defect on the right lobe. **b** Size of filling defect on liver scintiscan was remarkably decreased 6 months after cryosurgery

Case 4. A 48-year-old woman was detected by AFP mass screening. The first operation, on July 26, 1978, revealed a well-encapsulated tumor of 6×7×5 cm in the right lobe. A partial right hepatectomy was performed. Her AFP returned to normal 2 weeks after the operation, but rose again nearly 2 years later. A reoperation on July 7, 1980 revealed a recurrent tumor of 2.5 cm in diameter near the cut margin of the right lobe. HCC was confirmed by pathological study, and cryosurgery carried out. AFP declined to normal 2-weeks after cryosurgery and remained negative for 1 year and 1 month. The patient has survived for over 2 years and is still well, though her AFP subsequently reappeared above normal.

III. Discussion

A. Mechanism of Cryosurgery

According to our experimental and clinical findings, there is no doubt that irreversible coagulative necrosis can be obtained in both normal liver and cancer cells after cryosurgery with liquid nitrogen. The mechanism of frozen necrosis might be elucidated as follows: Intra- and extracellular ice crystals are formed during the repeated fast freezing and slow thawing process, which might lead to mechanical cell damage, rupture of nuclear and cellular membranes, alterations in the lipoprotein components of the cell membrane, change in PH, toxic concentration of electrolytes, polymerization, denaturation of proteins, vascular stasis and microthrombi resulting in ischemia of the tissues. Moreover, there is evidence that cryosurgery might also induce the creation of some specific antibodies (Ablin et al. 1976; Helpap et al. 1976; Nagasue 1975). Some reports suggested that the distant metastases from cancers of the prostate might shrink in size in some individuals following cryosurgery (Ablin and Reddy 1977; Ikeda 1976; Soanes et al. 1969, 1970). Our laboratory results also suggested that following the freezing of hepatoma-22 solid tumors, both original and reimplanted tumors were inhibited ($P<0.01$ in comparison with control group), and that there was some evidence of immune reaction after cryosurgery.

B. Factors Influencing Freezing Effects

1. Duration of Freezing

Gill showed that a cryoprobe at a given temperature (−80 to −180 °C) would produce 80%–90% of its maximum freezing effect within 15 min; however, the maximum effect would require approximately 2 h of freezing (Gill et al. 1970, Gill and Long 1971). According to our data, there is a balance between drop in temperature and extension of frozen area while the duration of freezing is 12–14 min. Therefore, it is our opinion that for practical purposes 15 min is sufficient for each freezing.

2. Repetitive Freeze-Thaw Cycles

Neel et al. (1971 b) demonstrated that the difference in the freezing rate between one and three cycles was highly significant ($P < 0.01$). Repetitive freeze-thaw not only increases the volume of frozen tissue but also profoundly reduces the rate of thawing. Our experiments of hepatoma-22 after cryosurgery showed that the rate of tumor cure was enhanced (with one and two cycles it was 35% and 48% respectively).

3. Blood Supply of Tissue

The experiments showed that the effects of one probe application with inflow occlusion approximated those of two to three freezes cycles without ischemia, and that the mean thawing time was increased by about 60% in the ischemia group (Neel et al. 1971 b). Hepatic artery ligation was performed before cryosurgery in six cases of our series, which produced a similar increase in thawing time.

4. Relationship Between Freezing and Necrotic Areas

It is generally accepted that all of the cells in a frozen area, including the marginal zone, can be destroyed. Smith and Fraser demonstrated that all liver cells could be devastated in the zone at a temperature of −15 °C. However, the distance from the margin of the frozen area to the zone at the temperature of −15 °C was only 0.1 cm (Fraser and Gill 1967; Smith and Fraser 1974). Our data also demonstrate that the frozen area is identical to the necrotic area. Therefore, the gross frozen area might represent the necrotic area.

C. Safety of Cryosurgery for HCC

The postoperative course of cryosurgery in all of the 35 patients was uneventful, there being no evidence of rupture of tumor capsule, bleeding, or bile leakage. The experiments showed that even the large blood vessels were frozen, that rupture of the devitalized vessel wall would never occur, and that the gallbladder as well as the bile ducts remained intact after they were moderately frozen. These results suggested that cryotherapeutic techniques could be safely applied to treat HCC (Zhou et al. 1979 a). However, Gage et al. (1967) reported that the common bile duct did not fare as well. Initially, edema of the wall caused partial luminal occlusion, and several days later stenosis developed. Among 13 dogs, one died of bile peritonitis following the development of a perforation in the duct wall. Therefore, great care should be exercised in treating HCC located near the hepatic hilum.

D. Evaluation of Cryosurgery for HCC

Surgery of HCC has two major problems that are pertinent to the development of visceral cryosurgical techniques. First, the technical difficulty of the operation for excision of cancers is chiefly related to the control of hemorrhage. Second, the majority of HCC are not suitable for surgical excision; consequently alternate methods of treatment are needed. In the cryosurgical techniques used no tissue was removed, but rather the frozen liver was left in situ to form a thin scar. Cryosurgery with liquid nitrogen can result in irreversible necrosis of cancer cells. As the procedure is safe and simple, it can be employed as one modality of treatment for nonresectable HCC. Cryosurgery can be considered the surgery of choice for nonresectable HCC in patients without jaundice, ascites, and noncompensated liver function, and the whole tumor mass can be involved in the frozen area. However, the effect of cryotherapy of HCC in prolongation of survival is far inferior to that of cryotherapy of superficial solid cancers (e.g., skin, cervix, head and neck). There are several reasons: (a) There may be inadequate freezing of a large tumor. Hence, cryosurgical technique should be further improved so as to extend the frozen area and in turn improve the ultimate outcome. (b) There may be difficulty in carrying out the reoperation for further freezing since the liver cancer is located in the abdomen. (c) Prognosis may also be influenced by the characteristics and multicentric development of HCC. For these reasons, it is doubtful that cryosurgery alone would be of benefit to the vast majority of HCC patients who are not candidates for conventional excisional surgery. Still, the technique is worth developing because benefit may be achieved by the combined method of treatment, i.e., a combination of cryosurgery with hepatic artery ligation and/or catheterization.

References

Ablin RJ, Reddy KP (1977) Cryosurgery of the monkey (macaque) prostate. II. Apparent immunopathologic alterations following cryostimulation. Cryobiology 14: 205–224

Ablin RJ, Soanes WS, Conder MJ, et al. (1976) Evaluation of cellular immunologic responsiveness in the clinical management of patients with prostatic cancer. II. effect of estrogen, cryosurgery and transurethral resection on thymic-dependent lymphocytic blastogenesis. Urol Int 31: 383–400

Cahan WG (1972) Cryosurgery for cancer. CA 22: 339–543

Cooper IS, Hirose T (1966) Application of cryogenic surgery to resection of parenchymal organs. N Engl J Med 274: 15–18

Dutta P, Montes M, Gage AA (1977) Experimental hepatic cryosurgery. Cryobiology 14: 598–608

Fraser SJ, Gill W (1967) Observation on ultra-frozen tissue. Br J Surg 54: 770–776

Gage AA, Fazekas G, Riley EE Jr (1967) Freezing injury to large blood vessels in dogs: With comments on the effect of experimental freezing of bile ducts. Surgery 61: 748–754

Gill W, Long WB (1971) The completeness of cellular destruction within a cryolesion. Br J Surg 58: 870–874

Gill W, Fraser SJ, Costa JD, et al. (1970) The cryosurgical lesion. Am Surg 35: 437–445

Grady ED, Nolan TR, Crumbley AJ, et al. (1973) Cryotherapy of implanted cancer in the rat liver. Oncology 28: 104–109

Healey WV, Priebe CJ Jr, Farrer SM et al. (1971) Hepatic cryosurgery, acute and long-term effects. Arch Surg 103: 384–392

Helpap B, Grouls V, Yamashita K (1976) The proliferative response of the spleen in cryosurgery. Cryobiology 13: 54–60

Holden HB, Mckelvie P (1972) Cryosurgery in the treatment of head and neck neoplasia. Br J Surg 59: 709–712

Ikeda K (1976) Immune response of distant lesions following cryosurgery in the experimental tumor system. Fukushima J Med Sci 22: 45–53

Nagasue N (1975) Release of lysosome enzyme beta-glucuronidase after hepatic cryosurgery. Arch Surg 110: 713–716

Neel HB, Ketcham AS, Hammond WG (1971 a) Ischemia-potentiating cryosurgery of primate liver. Ann Surg 174: 309–318

Neel HB, Ketcham AS, Hammond WG, et al. (1971 b) Cryonecrosis of normal and tumor-bearing rat liver potentiated by inflow occlusion. Cancer 28: 1211–1218

Rand RW, Rinfret AP, von Leden H (1968) Cryosurgery. Thomas, Springfield

Serra P, Brunschwig A (1955) Freezing of liver parenchyma with liquid nitrogen for hemostasis in excisional liver surgery. Cancer 8: 1234–1238

Shanghai Coordinating Group for Liver Cancer Research, China (1974) Primary liver cancer – a clinical analysis of 3254 cases (from 11 provinces, 21 hospitals of China). Tumor Prevent Treat Study 2: 207–215[1]

Smith JJ, Fraser J (1974) An estimation of tissue damage and thermal history in the cryolesion. Cryobiology 11: 139–147

Soanes WA, Gonder MJ, Ablin RJ, et al. (1969) Clinical and experimental aspects of prostatic cryosurgery. J Cryosurg 2: 23–31

Soanes WS, Albin RJ, Conder MJ (1970) Remission of metastatic lesions following cryosurgery in prostatic cancer: Immunological considerations. J Urol 104: 154–159

von Leden H, Cahan WG (1971) Cryogenics in surgery. Huber, Bern

Zhou XD, Tang ZY, Yu YQ, et al. (1979 a) Cryosurgery for liver cancer – experimental and clinical study. Chin J Surg 17: 480–433[1]

Zhou XD, Tang ZY, Yu YQ (1979 b) Cryosurgery in tumor of viscera (collective review). In: Application of new technique to prevent and treat tumor, edn I, Shanghai Scientific and Technological Literature Publishers[1], Shanghai, pp 5–9

1 Chinese

11 Highpower Nd: YAG Laser in the Treatment of Liver Cancer – Experimental Study and Clinical Application

Yu Ye-qin

Since the development of laser equipment in the 1960s, its use in the treatment of cancer on the head, face, and skin has been reported quite often (Goldman 1973; Liu et al. 1979; Goldman et al. 1982). However, reports on partial resection and vaporization of liver cancer by laser are scarce. Whatever has appeared in the literature has been experimental studies on animals, and only under lowpower laser (Mullins et al. 1968; Fidler et al. 1975; Hall et al. 1973; Orda et al. 1977; Orda and Ellis 1981). We have not yet seen any report about treatment of human liver cancer with laser. Since 1975, we have made experimental laser studies on animal liver (Zhou et al. 1980). Based on the gratifying experimental results we have tried to use the laser to treat clinical liver cancer since 1980, and the results appear to be very satisfactory (Yu et al. 1981).

I. Experimental Observations

We applied two types of laser (CO_2 and Nd:YAG) and four modes of power density to 26 dog livers for extirpation and vaporization with the following results.

A. Vaporization Effect on Dog Liver

Non-focus CO_2 laser for vaporization. Active oozing of the irradiated liver area could be observed when it was vaporized at 199 W/cm^2 power density. Laser energy was absorbed by blood and a thick layer of charring formed, so that the laser could not penetrate deeply enough. At 382–995 W/cm^2, the speed of vaporization was quicker and coagulation was better than in the former group; the charred layer was thinner, though there was still some oozing.

Non-focus Nd: YAG laser for vaporization. At 64–255 W/cm^2 power density, the speed of vaporization was slow and the layer of charring also thick. But at 764–1000 W/cm^2, the effect of vaporization was satisfactory; the irradiated liver tissue changed rapidly into gas and a hole was formed, the effects of coagulation and penetration being good. When the first hepatic portal was occluded the effects could be increased threefold.

B. Cutting Effect on Dog Liver

With the focused highpower Nd: YAG laser (0.87×10^3–1.28×10^4 W/cm^2) both hemostasis and cutting were superior to what was achieved with the CO_2 laser.

C. Morphology of Liver Tissue After Laser Irradiation

Under light microscopic observations immediately following focused laser irradiation (10^5–1.592×10^5 W/cm^2), a cross-section of the liver tissue could be divided into four layers. Owing to high temperature, the superficial layer produced a thin layer of necrosis and denatured protein. All structures of the liver cells were destroyed (about 20–40 μm thick). In the second layer there was complete cellular destruction with vacuolization (about 40–60 μm thick). In the third layer nonviable cells could be seen, but the structure of the cell was preserved. Liver cells were swollen and turbid (about 100–200 μm thick). The fourth layer showed normal liver tissue.

Pathological findings with the Nd:YAG laser and CO_2 lasers were similar, but the former produced a brown hole and almost no bleeding was observed. The extent and depth of the hole were directly correlated with laser energy, irradiation time, and the size of the light spot.

D. General Reactions After Laser Irradiation of Liver

After laser surgery, the ALT level was elevated to varying degrees in the majority of the animals, but returned to normal within 2 weeks. Neither serum bilirubin nor prothrombin time was changed. The white blood count was slightly increased in the majority of the dogs.

E. Complications

Three dogs died owing to unsatisfactory care and feeding, and the remaining dogs were killed for study after 2 months, with no secondary bleeding or bile leakage observed.

II. Clinical Application

Since 1980 we have used the Nd:YAG laser (power density 0.87×10^3–1.28×10^4 W/cm^2) to vaporize or cut human liver cancers. Eight subclinical liver cancers have been thus treated to date. During surgery bleeding was minimal and wound healing was good. Postoperative complications particularly related to the laser did not occur (Table 1).

Table 1. Data on eight operations with the Nd: YAG Laser

Case no.	Age	Discovery	Operation			Result of operation
			Date	Cancer site & size (cm) VL* CL^Δ OSR**	Pathological diagnosis	
1	51	No symtoms or signs AFP (+)	May 16, 80	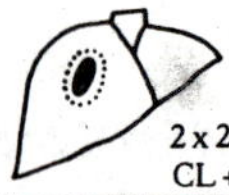 2x2x1.9 CL+VL	HCC	Well at 3 years; resumed his original work
2	60	AFP (+), radionuclide imaging: space-occupying lesion in left side of liver	May 17, 80	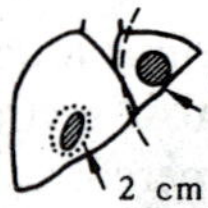 4x4x3.8 OSR; 2 cm in diameter VL	HCC	AFP (-). Died 21 months later as result of bleeding of the varices of esophagus
3	42	$5\frac{1}{2}$ years after left hemihepatectomy for cancer; AFP reelevated	June 30, 81	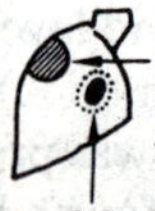 6x5.5x4.2 OSR locally +VL of the wound; 2.8x1.7 VL	HCC	Died from recurrence at 9 months
4	52	AFP (+)	July 1, 81	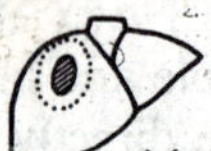 4.1x3.7x3.3 CL+VL	HCC	Well at 2 years
5	68	AFP (+)	July 2, 81	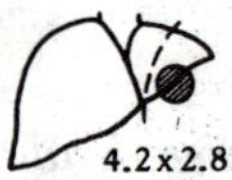 4.2x2.8x2 CL	HCC	Well at 2 years
6	56	17 days prior to laser surgery, during sigmoidectomy for cancer; two secondary liver cancer nodules were found	July 3, 81	1x1 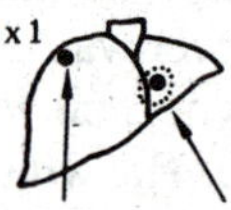 OSR; 1x1 VL.	Secondary liver cancer	Well at 2 years
7	48	Four years after partial hepatectomy for cancer; AFP reelevated	June 19, 82	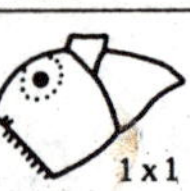 1x1 VL	HCC	Well at 1 year
8	50	AFP reappeared after left hemihepatectomy	July 26, 82	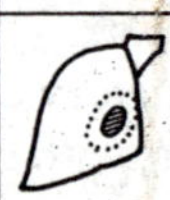 2x2x2 VL	HCC	Well at 6 months

*VL, Vaporization with laser; ^ΔCL, cutting with laser; **OSR, ordinary scalpel resection

III. Evaluation of Nd: YAG Laser for Treating Liver Cancer

A. Advantages

Hemostatic action is good. Under temporary occlusion of the first hepatic portal, the high temperature produced by the output of the Nd: YAG laser cuts and seals the small blood vessels and bile channels so that bleeding can be kept to a minimum. This good degree of hemostasis is valuable in liver surgery.

Multiple cancer nodules can be *vaporized* one after another *without excessive blood loss*. Cancer nodules of 1 cm in diameter can be completely vaporized into gas within 1 min. The procedure is very simple, and certainly superior to ordinary surgical extirpation with a scalpel.

In patients with associated severe cirrhosis, the laser can be used for *resection or vaporization of the lesion in situ*. The penetration of the continuous Nd: YAG solid laser is strong enough to resect the cirrhotic parenchyma. Therefore, a routine hemihepatectomy can be avoided, more normal liver tissue preserved, and the safety of the operation ensured. In recurrent cases where partial or hemihepatectomy was previously performed the remaining liver tissue is small, and eradication of the recurrent cancer nodule by laser is therefore more suitable.

Laser surgery is a *safe and simple procedure,* with no complications or operative mortality observed. The postoperative inflamatory reaction is minimum. The changes in the patient's liver function after laser surgery are similar to those observed after resection of a tumor of the same size with a surgical scalpel. Recovery after laser surgery is invariably good.

B. Disadvantages

The available devices are *bulky and cumbersome*. The light-conducting system must be further improved and substituted with a flexible fiberglass system for easier application.

The high-power Nd: YAG laser equipment is still *too expensive* for general use.

Although the laser devices have their disadvantages and need improving, we do believe that such a strong Nd: YAG laser is very promising and quite reliable. For the treatment of all relatively well localized liver cancers, especially subclinical small liver cancers, it can be recommended as a new modality.

References

Fidler JP, Hoefer RW, Polanyi TG, et al. (1975) Laser surgery in exsanguinating liver injury. Ann Surg 181: 74–80

Goldman L (1973) Applications of the laser. CRC, Cleveland, pp 173–197

Goldman L, Younger B, Perry E (1982) Surgery with the argon laser. Recent advances in instrumentation and techniques. J Dermatol Surg Oncol 8: 30–31

Hall RR, Beach AD, Hill DW (1973) Partial hepatectomy using a carbon dioxide laser. Br J Surg 60: 141–144

Liu DM, Yang XX, Wei XB (1979) Evaporation of malignant tumor by CO_2 laser. Laser 6: 52–55[1]

Mullins F, Jennings B, McClusky L (1968) Liver resection with continuous wave carbon dioxide laser – Some experimental observations. Am Surg 34: 717–722

Orda R, Ellis H (1981) Experimental study of hepatic, renal, and splenic wound healing following laser, diathermy, and scalpel incisions. Am Surg 47: 447–451

Orda R, Wiznitzer T, Goldwasser B, et al. (1977) Partial hepatectomies with a hand-held laser knife: An experimental study. Br J Surg 64: 857–861

Yu YQ, Tang ZY, Zhou XD, et al. (1981) Treatment of human primary hepatic cancer by highpower Nd: YAG laser. Kexue Tongbao 13: 826–828[1]

Zhou XD, Yu YQ, Tang ZY, et al. (1980) Experimental study of laser surgery on liver. Acta Acad Med Primae Shanghai 7: 216–221[1]

1 Chinese

12 Immunity to Subclinical Hepatocellular Carcinoma

Lin Zhi-ying, Tang Zhao-you

With the development of immunology there is a vast amount of data supporting the concept that tumors bear antigens different from those of the normal host tissue. Although a purified human malignant tumor antigen has not yet been separated, a great many experimental data in vivo and in vitro suggest that tumor-associated antigens are recognized by the immunological system of the host and provoke an immunologic reaction – cellular and humoral immunity that permits tumor rejection. In recent years, a great deal of effort has been spent on determining the nature of such immune responses to tumor-associated antigens, on searching for the manner in which these responses affect tumor growth, and on seeking methods of enhancing the antitumor mechanism to the host's benefit. On the other hand, the tumor embryonal antigens or tumor-associated antigens provide the basis for clinical diagnosis and immunotherapy. AFP, the tumor embryonal antigen, has been employed for early detection of SCHCC (Shanghai Coordinating Group for Research on Liver Cancer 1979). Anti-AFP antibodies (Kim et al 1980), anti-ferritin antibodies (Order et al 1981; Ettinger et al 1982), and monoclonal antibodies against tumor-associated antigens, such as the carriers with isotopes or effective drugs, permit recognition of tumor cell antigens, and the antibodies may be deposited in the tumor-bearing region, so the localization and treatment of HCC could be expected.

I. Tumor Antigens Related to Hepatocellular Carcinoma

The most valuable clinical use of the AFP assay lies in the screening of suspicious populations and in following up patients after therapy; serial monitoring of AFP may allow early detection of recurrence or measure response to chemotherapy in unresected patients (see Chapters 2, 3, 5, 6). Although not cell surface markers or tumor-specific antigens, AFP, ferritin, and carcinoembryonic antigen (CEA) are released from tumor cells presenting a high local antigen concentration, to provide a gradient between tumor and nontumor (Goldenberg et al. 1980) which leads us to consider the use of isotopically labeled antibodies to cancer-containing antigens for localization and therapy (Ettinger et al. 1979; Goldenberg et al. 1980; Kim et al. 1980; Order 1976; Order et al. 1981).

In recent years, the radio-labeled antibodies to AFP have been used for radioimmunodetection of hepatocellular carcinoma and other tumors containing AFP; meanwhile, specific AFP antiserum has been administered to clinical patients (Liu et al. 1983).

Ferritin is synthesized and secreted by hepatomas and other tumors, but it is intimately associated with tumor cells of hepatocellular carcinoma, although ferritin is also a normal tissue component in certain normal organs. Our data showed that the normal value obtained by RIA is 121.5 ± 56.5 ng/ml, ranging from 16 to 234 ng/ml. The concentrations of 12 of 18 patients (66.7%) with HCC were higher than 300 ng/ml. Serum ferritin is a useful tumor marker for HCC in patients producing low AFP, being raised in four of five patients with small HCC, suggesting its value in the early diagnosis of HCC (Kaneto et al. 1980). The elevated value of serum ferritin probably results from the production and secretion of specific isoferritin by the tumor. Acidic isoferritins have been shown in human HCC tissue, but the concentration of isoferritin is lower in HCC than in nontumor liver tissue, suggesting that the isoferritins synthesized by the tumor do not accumulate in the neoplasm but are secreted into the circulation (Niitsu et al. 1975; Bullock et al. 1980). They have also been isolated from fetal liver, representing a dedifferentiation of function of the malignant hepatocytes (Kew and Dusheiko 1981).

Knowledge of the surface antigenic structure of several types of human cancer has advanced with research into mouse monoclonal antibodies, and application of these reagents to cancer diagnosis and therapy is developing (Cote et al. 1983). Up to now, monoclonal antibodies specific for human AFP have been derived by the mouse-to-mouse hybridoma technique. The human AFP-specific antibody has now been shown to be a monoclonal IgG1 subclass, with extremely high avidity for human AFP (Tsung et al. 1980), which will be used for the diagnosis of human HCC.

II. Antitumor Immune Mechanism and Development of HCC

Immune responses elicited against tumor antigens are highly complex. They include natural killer cells, the generation of sensitized lymphocytes, activated macrophages, and antibody formation. These responses are part of an immunologic network subject to a series of feedback mechanisms involving the suppressor T cells and macrophages. Meanwhile, the growing tumors can produce humoral factors including circulating tumor antigen and immune complexes which interfere with all mediated immunity. It is possible that tumor rejection involves multiple effector mechanisms.

In China, more than 80% of patients with HCC have a background of chronic hepatic disease, macronodular cirrhosis in most cases, even in patients with SCHCC. William (1975) suggested that the significant decrease in spontaneous rosette-forming T cells with seep erythrocytes occurred in patients with macronodular cirrhosis and liver cancer. It may be that the frequent development of PLC is a result of severe deficiency of the anti-tumor mechanism in patients with macronodular cirrhosis. Littmann et al. (1977) suggested that AFP in the serum of patients with viral hepatitis may be the serum factor suppressing the cellular immune response to the hepatits virus, causing persistency of the disease. In addition, although the cytolytic action of T cells and natural killer cells can nonspecifically destroy the tumor cells, their activity is limited and may be overcome by progressive tumors. The number of T cells in peripheral blood lymphocytes (PBL) and lymphocyte-response to PHA were significantly decreased in patients with liver cancer, as was natural killer activity. These results suggest that the antitumor mechanism is impaired in patients with liver cancer; this may be one etiological factor in the genesis of hepatocellular carcinoma in liver cancer (Morizane et al. 1980).

III. Cell-mediated Immunity and Its Clinical Applications in Subclinical and Clinical Hepatocellular Carcinoma

A. In Vivo Study

Skin Delayed Hypersensitivity Test

In our group we used old tuberculin (OT) combined with streptokinase-streptodornase (SK-SD) and phytohemagglutinin (PHA) antigens to detect delayed hypersensitivity of the skin in order to measure cellular immunity in vivo. Positive rates were coincident with the stage of disease (Lin et al. 1979).

We (Lin and Tang 1979) observed the OT test in patients with histologically proven HCC, the OT-positive rates being 85.4% in patients with SCHCC and 61.8% in those with CHCC. The data on 210 patients with HCC showed that the positive rates of the OT test were 93.7% in the early stage, 65.4% in the moderate stage, and 48.9% in the late stage. The differences among them were statistically significant. The overall postive rate of the OT test was 66.2%, being lowest in the group over 60 years of age. The survival period for OT-positive patients was longer than that for OT-negative ones. Some of the patients were periodically monitored by the OT test, and the results show that persistently positive reactions or the conversion of negative to positive reactions usually denote a good prognosis, and vice versa. Serial observations of the OT test corresponded with the clinical status in 71.1% of the patients.

Table 1. OT test and lymphocyte transformation in patients with HCC

	OT test		Lymphocyte transformation	
	SCHCC	CHCC	SCHCC	CHCC
No. of patients	76/89	173/280	15/16	23/40
Positive (%)	85.4	61.8	93.8	57.5
P value		<0.001		<0.01

Table 2. Relationship between the changes of OT test and survival rates

Change of OT	*n*	1-year survival		2-year survival		3-year survival	
		n	%	*n*	%	*n*	%
+→+ −→+	54	28/54	51.9	15/51	29.4	12/49	24.5
+→− −→−	38	7/37	18.9	4/30	13.3	2/30	6.7
P value		<0.001		>0.05		<0.01	

Among patients with positive reactions, the rate of AFP conversion to normal was higher and the recurrence rate within the first year lower as compared with those with negative reactions. In consideration of these results, we are of the opinion that the OT test is of some value in the evaluation of the clinical course, including prognosis and outcome of treatment.

B. In Vitro Tests

1. Lymphocytes

T-lymphocytes represent a heterogeneous population of cells with different functions. The two subsets helper T cells and suppressor T cells are components of a homeostatic mechanism controlling immune responses. Of particular importance in tumor immunity is the killer T cell population, which is involved in recognition and lysis of aberrant or tumor cells.

1. E-Rosette-Forming Cells (ERFC)
   It has been established that human PBL can bind spontaneously with uncoated SRBC to form a characteristic rosette configuration. These ERFC have been identified as T-lymphocytes; they constitute about 60%–70% of the total number of T-lymphocytes in human PBL.
   Our study (Lin et al. 1979) indicated that patients with HCC have a percentage of ERFC lower than that of healthy controls (Table 3, Fig. 1). The percentage of ERFC in patients with HCC after chemotherapy can return to normal, and the percentage of ERFC in patients who survived longer than 6 months was higher than that in patients who survived less than 6 months (Kan 1978; William 1975; Zuberi 1980).

2. Subpopulation of T-Lymphocytes
   – Active E-Rosette-Forming Cells
   Wybran and Fudenberg (1973) established another population called the active ERFC (EaRFC), which was found after a short incubation between PBL and SRBC, representing a subpopulation of the total ERFC having an active immunocompetence. The EaRFC may reflect the quality as well es the quantity of the immune response (Kerman et al. 1976). A remarkable decrease in EaRFC was found in patients with HCC as compared with healthy controls (Lin et al. 1979).

Table 3. E-rosette-forming cells in PLC

References	PLC		Control	
	No. of cases	% Rosettes (mean ± SE)	No. of cases	% Rosettes (mean ± SE)
William (1975)	8	36.78 ± 5.8	12	54.40 ± 7.9
Kan (1978)	21	43.00 ± 3.9	18	68.20 ± 1.5
Zuberi (1980)	8	8.60 ± 1.5	16	36.60 ± 3.5
Lin (1979)	24	50.00 ± 2.4	22	65.90 ± 1.2

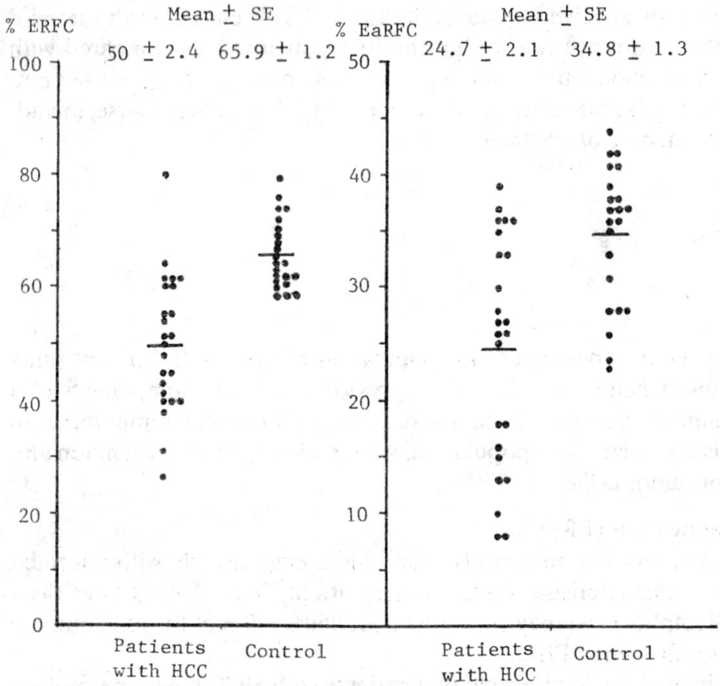

Fig. 1. ERFC and EaRFC in peripheral blood of patients with HCC as compared with healthy controls; the values are significantly lower in patients than in controls ($P < 0.01$)

Table 4. Percentage of ERFC and EaRFC in HCC

	Control	SCHCC after radical resection	CHCC, stage II	CHCC, stage III
No. of patients	52	14	10	13
ERFC (%)	54.8 ± 6.7	58.9 ± 3.3	41.3 ± 5.3	43.5 ± 4.3
P value			< 0.01	< 0.01
EaRFC (%)	30.1 ± 8.2	31.9 ± 2.3	17.5 ± 4.1	20.3 ± 3.7
P value			< 0.01	< 0.01

Obviously, the percentages of ERFC and EaRFC which returned to normal were limited in the group of SCHCC patients after radical resection. The percentages of ERFC and EaRFC were noticeably decreased with the deterioration of the patients' condition. There were statistically significant differences between patients with stage II or stage III disease and the radical resection group (Lin et al. 1981; see Table 4).

T Helper Cells and T Suppressor Cells

On the basis of T cell receptors binding Fc fragments of IgM or IgG, the human lymphocytes may be separated into two subsets; the former is T_μ and the latter is T_γ. Studies of "helpers" and "suppressors" have shown that helper cells are comprised mainly of T_μ cells, suppressor cells of T_γ cells (Moretta et al. 1980). Recently, Yao et al. (1983) reported that T_γ and T_μ in 15 patients with HCC amounted to 19.5% ± 8.7% and 26.8% ± 11.8%, as compared with 11.2% ± 4.9% and 33.8% ± 11.8% in 35 normal persons. T_γ was significantly higher in HCC cases than in normal controls, especially in the late stage, T_γ being as high as 29.3% ± 3.2%.

Shimbo (1977a, b) used a double-rosette method to examine T lymphocytes bearing IgG Fc receptors (FcR^+T, T_γ) as T suppressor cells, and found a markedly increased number of T lymphocytes bearing Fc receptors in patients with untreated liver cancer, thyroid cancer, and angiosarcoma. Our data (Lin et al. 1981) also showed that the percentage of T lymphocytes bearing Fc receptors in patients with HCC is much higher than that in healthy controls, being 11.3% ± 1.3% and 2.6% ± 0.2% respectively ($P<0.01$). Recent evidence indicates that the T_γ subset is clearly a heterogeneous population of cells; hybridoma technology has provided a reliable, defining, functional T cell subset (Moretta et al. 1980; Reinberg and Schlossman 1980). The significance of the T_γ subset will be further investigated.

Clinical Applications of Lymphokine Detection

Lymphocyte Transformation

Lymphocyte transformation (LT) was detected morphologically in 16 patients with SCHCC and 40 with CHCC, the percentages above normal level being 93.8% and 57.5% respectively. The technique of incorporation of ^{3}H-thymidine was undertaken for 24 patients with PLC (Lin et al. 1979). The value of cpm and stimulation index estimated by incorporation of ^{3}H-thymidine were close to normal in the SCHCC group after radical resection, intermediate in the recurrent group, and lowest in the late-stage group (Table 5). The recovery of cell-mediated immunity in the radical resection group may be due to the elimination of the immune suppressor factor following the removal of the tumor. The cell-mediated immunity of HCC was definitely suppressed, as shown by various in vitro and in vivo tests. The technique of incorporation of ^{3}H-thymidine coincides well with the results of in vivo skin tests (Table 6).

Kan (1978) indicated that PHA-lymphocyte transformation was lower in patients with PLC than in the control group, being 34.3% ± 2.6% and 56.6% ± 2.8% respectively. The lymphocyte transformation was normal in patients with long survival after effective chemotherapy; the test for lymphocyte transformation is usually more sensitive than the test for ERFC.

Lymphocyte Microcytotoxicity Test

In giving the microcytotoxicity test of peripheral blood lymphocytes in patients with HCC, we used ^{125}I-iododeoxyuridine (^{125}IudR)-labeled human HCC cell line 7402 as the target cell. The lymphocytes showed obvious cytotoxicity against the 7402 target cell in about 40% of patients with HCC, but in only 10% of normal individuals. Lymphocyte cytotoxicity was present in patients in a moderate stage of diesease. After removal of the tumor, AFP declined and the patients' condition improved (Tumor Research Group, Shanghai Institute of Experimental Biology, Academia Sinica, 1977).

Leukocyte Adherence Inhibition

The leukocyte adherence inhibition (LAI) technique was first described in 1972 by Halliday and Miller. Recently it has provided the specific technique for the im-

Table 5. Assay of lymphocyte transformation by incorporation of ^{3}H-thymidine in HCC

	Control	SCHCC after radical resection	Recurrence of HCC	Late-stage HCC
No. of patients	9	6	5	7
No. PHA (cpm)	118 ± 23.3	152 ± 35.1	228 ± 47.3	848 ± 457
PHA 25μg (cpm)	1760 ±549	1904 ± 524	1734 ± 251	1148 ± 485
SI	15.9± 5.2	14.73± 4.1	4.7± 1.1	2.61± 0.9[a]
100μg (cpm)	8618 ±804	9154 ±2372	4606 ±1686	4864 ±2487
SI	82.8± 8.2	70 ± 17.8	25.6± 12.2[b]	8.95± 3.9[c]

Each group as compared with controls and SCHCC group after radical, resection
[a] $P<0.05$, $P<0.05$
[b] $P<0.01$, $P<0.05$
[c] $P<0.01$, $P<0.01$

Table 6. Relationship between combined skin tests, (OT, SK-SD, PHA) and lymphocyte transformation

	Combined skin tests (OT, SK-SD, PHA)			
	3/3 positive	2/3 positive	1/3 positive	0/3 positive
Lymphocyte transformation (SI)				
PHA 25 μg (18)[a]	11.6 (8)	4.1 (6)	2.5 (2)	1.37 (2)
100 μg (18)	63.5 (8)	16.1 (6)	9.5 (2)	2.65 (2)

[a] No. of patients

Table 7. Positive rates of lymphocyte transformation in patients with small and large HCC after treatment

Treatment	Small HCC	Large HCC
Resected	100% (9/9)[a]	66.7% (6/9)
Nonresected	80% (4/5)	28.5% (6/21)
Total	92.9% (13/14)	40% (12/30)

[a] No. of patients

munodiagnosis of HCC (Halliday et al. 1974; Kumagai et al. 1980). The patient's blood leukocytes are tested in vitro for cell-mediated immunity against tumor associated antigens and the serum is tested for a blocking factor which interferes with the immunological reaction; both of these were positive in patients with PLC but negative in those with other liver diseases and secondary liver cancer. A positive result was obtained about 3 years before the clinical appearance of tumor

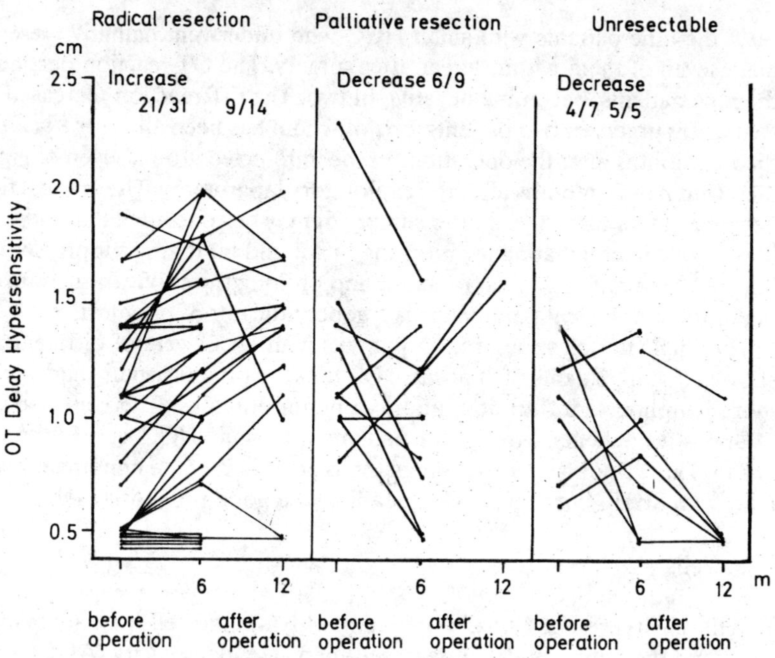

Fig. 2. Sequential determination of OT delayed hypersensitivity in patients with small HCC after radical resection, palliative resection, and those who were not resectable

in two patients. LAI was tested in four patients with PLC 17 times, and was positive for 17 times (100%)(Ge 1977). However, Dusheiko et al. (1979) observed that only 17 of 36 patients gave positive LAI results; therefore, the technique is of limited value in the diagnosis of HCC. Large tumor burden and the antigenic heterogeneity in patients with HCC may be responsible for abrogation of the immune response.

Cell-mediated Immunity and Pathological Findings in Small HCC.

Almost all small HCC (< 5 cm in diameter) cases are in the subclinical stage. In the resected group a normal lymphocyte transformation rate was seen in 100% of 14 patients with small HCC, but in 66.7% of patients with large HCC. In the nonresected group, the lymphocyte transformation rates in small HCC and in large HCC were 80% and 28.5% respectively. The difference was significant, which suggests that the immune function of the patients recovers easily after resection of the tumor (Table 7).

The OT skin test was given to 48 patients with small HCC 6 months and 1 year after exploratory surgery (31 radical resection; nine palliative resection; eight cryosurgery, local chemotherapy, ligation, cannulation of hepatic artery; Fig. 2). Of the 31 patients who underwent radical resection, 21 showed a stronger OT reaction after surgery than before. Of these 31, only three died of tumor, 21, 36, and 72 months after surgery.

Of the nine patients with small HCC who underwent palliative resection, eight died, seven of them within 1 year after surgery. The OT reaction declined in six of the nine patients, becoming negative in two. The OT reaction increased during the year after surgery in two patients, one of whom has been alive for 8 years; the other died 22 months after the operation. In the unresected group, seven of eight patients died within 6–26 months after the exploratory laparotomy. The OT reaction became negative in five cases 1 year after surgery. It may be concluded that radical resection plays a role in eliminating the blocking factor and inhibiting suppressor cells. It can improve the immunological function and prolong the survival; therefore, monitoring of immunological parameters is a good indicator of prognosis.

The single nodules found in 19 patients with HCC were of different sizes. HCC showed that in patients with positive OT tests the tumors usually had encapsulation, more lymphocyte infiltration, and less tumor embolus. The converse was true in OT-negative patients. Most of the patients with small HCC were in the OT-positive group. These findings provide the pathological basis of the immune function of patients with SCHCC or small HCC, leading to a good prognosis (Table 8).

2. K Cells

K cells may represent a small population of lymphoid cells that are neither T nor B cells, and the antibody-dependent, cell-mediated cytotoxicity (ADCC) mechanism in tumor rejection is not clear. They may play a role in the lysis of target cells during direct contact, mediated by antibodies bound to target cells, all surface antigens, and K-cell Fc receptors. In fact, it is possible that any cell possessing surface Fc receptors may play the role of a K cell, including macrophages and polymorphs. By using a modified Calder assay, we detected ADCC in patients with HCC (Zheng et al. 1980) (Table 9).

Table 8. The relationship between OT test and pathological findings of single-nodule HCC

Pathological findings	OT test – positive	OT test – negative
No. of patients	14	5
Well-encapsulated	38.4% (5/13)	25.0% (1/4)
Tumor embolus	35.7% (5/14)	60.0% (3/5)
Lymphocyte infiltration	30% (3/10)	0 (0/4)

Table 9. Cytotoxic index of ADCC in HCC

	Controls	SCHCC after radical resection	CHCC, stage II	CHCC, stage III
No. of patients	15	14	12	10
Cytotoxic index of ADCC	69.3±2.6	70.3±4.3	47.4±2.9	42.6±4.6
P value			<0.01	<0.01

The cytotoxicity in patients with HCC after radical resection returned to the normal level, (almost all of them were subclinical HCC patients before surgery); however, ADCC was still significant at a low level in stage-II and stage-III HCC patients (Lin et al. 1981). ADCC activity reguires excess antibodies, because the existence of free antibody sites is necessary for K cells to recognize the tumor cells. In large tumors, antigens are usually in excess and block these free sites; K cell action is inhibited, and the action can be released after the tumor is removed with the loss of large numbers of antigens.

3. Natural Killer Cells

(a) Biological Characteristic and Function

Natural killer (NK) cells are a small subpopulation of lymphocytes or cytotoxic effector cells with a set of cell surface markers, $Fc_\gamma R$, low-affinity receptors for SRBC in normal individuals, and certain morphological characteristics. Timonen et al. (1979) found that the majority of human lymphocytes binding to NK-sensitive target cells are large granular lymphocytes (LGLs). These may be responsible for the cytotoxic activity, because about 50% of the LGLs conjugate with K_{562} and most of these conjugate-forming LGLs have the power to kill the attached target cells (Herberman 1981).

An NK-cell population can kill syngeneic, allogeneic, or xenogeneic tumor cells. NK cells show cytotoxicity of their spontaneous reactivity in the absence of any previous sensitization; therefore, the in vivo function of NK cells is an antitumor mechanism, especially in the early stage of tumor development. The tumor-cell clearance can be reduced by anti-NK_1, providing direct evidence that NK cells may eliminate tumor cells in vivo (Pollack and Hallenbeck 1982). The NK-cell activity of human blood lymphocytes was examined against the human target cell line K_{562} by using the ^{125}IudR or ^{51}Cr release assay.

(b) Factors Affecting Level of NK-Cell Activity

Morizane et al. (1980) observed that the NK activity was significantly decreased in patients with liver cancer, showing the impairment of anti-tumor mechanism in these patients. Another report (Son et al. 1982) showed that lymphocytes from patients with HCC demonstrated the decrease of natural cytotoxicity, which was not seen in normal individuals or in those with nontumor liver diseases. Morimoto (1982) observed natural cytotoxicity in patients with various liver diseases; it was found to be the same for each disease studied except in four patients in the end-stage of hepatoma, who showed significant decreases. Our data showed that the natural cytotoxicity in patients with subclinical HCC was within the normal level, but that it was significantly decreased in late-stage patients (Fig. 3).

Natural cytotoxicity may decrease in patients with ovarian cancer at stages III and IV, 24 h after surgery, and recover within 7–9 days. It is also depressed by chemotherapy and is not related to tumor advancement. NK activity appears to fluctuate with tumor burden if the disease is in remission, if its activity is lower than that in relapse, and if it is correlated more with tumor burden than with chemotherapy (Forbes et al. 1981; Lukomska et al. 1983).

As surgery usually inhibits NK activity, we did not measure the NK activity of patients with HCC immediately after an operation, but rather 2 weeks after, and

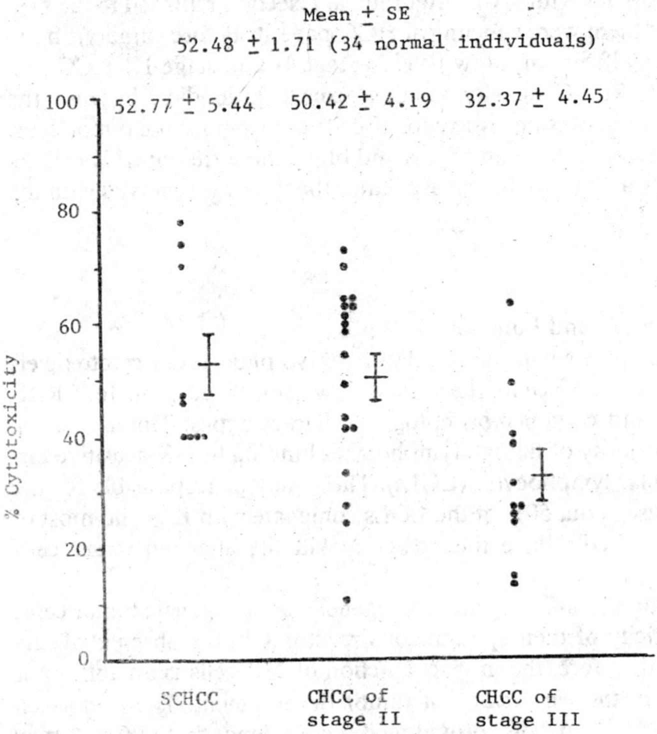

Fig. 3. NK activity in patients with SCHCC and CHCC. The percentage of natural cytotoxicity is lowest for those with stage-III CHCC, as compared with SCHCC ($P<0.01$), stage-II CHCC ($P<0.01$), or normal individuals ($P<0.001$)

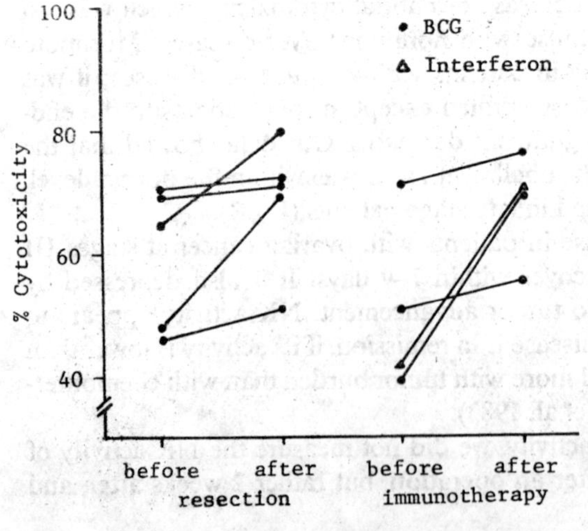

Fig. 4. The percentages of NK cytotoxicity increase after tumor resection and immunotherapy

compared it with that before. We found that NK activity after surgery was within the normal range and even higher than that before operation (Fig. 4).

In addition, immune adjuvants, bacille Calmette Guérin (BCG) or *Corynebacterium parvum,* or tumor cells susceptible to NK activity could induce a rapid and strong augmentation of reactivity. In some patients, administration of polycytidylic acid resulted in an increase of cytotoxicity, and anti-interferon antibodies decreased the NK activity below the spontaneous levels. So interferon might be important in the spontaneous activation or at least the maintenance of NK cells. According to our data, three patients received BCG inoculations and one received interferon; the NK cytotoxicity in all of them was higher after immunotherapy than before.

4. Macrophages

Several studies demonstrated the ability of macrophages to phagocytose and destroy tumor cells.

The nonimmunoglobulin-arming factor, probably derived from T cells, and the specific macrophage-arming factor (SMAF) may activate macrophages toward tumor cells. In addition, macrophages activated by various stimulants, including such bacteria as BCG, exert a cytolytic action against most tumor cells in vitro. It is possible that activated macrophages contribute to the destruction of tumor cells in the tumor. However, the fact that this action is not specific for rejection antigens suggests that its significance in vivo is probably minimal, except if it is triggered by specific lymphokines derived from sensitized T cells.

The cooperation between lymphocytes and macrophages is seen in antitumor immune responses; macrophages may be shown to be cytostatic or cytotoxic in the presence of certain factors derived from sensitized lymphocytes. Macrophage suppressors may also effect resistance against the tumor in the antitumor immune response.

Cameron and O'Brien (1982) reported that macrophage cytotoxic function might be normal in some patients with cancer; however, in some cases macrophages were ineffective in vivo, and the cytotoxicity might be inhibited by factors in autologous plasma.

5. B Lymphocytes

The proportion of B lymphocytes in human peripheral blood lymphocytes is 20%–30%. B lymphocytes in patients with HCC were measured by using surface membrane immunoglobulin (sIg) and compared with those in healthy controls (Table 10). We found that the percentages and absolute numbers of B lymphocytes in patients with HCC were higher than those in normal controls ($P<0.01$) (Lin et al. 1979).

Antitumor immunity of B lymphocytes: The role of B lymphocytes in cytotoxic responses to tumors appears to be confined to the production of tumor-specific antibodies, which may act in combination with K cells to mediate this form of cytotoxicity – ADCC. Sometimes the antibody may combine with free tumor antigen as a blocking factor to inhibit ADCC or cytolytic T lymphocytes. Recent data on the interaction of T and B lymphocytes indicate that the antibodies produced by B lym-

Table 10. Percentages and absolute values of B lymphocytes in HCC

	Control	HCC	*P* value
No. of patients	18	24	
sIg (%)	11.2± 0.4	16.1± 1.1	<0.01
No./mm³	181.0±12.5	243.8±29.0	<0.01
sIgM (%)	8.4± 0.4	9.5± 0.5	
No./mm³	136.0±80.0	149.7±14.0	

Table [illegible]rious immunotherapies compared with nonimmunotherapy of HCC

Immunotherapy	No. of patients	1-year survival			
		SCHCC	*P* value[b]	CHCC stage II	*P* value[b]
BCG	204	72% (18/25)[a]	N.S.[c]	25% (37/143)	<0.01
Tumor vaccine	84	57.1% (4/7)	N.S.	26.8% (15/56)	<0.05
Immune RNA	27	72.7% (8/11)	N.S.	56.3% (9/16)	<0.01
Control	349	37.5%(3/8)		13.4% (22/164)	

[a] No. of patients
[b] Different group of immunotherapy as compared with control
[c] No significance

Table 12. Comparison of conventional therapy with or without immunotherapy (matched study)

Conventional treatment	No. of patients	1-year survival			3-year survival		
		Immuno-therapy (%)	Control <(%)	*P* value	Immuno-therapy (%)	Control <(%)	*P* value
Radical resection	18	93.3	86.7		63.7	20	<0.05
Palliative resection	22	40.9	4.8	<0.01	10		
Cryosurgery	4	25					
Catheterization or ligation of hepatic artery	24	27.3	8.7	<0.05			
Radiotherapy	20	25	5.0			5.3	
Chemotherapy and herbs	50	12	4.1		2.2		
Total	138	30.8 (41/133)	14.4 (19/132)	<0.01	8.8 (10/114)	3.5 (4/116)	>0.05

phocyte cells require the help of T cells (helper cells); with virally induced tumors especially antibodies can neutralize excess viral particles, reduce transformation of cells, and limit tumor growth.

IV. Immunotherapy in Patients with HCC

Since 1970 we have used several kinds of immunological preparations for patients with HCC and compared them with controls in a nonimmunotherapy group (Table 11). We found preliminary clinical improvement and raised survival rates in HCC patients given immunotherapy (Lin and Tang 1981).

In order to compare the effects with and without immunotherapy, we observed two strictly matched groups of HCC patients in which the sex and age of patients, the size of tumors, the mode of surgery, extent of resection, extent and degree of cryosurgery, total dose of radiotherapy, and total dose and route of chemotherapy were similar (Table 12).

We compared the 3-year survival rates in the radical resection group and the 1-year survival rates in the palliative resection group; survival rates were significantly higher for those given immunotherapy than for those without immunotherapy. This demonstrated that surgical resection combined with immunotherapy is of benefit in eliminating residue tumors and decreasing recurrence rates. For patients who underwent hepatic artery cannulation or ligation the 6-month and 1-year survival rates were obviously higher when immunotherapy was given than when it was withheld. In the chemotherapy group only the 6-month survival rate was somewhat increased with immunotherapy (Lin and Tang 1981). Currently all SCHCC patients receive immunotherapy after resection, and we will later make a comparison at random.

A. Nonspecific Active Immunotherapy

1. BCG

Experimental evidence from guinea pig L_{10} and human melanoma showed that there was a common antigen existing in BCG and tumor cell, suggesting that the microbial preparation probably has the special role of resisting tumor. BCG may affect the activation of NK cells and macrophages – through the release of interferon – and stimulate the increase of the T-lymphocytes and K cells. Adjuvant immunotherapy with BCG has been used for patients with various tumors, including HCC (Balasegaram 1975).

The BCG was given by intradermal injection in our hospital; the 1-year survival rate for patients with CHCC (stage II) was higher than that of the control group ($P<0.01$; Table 11). The OT test became positive or it remained positive in the course of BCG therapy, the median survival time being longer than that for those with a changing or persisting negative reaction (6.7 versus 4.5 months) (Lin et al. 1975). There have been some reports about the different routes of administration and about toxicity or side effects of BCG and its derivative (Sparks 1976). However,

BCG has been used intradermally up to now, with only low fever and ulcer experienced as side effects. Kokoschka (1977) also reported that he had seen neither severe side effects nor involvement of the liver or other organs with the bacillus.

2. Corynebacterium parvum

The mechanism of *C. parvum* (CP) is that it stimulates the mononucelar macrophage system, the activated macrophages releasing the enzyme lysosome and destroying the tumor cells (Gupta et al. 1978). The activated CP inhibits the immunity of T lymphocytes and the reaction to mitogen PHA. The activated macrophages may be responsible for decreasing the reaction of T lymphocytes. CP can also increase the activation of NK cells. CP is an adjuvant which can activate B cells and increase humoral immunity. We have used it effectively to control the carcinomatous pleural effusions of liver cancer. Recently it was reported that carcinomatous pleural effusions contain two kinds of suppressor cells for NK activity, macrophages and nylon wool-nonadherent lymphocytes, that may impair NK activity in the effusions (Uchida and Micksche 1981).

3. Interferon

There is almost no therapeutic use of interferon for cancer patients owing to the limited supply of the agent, which would otherwise be of significance in the enhancement of NK cells (Son et al. 1982). We used interferon II in a patient with HCC after ligation and catheterization of the hepatic artery; the NK cell cytotoxicity was elevated from 41.79% to 69.76% after administration of 1×10^6 units/day for 2 weeks.

B. Specific immunotherapy

The allogeneic or xenogeneic liver cancer cells were modified by chemotherapy or radiation plus an incomplete adjuvant, such as a tumor vaccine. These vaccines were injected periodically into recipients after resection or intensive chemotherapy. BCG was administered concurrently with the vaccine in some patients. We found the effect of tumor vaccine plus BCG better than that of tumor vaccine or BCG alone (Lin and Tang 1975).

C. Adoptive Immunotherapy

Adoptive immunotherapy may involve the lymphocyte transfer factor and immune RNA extracted from sensitized lymphocytes. We injected 14 HCC patients with immune RNA after resection; eight of them were SCHCC cases, and seven of the 14 underwent radical resection. In a control group of 13 patients eight were SCHCC cases, and in ten of 13 cases the tumors were radically resected (Fig. 5). Immune RNA was administered for at least half a year, the longest period being 26 months. The recurrent rate for patients who had undergone radical resection in the treated group was 57.1%; for those in the control group it was 80%. The period of recur-

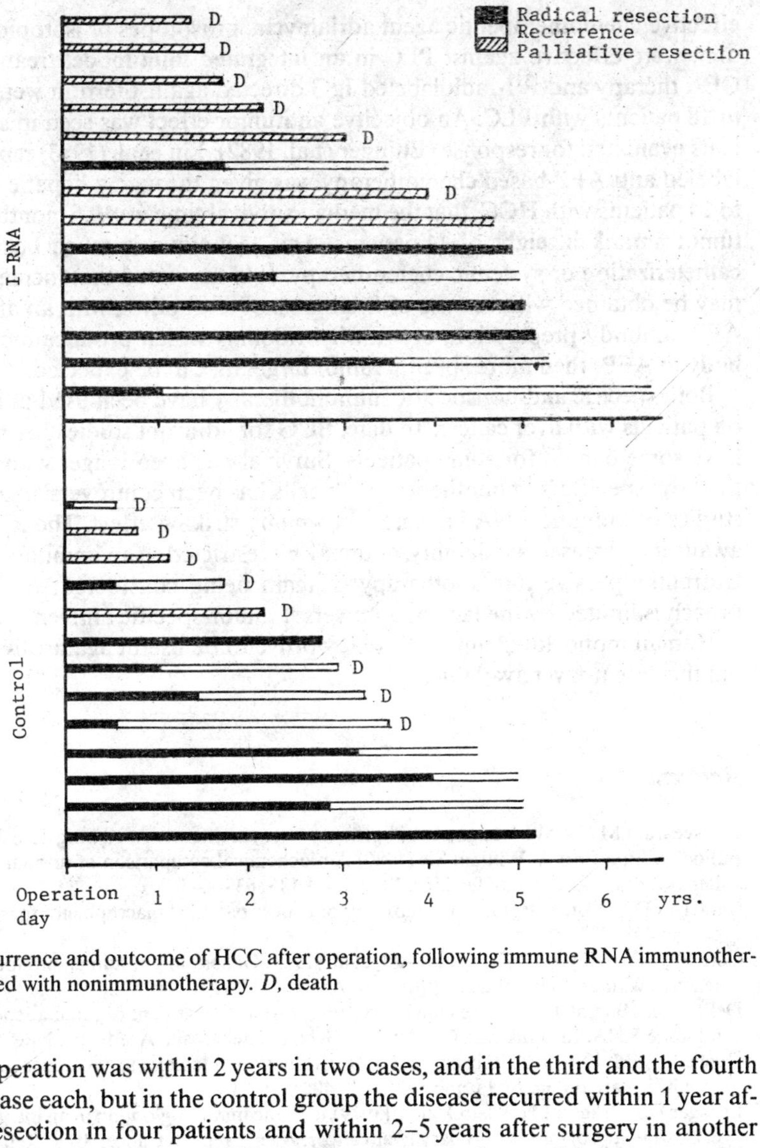

Fig. 5. The recurrence and outcome of HCC after operation, following immune RNA immunotherapy as compared with nonimmunotherapy. *D*, death

rence after operation was within 2 years in two cases, and in the third and the fourth year in one case each, but in the control group the disease recurred within 1 year after radical resection in four patients and within 2–5 years after surgery in another four. It is possible that immune RNA therapy after resection could postpone recurrence, and that immune RNA can change the natural course of tumors with poor prognoses (Dekernion 1976).

D. Passive Immunotherapy

Passive immunotherapy is the transfer of antitumor antibodies from an immune donor to a recipient with a malignant tumor. A few recent reports have demonstrated that the antibody of AFP and specific antibodies, such as the carriers of an effective chemotherapeutic agent adriamycin, or isotopes or isotopic immunoglobulin, were effective against PLC in an integrated multimodel treatment program. CEA therapy and ^{131}I-radiolabeled IgG directed against ferritin were administered to 18 patients with PLC. An objecitve antitumor effect was seen in six of nine patients evaluated for response (Ettinger et al. 1982). Liu et al. (1983) reported that ^{131}I-labeled anti-AFP-based chemotherapy was given through a hepatic artery catheter to 14 patients with HCC, that the median survival time was 9.5 months, and that the tumor shrank in eight of 11 patients. This technique is much better than single catheterization or systemic chemotherapy. It is suggested that increased specificity may be obtained with the use of fragments of antibodies, with an affinity-purified AFP antibody preparation, or with hybridomas which produce monoclonal antibody to AFP; then more specific tumor targeting can be expected.

Both specific and nonspecific immunotherapy have been used in limited studies on patients with liver cancer. To date, BCG for adjuvant studies has been proved to have some benefit for some patients. Survival has been longer with these types of therapy; specific immunotherapy with cells has been controversial, and the limited studies of immune RNA have not shown any striking effect. The use of interferon awaits its increased availability, and may be restricted to an immunoregulating role. Currently, passive immunotherapy is again being considered; however, this approach is limited by the lack of a universal tumor-specific antigen.

Human monoclonal antibodies may prove to be useful against liver cancer cells but they are not yet available.

References

Balasegaram M (1975) Management of primary liver carcinoma. Am J Surg 130: 33–37

Bullock S, Bomford A, William SR (1980) A biochemical comparison of normal human liver and hepatocellular carcinoma ferritins. Biochem J 185: 639–645

Cameron DJ, O'Brien P (1982) Cytotoxicity of cancer patients' macrophages for tumor cells. Cancer 50: 498–502

Cote RJ, Morrissey DM, Houghton AN, et al. (1983) Generation of human monoclonal antibodies reactive with cellular antigens. Proc Natl Acad Sci USA 80: 2026–2030

Dekernion JB et al. (1976) The clinical experience in the treatment of renal adenocarcinoma with immune RNA. In: Fink MA (ed) Immune RNA in neoplasia. Academic, New York, p 259

Dusheiko GM, Kew MC, Rabson AR (1979) Evaluation of leukocyte adherence inhibition in hepatocellular carcinoma. Br J Cancer 40: 397–402

Ettinger DS, Dragon LH, Klein J, et al. (1979) Isotopic immunoglobulin in an integrated multimodel treatment program for primary liver cancer: A case report. Cancer Treat Rep 63: 131–134

Ettinger DS, Order SE, Wharam MD, et al. (1982) Phase I–II study of isotopic immunoglobulin therapy for primary liver cancer. Cancer Treat Rep 66: 289–297

Forbes JT, Greco FA, Oldham RK (1981) Human natural cell-mediated cytotoxicity. II. Levels in neoplastic disease. Cancer Immunol Immunother 11: 147–153

Ge XR (1977) Research progression of leukocyte adherence inhibition test. Shanghai Med J 1: 182–189[1]

Goldenberg DM, Kim EE, Deland F, et al. (1980) Clinical studies on the radioimmunodetection of tumors containing alphafetoprotein. Cancer 45: 2500–2505

Gupta JD, Morahan PS, Kaplan AM (1978) *Corynebacterium parvum* induced resistance to a methylcholenthrene fibrosarcoma. J Reticuloendotheliel Soc 23: 1–9

Herberman RB (1981) Natural killer (NK) cells. In: Sell KW, Miller WV (eds) The lymphocyte. Alan R. Liss, New York, (Progress in clinical and biological research. V. 58 pp 33–43)

Halliday WJ, Miller S (1972) Leukocyte adherence inhibition: A simple test for cell-mediated tumor immunity and serum blocking factors. Int J Cancer 9: 477–483

Halliday WJ, Halliday JW, Campbell CB, et al. (1974) Specific immunodiagnosis of hepatocellular carcinoma by leucocyte adherence inhibition. Br Med J 2: 249–352

Kan D (1978) Cellular immunity in hepatocellular carcinoma. Acta Hepatol Jpn 19: 175–182

Kaneto A, Kubo Y, Nagasaki Y, et al. (1980) Clinical evaluation of serum ferritin in hepatocellular carcinoma and liver cirrhosis. Acta Hepatol Jpn 21: 745–753

Kerman RH, Smith R, Stefani SS, et al. (1976) Active T-rosette-forming cells in the peripheral blood of cancer patients. Cancer Res 36: 3274–3278

Kew MC, Dusheiko GM (1981) Paraneoplastic manifestations of hepatocellular carcinoma. In: Berk PD, Chalmess TC (eds) Frontiers in liver disease. Thieme-Stratton, New York, pp 305–318

Kim EE, Deland FH, Nelson MO, et al. (1980) Radioimmunodetection of cancer with radiolabeled antibodies to L-fetoprotein. Cancer Res 40: 3008–3012

Kokoschka EM (1977) Active specific and active nonspecific immunotherapy of patients with malignant melanoma. Oncology 34: 229–233

Kumagai N, Morizane T, Nakamura T, et al. (1980) Specific immunodiagnosis of hepatoma by tube leukocyte adherence and application of "repeated LAI assay". Acta Hepatol Jpn 21: 1188–1195

Lin ZY, Tang ZY (1975) Preliminary report of active immunotherapy in primary liver cancer. Tumor Prevent Treat Study 4: 54–57[1]

Lin ZY, Tang ZY (1979) Delayed hypersensitivity reaction to old tuberculin and the prognosis of primary carcinoma of the liver. Acta Acad Med Primae Shanghai 66: 103–110

Lin ZY, Tang ZY (1981) The immunostatus and immunotherapy of patients with primary liver cancer. In: Tang ZY (ed) Primary liver cancer. Shanghai Science and Technique Publisher, Shanghai, pp 319–331[1]

Lin ZY, Tang ZY Chen KJ, et al. (1979) Preliminary study on cell-mediated immunity in primary carcinoma of the liver. Acta Acad Med Primae Shanghai 6: 1–7

Lin ZY, Chao YZ, Tang ZY, et al. (1981) Detection of cell-mediated and humoral immunity in primary liver cancer. Shanghai J Immunol 1: 34–36[1]

Littmann BH, Alpert E, Rocklin RE (1977) The effect of purified fetoprotein on in vitro assays of cell-mediated immunity. Cell Immunol 30: 35–42

Liu YK, Yand KZ, Wu YD, et al. (1983) Treatment of advanced primary hepatocellular carcinoma by ^{131}I-anti-AFP. Lancet I: 531–532

Lukomska B, Olszewski WL, Engeset A, et al. (1983) The effect of surgery and chemotherapy on blood NK-cell activity in patients with ovarian cancer. Cancer 51: 465–469

Moretta L, Feuci AS (1980) Subpopulations of human T lymphocytes. Immunol Today 1: 3–4

Moretta L, Mingari MC, Moretta A, et al. (1980) T-cell Fc receptors as markers of function in human lymphocyte subsets. In: Fougerean M, Dansset J (eds) Immunology. Academic, New York, p 223

Morimoto T (1982) Natural killer activity of peripheral blood lymphocytes from patients with various liver deseases. Acta Hepatol Jpn 23: 132–140

Morizane T, Watanabe T, Tsuchimoto K, et al. (1980) Impaired T cell function and decreased natural killer activity in patients with liver cirrhosis and their significance in the development of hepatocellular carcinoma. Gastroenterol Jpn 15: 226–232

Niitsu Y, Ohtsuka S, Kohgo Y, et al. (1975) Hepatoma ferritin in the tissue and serum. Tumor Res 10: 31–41

Order SE (1976) The history and progress of serologic immunotherapy and radiodiagnosis. Radiology 118: 219–223

Order SE, Klein JL, Leichner PK (1981) Antiferritin IgG antibody for isotopic cancer therapy. Oncology 38: 154–160

Pollack SB, Hallenbeck LA (1982) In vivo reduction of NK activity with anti-NK_1 serum: Direct evaluation of NK cells in tumor clearance. Int J Cancer 29: 203–207

Reinberg EL, Schlossman SF (1980) Current concepts in immunology regulation of the immune response-inducer and suppressor T-lymphocyte subsets in human being. J Exp Med 151: 969–974

Shanghai Coordinating Group for Liver Cancer Research, China (1979) Diagnosis and tratment of primary hepatocellular carcinoma in early stage – report of 134 cases. Chin Med J [Engl] 92: 801–806

Shimbo T, Yata J, Nakagawa J, et al. (1977a) Method to identify human T lymphocytes bearing Fc receptors and studies of these T-lymphocytes in various dieseases. Clin Immunol 9: 141–145

Shimbo T, Yata J, Hiei U, et al. (1977b) The significance of human T cells bearing IgG-Fc receptor in patients with malignant solid tumor. Clin Immunol 9: 487–493

Sen K, Kew MC, Rabson AR (1982) Depressed natural killer cell activity in patients with hepatocellular carcinoma:In vitro effects of interferon and levamisole. Cancer 50: 2820–2825

Sparks FC (1976) Hazards and complications of BCG immunotherapy. (Symposium on immunotherapy in malignant disease.) MCNA 60: 499–509

The Tumor Research Group, Shanghai Institue of Experimental Biology, Academia Sinica (1977) Assay of lymphocyte microcytotoxicity useing ^{125}I-iododeoxyuridine-labeled human liver cancer cell line. The Short Report of Shanghai Tumor Prevent Treat Study 1: 23–28[1]

Timonen T, Saksela E, Ranki A, et al. (1979) Fractionation, morphological and functional characterization of effector cells responsible for human natural killer activity against cell-line targets. Cell Immunol 48: 133–148

Tsung YK, Milunsky A, Alpert E (1980): Derivation and characterzation of a monoclonal hybridoma antibody specific for human alphafetoprotein. J Immunol Method 39: 363–368

Uchida A, Micksche M (1981) Suppressor cells for natural killer activity in carcinomatous pleural effusion of cancer patients. Cancer Immunol Immunother 11: 255–263

William AO (1975) Impairment of rosette-forming T lymphocytes in cirrhosis and liver cancer. N Engl Med J 293: 1100

Wybran J, Fudenberg HH (1973) Thymus-derived rosette-forming in various human disease states: cancer, lymphoma, bacterial and viral infection and other disease. J Clin Invest 52: 1026–1032

Yao XH, Li DG, Gu HD (1983) Changes of T-cell subpopulation in patients with hepatoma. Shanxi Med J 12: 48–50[1]

Zheng XR, Weng HZ, Chen KQ, et al. (1980) A preliminary report of determination of antibody-dependent cell-mediatet cytotoxocity and its clinical application. Shanghai Med J 3: 59–62[1]

Zuberi SJ (1980) Immunological studies in primary liver cancer in Karachi. Ann Acad Med 9: 203–209

[1] Chinese

13 Erythrocyte Sodium Pump Activity and Hepatocellular Carcinoma

Ye Sheng-long, Tang Zhao-you

Hepatocellular carcinoma is a common and grave malignancy in China. The sufferers frequently exhibit significant metabolic disturbances, especially cachexia in the late stage. Although advances have been made in HCC research in recent years (Foster 1982; Okuda and Ohnishi 1982; Tang et al. 1982), the knowledge of pathophysiological and biochemical alterations in HCC patients is so far insufficient.

In the past two decades, remarkable progress has been made in the research of sodium-potassium pump (sodium pump). A relationship between tumor and sodium pump was recently noticed (Kolata 1981). The structural and functional changes of tumor cells are closely related to sodium pump (Racker 1976 a). The visible metabolic disturbances in HCC patients may be due to the change of sodium pump function caused by malignant tumor, and may reflect the interaction of tumor and host. It may be of significance theoretically and practically to probe into sodium pump function in HCC patients.

In this chapter we attempt to review the major aspects of sodium pump and its relation to some disorders, and to study the alteration of erythrocyte sodium pump activity in HCC patients.

I. General Considerations About Sodium Pump

A. Sodium Pump and Na,K-ATPase

Sodium pump is a molecular machinery for the active transport of sodium (Na^+) and potassium (K^+) in the membrane of human and all animal cells. Much of the metabolic energy produced by the body is used to establish high intracellular concentrations of potassium and low sodium, and the reverse of the relative concentrations of these ions in the extracellular fluids. The extrusion of sodium requires its movement against a gradient of concentration (higher outside than inside) and electrical potential (more negative inside than outside); therefore, energy is needed to overcome this electrochemical gradient (Sweadner and Goldin 1980). It was not until 1957 that Skou discovered the sodium-potassium-dependent adenosine triphosphatase (Na,K-ATPase) in crab nerves and identified an ouabain-inhibitable enzymatic activity which hydrolyzes ATP when stimulated simultaneously by sodium and potassium ions. He further demonstrated that the Na,K-ATPase was similar to the sodium pump in many respects (Skou 1965). Since then, a considerable amount of investigation has been carried out in this field. At present, it can be confirmed without any doubt that the Na,K-ATPase is actually the sodium pump in vivo responsible for the active transport of sodium and potassium (Robinson and Flashner 1979; Schwartz et al. 1980; Wallick et al. 1979).

B. Characteristics

Sodium pump, or Na,K-ATPase, is ubiquitous in all animal cells (Stekhoven and Bonting 1981). In spite of its wide range of activity with different cells, the enzyme has the following basic characteristics (Dahl and Hokin 1974; Glynn and Karlish 1975; Schwartz et al. 1975; Stekhoven and Bonting 1981; Wallick et al. 1979):

1. It is embedded in the plasma membrane, composed of protein and lipids.
2. It catalyzes the hydrolysis of ATP, the primary substrate for the enzyme, into ADP and inorganic phosphate (Pi). Other nucleotides may be hydrolyzed at much lower rates, from 15% to 0.5% of the activity with ATP, in the following decreasing order of activity: CTP > ITP > GTP > UTP > TTP.
3. The requirement for the presence of both Na^+ and K^+ is the most characteristic property of the enzyme. Na^+ is absolutely required, whereas K^+ can be replaced by Tl^+, Rb^+, Cs^+, and NH_4^+, and only poorly by Li^+.
4. The reaction is specifically inhibited by cardiac glycosides; ouabain is widely used because of its highest sensitivity.
5. The most available pH for sodium pump is about 7.5.
6. The ratio of sodium and potassium transport is tightly coupled with three sodium ions pumping out vs. two potassium ions pumping in per ATP hydrolysis. Two of the sodium ions are presumably exchanged for potassium ions, and the remaining one is transported electrogenically.
7. The Mg^{++} required by the enzyme may be replaced by other divalent cations such as Mn^{++} or Co^{++}, the efficiency being only one-tenth. On the other hand, Fe^{++}, Ca^{++}, Zn^{++}, Cu^{++}, Ba^{++}, Sr^{++}, and Be^{++} inhibit the hydrolysis of ATP.

C. Structure and Mechanism

Na,K-ATPase purified from a variety of tissues contains two different protein subunits. The large one, called α, has a molecular weight of approximately 95000, spanning the membrane completely. It possesses the active site for ATP hydrolysis and the site for inhibition by cardiac glycosides. The smaller subunit, called β, is a glycoprotein with a molecular weight of 40000. It was conjectured that the complete structure might be $\beta\alpha\alpha\beta$ (Schwartz et al. 1980; Stekhoven and Bonting 1981; Sweadner and Goldin 1980; Wallick et al. 1979).

It was reported recently that a protein with a low molecular weight of 13500, termed γ protein, had been isolated from some Na,K-ATPase and shown to be located at approximately the ouabain binding site on the α subunit (Schwartz et al. 1980).

The exact molecular mechanism of active transport by sodium pump remains unclear. It is generally accepted that the enzyme complex does not rotate or diffuse across the membrane. The total process of ATP hydrolysis catalyzed by sodium pump is a step-by-step continuous reaction involving multiple ions. The energy from ATP hydrolysis gives rise to active transport by causing conformational changes in the enzyme. In the presence of Na^+ and K^+, phosphate production can be resolved into two phases, i.e., an initial burst and a late steady-state phase. Total reactions may be a cyclical process. The binding of enzyme and sodium causes phosphorylation and change of conformation, so that sodium is moved out of the membrane, potassium is bound, the phosphorylated intermediate is hydrolyzed, and the conformation returns to the initial status. Owing to this cycle, the electrochemical gradient can be maintained.

D. Functions

The fundamental function of the sodium pump is to extrude sodium and accumulate potassium in all cells, and to transport sodium between epithelial cells (Smith and Edelman 1979), thus maintaining the electrochemical gradient between the inside and outside of the membrane and ensuring the normal physiological functions and metabolic requirements of the body cells. Sodium pump may play an important role in energy metabolism. The basal rate of fuel consumption depends on ATP hydrolysis to provide energy for those synthetic, mechanical, and osmotic processes necessary to keep the body alive. Although distributed in a variety of cells, the enzyme catalyzes the same hydrolytic process. Various secondary transport systems are inserted into different cell membranes, carrying out different functions with the energy of the sodium gradient produced by the enzyme (Sweadner and Goldin 1980). It is believed that the uptake of nutrition in the small intestine or other organs (Charney and Donowitz 1978; Giese 1979), the reabsorption of sodium chloride in the kidneys (Sweadner and Goldin 1980), the maintainance of bile production and other functions in the liver (Erlinger and Dumeaux 1974; Van Dyke et al. 1982), the secretion of pancreatic juice (Ridderstap and Bonting 1969), the formation of cerebrospinal fluid (Vates et al. 1964), and the balance of contractile force in cardiac muscles (Sweadner and Goldin 1980), are all correlated to sodium pump.

E. Regulation and Modification

It has been recognized that several endogenous factors may regulate the activity of sodium pump in vivo, while a variety of drugs and other factors are also capable of affecting sodium pump activity. Some of them had been thoroughly studied.

1. Cardiac Glycosides

Cardiac glycosides bind with high specifity to the sodium pump and strongly inhibit it, so they have been used to determine the presence and function of the pump in different tissues. Most widely used is ouabain. It inhibits binding of ATP and dephosphorylation of the phosphointermediate by reacting only at the outermembrane side (Stekhoven and Bonting 1981). Treatment of congestive heart failure with cardiac glycosides to increase the force of myocardial contraction might be based on inactivation of a portion of the Na,K-ATPase of heart muscle (Wallick et al. 1977), reducing the sodium concentration gradient across the cell membrane and, in turn, the magnitude of exchange-coupled calcium efflux; the overall effects are increases in the net intracellular calcium concentration and in muscular contractility (Brody and Akera 1977; Sweadner and Goldin 1980).

2. Vanadates

Vanadates cause a slow inhibition of purified Na,K-ATPase by binding to a Pi phosphorylation site (Stekhoven and Bonting 1981; Sweadner and Goldin 1980). The inhibition requires Mg^{++} at the intracellular surface and K^{+} at the extracellular surface. Sufficient quantities of vanadates are present in the body to inhibit roughly half the sodium pump activity, but the inhibition by vanadates may be completely reversed by high concentration of norepinephrine; thus they may serve as physiological modulators of sodium pump activity (Wallick et al. 1979).

3. Sulfhydryl Reagents

There are 36 sulfhydryl (SH) groups per mole of Na,K-ATPase, 34 on the α-subunit and only 2 on the β-subunit. Agents modifying the SH groups inhibit sodium pump activity. Owing to the existence of various essential as well as nonessential SH groups, there may be noticeable differences in the inhibitory effects of different reagents on overall or partial reaction (Stekhoven and Bonting 1981). The SH reagents which have been reported as able to inhibit sodium pump include chlorpromazine and derivatives, ethacrynic acid, N-ethylmaleimide (NEM), P-chloromercuribenzoate (PCMB), 5,5′-dithiobis-2-nitrobenzoic acid (DTNB), dinitrofluorobenzene (DNFB), and ethylmercurithiosalicylate (Glynn and Karlish 1975; Robinson and Flashner 1979; Schwartz et al. 1975; Skou 1965; Stekhoven and Bonting 1981).

4. Oligomycin

Oligomycin, a specific inhibitor of oxidative phosphorylation in mitochondria, may inhibit Na,K-ATPase reversibly; it inhibits the hydrolysis of ATP in the presence of sodium, potassium, and magnesium, reducing the rate of the enzyme reaction. The inhibition is incomplete even at a high concentration of oligomycin. The relative efficacy of the inhibition produced by oligomycin may decrease if ouabain is present, whereas the inhibition increases with a decline in temperature (Blostein 1970; Cavieres 1977; Robinson and Flashner 1979; Schwartz et al. 1975; Skou 1965; Stekhoven and Bonting 1981).

5. Thyroid Hormone

Thyroid hormone causes an increase in Na,K-ATPase activity. Injection of triiodothyronine (T_3) produced a significant rise of Na,K-ATPase activity in skeletal muscle, kidney, and liver, and a slight rise of that in heart muscle, while it had no demonstrable effect on that in the cerebral cortex. Thyroid hormone might cause an increase in sodium transport-dependent respiration via Na,K-ATPase.

It is generally considered that the hormone-induced increase in ATPase activity was due to an increase in the number of sodium pump units, either by the unmasking of preexisting precursors or by the biosynthesis of new enzymes (Himms-Hagen 1976; Ismail-Beigi 1977; Lin and Akera 1978; Sterling 1979; Sweadner and Goldin 1980).

6. Catecholamines

It has been reported that catecholamines increase sodium pump activity. Sometimes this action is blocked by alpha- or beta-adrenegic receptor blockers. Catecholamines can form a tight complex with the vanadate ion and effectively neutralize it, thus playing a regulatory role in vivo (Schwartz et al. 1975; Sweadner and Goldin 1980).

In addition to those mentioned above, a variety of other factors which regulate or influence sodium pump have been reported by numerous investigators: mercurial diuretics, diphenylhydantoin (DPH), hydroxylamine, fusidic acid, dimethyl sulfoxide (DMSO), phlorizin, suramin, vasodilators (minoxidil, diazoxide, hydralazine), prostaglandins, amiodarone, ascorbic acid, azasteroids, carbodiimides, insecticides, *Erythrophloeum* alkaloids, diketocoriolin B, AY 22241 (actodigin), harmaline (Schwartz et al. 1975); beryllium, fluoride, dicyclohexylcarbodiimide (DCCD) (Glynn and Karlish 1975); aldosterone, vasopressin (Sweadner and Goldin 1980; Weiner and Maffly 1978); butanedione, detergent, organic solvents, phospholipase (Stekhoven and Bonting 1981); cAMP-dependent protein kinase, endorphins, enkephalins (Schwartz et al. 1980); glucocorticoids (Kaji et al. 1981); bilirubin (Kashiwamata et al. 1979); flavonoids (Suolinna et al. 1975); endotoxin (Tenney and Rafter 1968); aminolevulinic acid (Becker et al. 1971); methanethiol (Quarfoth et al. 1976); adriamycin (Gosalvez et al. 1979); estrogen (Davis et al. 1978); glucagon and insulin (Fehlmann and Ereychet 1981; Resh et al. 1980); phenobarbital (Simon et al. 1977); ethanol (Ricci et al. 1981); anesthetics, radiation, heavy metal, acetylcholine, thyrotropin (Giese 1979).

II. Disorders Related to Sodium Pump

With a variety of illnesses there might be membrane abnormality in one or more organs. Some have been considered dysfunctions of sodium pump in view of its wide distribution and special characteristics, and they might be reflected in peripheral blood cells. In this section, we briefly review some disorders which were reported in literature to be related to sodium pump, putting emphasis on the relation between tumor and sodium pump.

A. Some Disorders Manifesting Dysfunction of Na,K-ATPase

Discussed below are some of the disorders which may be correlated with Na,K-ATPase, except for tumors and liver diseases, which will be reviewed separately.

1. Hypertension

In erythrocytes of essential hypertension patients, an abnormally low sodium-potassium net flux ratio was confirmed, while in those of secondary hypertension and normotensive patients the ratio was similar to that for controls (Garay et al. 1980). Wambach et al. (1979) found increased Na,K-ATPase activity in erythrocyte ghosts of essential hypertension patients, and reported different erythrocyte Na,K-ATPase activities in various types of hypertension (Wambach et al. 1980). However, Swarts et al. (1981) failed to show a difference in erythrocyte Na,K-ATPase activity between hypertensive and normotensive subjects.

2. Uremia

Uremia patients were reported to have a high intracellular Na^+ content and a transport abnormality including depressed activity of Na,K-ATPase in erythrocytes (Cole 1973; Smith and Welt 1970) and in leukocytes (Edmondson et al. 1975). Effective treatment might reverse the abnormal alteration of the Na,K-ATPase activity (Smith and Welt 1970; Edmondson et al. 1975).

3. Obesity

Obese animals had a decreased Na,K-ATPase activity of cell membranes in liver, kidney, and skeletal muscle (Bray et al. 1978; Lin et al. 1978; York et al. 1978). It was recently found that both the number of sodium pump units and cation transport activity of the pump were reduced in erythrocytes from obese human subjects, suggesting a possible role of sodium pump abnormalities in the pathophysiology of obesity (De Luise et al. 1980). On the other hand, liver homogenates from obese subjects were found to have more Na,K-ATPase activity than those from normal controls (Bray et al. 1981). There was no satisfactory explanation for the different results.

4. Affective Disorders

The Na,K-ATPase activity of erythrocytes of manic patients in acute phase was higher, but that in normal phase was not higher, than that of normal subjects, indicating a correlation between changes in clinical phases of mania and erythrocyte Na,K-ATPase activity (Akagawa et al. 1980). The Na,K-ATPase activity of erythrocytes decreased in depressive patients and increased with lithium treatment or improvement of depression (Hesketh et al. 1977).

5. Thyrotoxicosis

Thyroid hormone stimulates the sodium pump activity of liver and kidney in experimental animals (Ismail-Beigi 1977). The activity decreased with hypothyroidism and increased with hyperthyroidism (Gambert et al. 1981). On the other hand, patients with hyperthyroidism were reported to have a high erythrocyte sodium concentration associated with a decrease in the rate constant for ouabain-sensitive Na efflux (Smith and Samuel 1970). Furthermore, it was demonstrated that both the number of sodium pump units and the cation transport activity of the pump in erythrocytes were reduced in hyperthyroidism, and that these changes were reversible with control of the hyperthyroidism. On the other hand, hypothyroid individuals showed changes which were the reverse of those seen in hyperthyroidism (De-Luise and Flier 1983).

6. Cystic Fibrosis

Patients with cystic fibrosis were shown to have a defect in sodium transport of erythrocytes which resulted from decrease in both ouabain-sensitive ATPase activity and ethacrynic acid-sensitive sodium efflux (Balfe et al. 1968). Cystic fibrosis fibroblasts in culture produced a substance or a group of substances, which was suggested to have had an inhibitory effect on membrane sodium pump (Schmoyer and Baglia 1974). Yet different results were also reported (Applegarth et al. 1977).

7. Other Disorders

It was reported that related to the alteration of erythrocyte sodium pump function were many other disorders such as myotonic dystrophy (Hull and Roses 1976), Bartter's syndrome (Haljamäe et al. 1975), pre-eclampsia (Kuhnert et al. 1977), lead poisoning (Hasan et al. 1967), chronic alcoholism (Israel et al. 1970), and hypokalemia (Parker and Welt 1972; Parker et al. 1978).

B. Sodium Pump Activity in Liver Diseases

Liver cells have high Na,K-ATPase activity in plasma membranes. It has been known that sodium pump played an important role in bile production (Erlinger and Dhumeaux 1974; Van Dyke et al. 1982) and bile acid-independent bile flow (BAIBF) was thought to be modulated mainly by Na,K-ATPase located in hepatocyte plasma membranes. Inhibitors of Na,K-ATPase decrease BAIBF (Erlinger and Dhumeaux 1974); the pathogenesis of some cholestasis in liver might be related to the decreased Na,K-ATPase activity (Van Dyke et al. 1982).

It was found that the sodium pump activity of erythrocytes or leukocytes decreased in fulminant hepatic failure (Alam et al. 1978), acute viral hepatitis (Banbassat et al. 1980), and advanced cirrhosis (Sewell et al. 1981). Incubation of cells from patients with fulminant hepatic failure in the serum of normal subjects resulted in a reversal of the change in Na,K-ATPase activity; on the other hand, incubation of normal cells in serum from patients achieved an inhibition of Na,K-ATPase activity. This suggested that a circulating toxin might be involved in the defective sodium pumping mechanism (Alam et al. 1978). The decreased activity of sodium pump in liver diseases might be the indication of damaged hepatocyte membranes (Banbassat et al. 1980).

C. Change of Sodium Pump Activity Associated with Tumor Tissues

Sodium pump is now considered a marker enzyme for plasma membrane because of its specificity of localization (Stekhoven and Bonting 1981). Attention has been paid to the relation between sodium pump and tumor in view of the alteration of structure and function in tumor cell plasma membranes (Kolata 1981; Racker 1976a).

1. Tumor Metabolism Involved with Na,K-ATPase

There is a dominant metabolic distinction between malignant tumor tissues and normal tissues. A high aerobic glycolysis was associated with progression in malignant growth capacity (Burk et al. 1967). The glycolysis pathway was demonstrated to be subject to regulation of Na,K-ATPase activity in intact cells (Whittam and Ager 1965), the regulative point of the pathway was recognized to be the sequence of reaction catalyzed by phosphoglycerate kinase (PGK) (Eckel et al. 1966). The high aerobic glycolysis in several tumor cells was considered to result from high Na,K-ATPase activity (Suolinna et al. 1974). For example, in Ehrlich ascites tumor cells, the Na,K-ATPase of the plasma membrane sustained high aerobic glycolysis (Scholnick et al. 1973). Certain bioflavonoids inhibit the glycolysis of a variety of tumor cells by inhibiting the activity of Na,K-ATPase of the plasma membranes (Suolinna et al. 1975).

2. Investigation with Experimental Tumors

Numerous papers have been published concerning Na,K-ATPase of cellular membranes in experimental tumors, but with differing results. Increased Na,K-ATPase activity was displayed in plasma membrane isolated from rat hepatoma (Emmelot and Bos 1969a) and mouse mammary epithelium neoplastic cells (Shen et al. 1978), being considered to facilitate nutrient transport with neoplastic transformation (Shen et al. 1978), whereas a significant decrease in special activity of plasma membrane Na,K-ATPase was recorded from Morris hepatoma 5123tc, which displayed a slow growth and minimal deviation, indicating a significantly decreased metabolism of purine, pyrimidine, and nucleotides (Barclay and Terebus-Kekish 1973). On the other hand, individual differences of enzyme activity were exhibited in mouse transplanted hepatoma strains (Emmelot and Bos 1969b) and rat ascites hepatoma (Koizumi et al. 1976). Normal concentration of plasma membrane Na,K-ATPase was presented in both line-10 and line-1 guinea pig hepatoma (Dau 1978). It was recently found, by the utilization of energy-dispersive X-ray microanalysis, that intracellular sodium concentration of tumor cells increased significantly (Cameron et al. 1980). Pietrzyk et al. (1978) indicated a strong positive correlation between cellular sodium content and electrogenic pumping activity, suggesting that intracellular activity of this ion regulated the rate of the electrogenic pump. Yu and Gu (1983) and the authors (Ye and Tang 1983) independently investigated erythrocyte sodium pump activity in BERH-2 transplantable hepatoma rats (Chiang et al. 1978) and found markedly increased erythrocyte sodium pump transport activity in HCC-bearing rats, suggesting a disturbance of energy metabolism in the host.

3. Sodium Pump in Human Tumors

To date, there are only a few reports concerning membrane Na,K-ATPase activity in human tumors. Knowles and Kaplan (1981) demonstrated a very high Na,K-ATPase activity in purified plasma membranes from several transplantable human tumors, including melanomas, astrocytomas, and oat cell carcinomas. In the meantime, a lower activity for Na,K-ATPase was exhibited in acute lymphoblastic leukemia (Losa and Morell 1979) and kidney adenocarcinoma (Zaheer et al. 1981).

The mechanism of differences of Na,K-ATPase activity among human, as well as experimental tumors is so far unclear, and remains to be investigated further.

III. Activity of Erythrocyte Sodium Pump in HCC Patients

Few papers have been published concerning the alteration of sodium pump activity in cancer patients. In view of the close correlation of sodium pump to energy metabolism, and the evident metabolic disturbance in HCC patients, we inferred that change of erythrocyte sodium pump activity might take place in HCC patients. Using an ^{86}rubidium transport assay which was modified from DeLuise's method (De-Luise et al. 1980), we examined 101 HCC patients and compared them with cirrhosis patients and healthy subjects at the authors' hospital. It was manifested that alteration of erythrocyte sodium pump activity did occur in HCC patients (Ye et al. 1983).

A. Comparison with Cirrhosis Patients and Healthy Individuals

HCC patients were examined before antitumor therapy and classified into different groups, namely, early (subclinical), moderate, and late stages of disease.
The criteria for staging were:
Subclinical (early) – without obvious symptoms or signs of liver cancer.
Late – with obvious cachexia, jaundice, ascites, or distant metastases.
Moderate – between the criteria of early and late stages.
The results of measurement showed that the worse the patients' condition, the higher the erythrocyte sodium pump activity, and that it was much higher in late stage than in either moderate or early stage HCC (Table 1).

Table 1. Erythrocyte sodium pump activity of HCC Patients at Different Stages

Disease stage	No. of cases	Mean ± SE (mmol/l RBC/h)	*P* value
Subclinical (early)	3	0.4123 ± 0.0391	< 0.05
Moderate	44	0.5215 ± 0.0133	< 0.001
Late	16	0.7167 ± 0.0506	

Analysis of HCC patients in moderate and late stage who were examined before treatment revealed no statistical difference (Table 2) between the activity in cirrhotic type (with obvious clinical and laboratory evidence of cirrhosis) and that in simple type (without obvious clinical and laboratory evidences of cirrhosis).

Compared with that in cirrhosis patients and healthy controls, the erythrocyte sodium pump activity of HCC patients in both moderate and late stages was higher, but the activity in cirrhosis patients was lower than that in healthy controls. However, there were no statistical differences between patients with SCHCC and cirrhosis or healthy persons (Table 3).

Table 2. Erythrocyte sodium pump activity of patients with CHCC of different types and at different stages

Disease type		No. of cases	Mean ± SE (mmol/l RBC/h)	*P* value
Moderate stage	Simple	38	0.5193 ± 0.0138	> 0.05
	Cirrhotic	6	0.5351 ± 0.0465	
Late stage	Simple	8	0.6968 ± 0.0831	> 0.05
	Cirrhotic	6	0.7044 ± 0.0813	
Moderate and late stage	Simple	46	0.5503 ± 0.0204	> 0.05
	Cirrhotic	12	0.6197 ± 0.0514	

Table 3. Comparison of erythrocyte sodium pump activity in HCC patients with that in patients with cirrhosis and in normal controls

Group		No. of cases	Mean ± SE (mmol/l RBC/h)	*P* value[a]
HCC	Total	63	0.5658 ± 0.0194	< 0.001
	Moderate and late stage	60	0.5735 ± 0.0198	< 0.001
	Moderate stage	44	0.5215 ± 0.0133	< 0.001
Subclinical stage		3	0.4123 ± 0.0391	> 0.05
Healthy		23	0.4503 ± 0.0130	
Cirrhosis		13	0.3853 ± 0.0125	< 0.01

[a] Compared with healthy controls

Table 4. Comparison of erythrocyte sodium pump activity between cirrhosis and cirrhotic-type HCC

Group		No. of cases	Mean ± SE (mmol/l RBC/h)	*P* value[a]
Cirrhotic-type HCC	Moderate stage	6	0.5351 ± 0.0465	< 0.001
	Moderate and late stage	12	0.6197 ± 0.0514	< 0.001
Cirrhosis		13	0.3853 ± 0.0125	

[a] Compared with cirrhosis cases

Considering the coexistence of cirrhosis in HCC, we compared HCC patients of the cirrhotic type with cirrhosis patients, the result indicating an obviously high activity in HCC patients despite their cirrhosis (Table 4).

B. Alteration of Pump Activity in CHCC Patients Before and After Various Therapies

Serial observations of erythrocyte sodium pump activity prior to and after treatment in patients with moderate and late stage HCC showed that in cases where the tumor was resected without emboli in the portal vein and without residue visible to the naked-eye, the activities of erythrocyte sodium pump decreased entirely after surgery, but that in patients who underwent palliative treatment with the tumor bulk remaining – including partial removal of tumor, ligation and/or catheterization of hepatic artery, chemotherapy, and traditional Chinese herbs – the activities differed from case to case, either increasing or decreasing after treatment (Fig. 1).

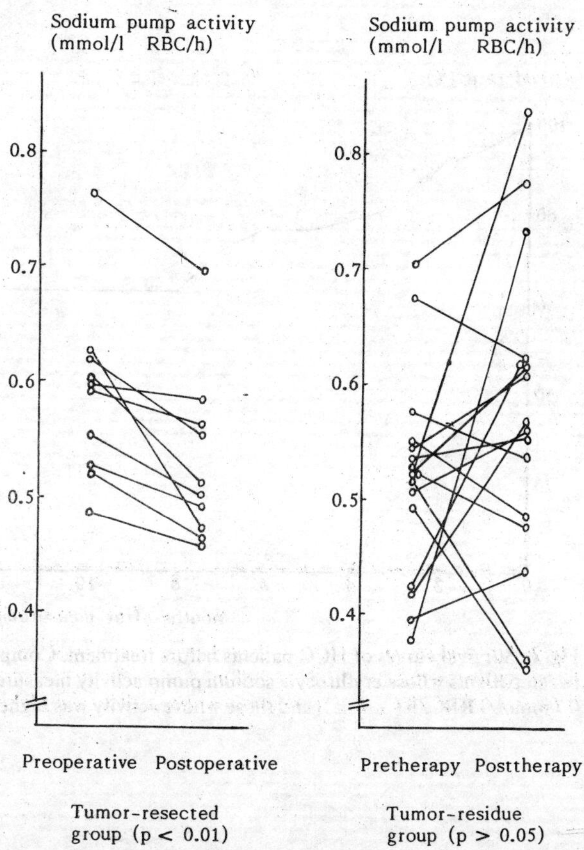

Fig. 1. Alteration of erythrocyte sodium pump activity in HCC patients, prior to and following treatment. *P* values are for comparison within group

C. Relation to Prognosis

Three-month mortality after measurement of erythrocyte sodium pump activity was investigated in HCC patients both before and after treatment. It was found statistically that the higher the sodium pump activity, the poorer the prognosis (Table 5). It might be more clearly manifested by using the life table method (Figs. 2 and 3).

Table 5. Relation of prognosis to erythrocyte sodium pump activity in HCC patients

Sodium pump activity		Cases *n*	3-month mortality *n*	3-month mortality %	*P* value
Before treatment	>0.7	12	10	83.3	<0.001
	<0.7	42	10	23.8	
	>0.6	18	12	66.7	<0.01
	<0.6	36	8	22.2	
After treatment	>0.7	5	4	80.0	<0.02
	<0.7	47	9	19.2	
	>0.6	18	9	50.0	<0.01
	<0.6	34	4	11.8	

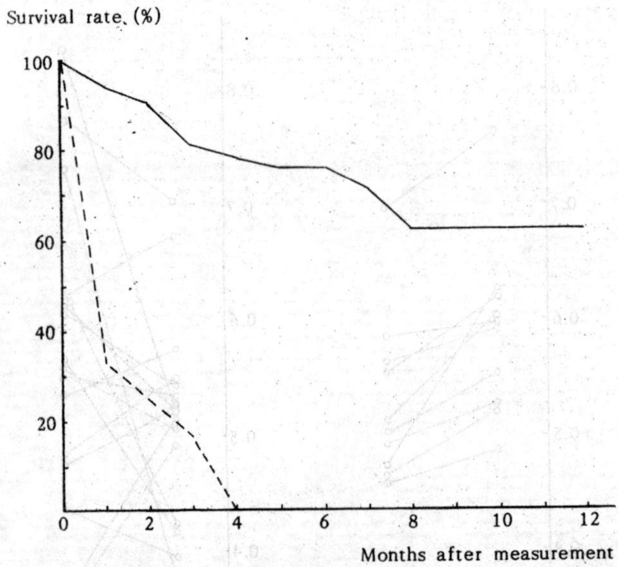

Fig. 2. Survival curves of HCC patients before treatment. Comparison, using life table method, between patients whose erythrocyte sodium pump activity measured before treatment was lower than 0.7 mmol/l RBC/h (______) and those whose activity was higher than 0.7 mmol/l RBC/h (– – – –)

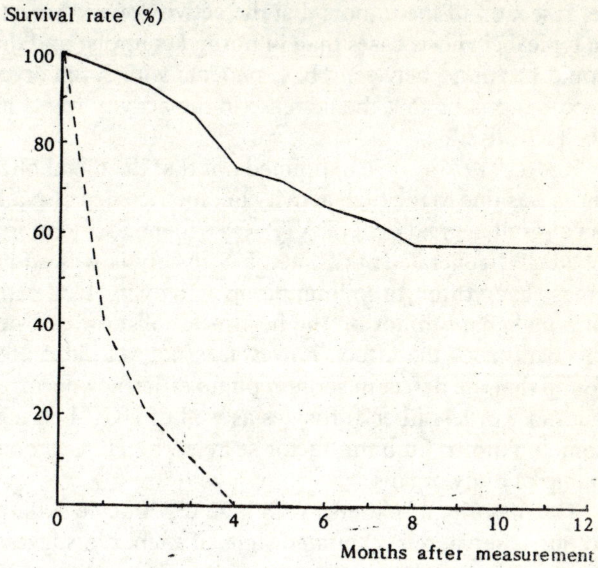

Fig. 3. Survival curves of HCC patients after treatment. Comparison, using life table method, between patients whose erythrocyte sodium pump activity measured after treatment was lower than 0.7 mmol/l RBC/h (———) and those whose activity was higher than 0.7 mmol/l RBC/h (- - - -)

IV. Significance and Mechanism of Sodium Pump Activity in HCC

A. Effects of Sodium Pump on Energy Metabolism

Sodium pump actively transports sodium and potassium ions across plasma membrane, utilizing metabolic energy released from ATP hydrolysis, and carries out various physiological functions of the body; therefore, it is closely related to energy metabolism. A widely accepted concept is that the Na,K-ATPase activity controls a major part of the basal metabolic rate (BMR) (Himms-Hagen 1976). Na,K-ATPase is the main enzyme in the cellular thermogenesis of BMR. It was established, according to oxygen expenditure, that the energy required to maintain normal function of sodium pump accounted for 35%–50% or more of the total energy consumption of the body in a basal metabolic state (Himms-Hagen 1976). It was 35%, 40%, and 52%, for example, in liver, kidney cortex, and brain slices respectively, and even accounted for 85% of energy metabolism in tumor cells (Young 1977). The increased heat production in some malignant tumors can probably be attributed to increased energy requirements for growth (Himms-Hagen 1976). As the activity of sodium pump in erythrocytes is far lower than that in excitatory and secretory tissues (Cavieres 1977), a change indicates that a remarkable alteration of the body metabolism has occurred.

B. Possible Mechanism of Alteration of Sodium Pump Activity in HCC Cases

It was shown in the above-mentioned investigation that the activity of erythrocyte sodium pump in HCC patients increased with the seriousness of the disease, being highest in the late stage; that sodium pump activity declined to a certain degree after resection of the tumor; that the activity of erythrocyte sodium pump was lower in typical cirrhosis cases than in normal controls; and that no significant difference could be found between HCC patients with simple type and those with cirrhotic type, suggesting that the increase in the activity was a host reaction resulting from the HCC itself.

Racker (1976a, 1976b) pointed out that the metabolic disturbance with some tumors was due to the high activity but inefficiency of Na,K-ATPase in tumor tissues. As a result, a great deal of ATP was expended and more ADP and inorganic phosphate (Pi) generated; thus, aerobic glycolysis was enormously enhanced. The increase in erythrocyte sodium pump activity in HCC patients showed that the effect of a malignant tumor on the host metabolism was systemic rather than local. The mechanism of the effect, however, is not yet clear. Recently, Yu and Gu (1983) found that the defect in sodium pump efficiency occurred not only in tumor tissues but more or less in erythrocytes as well of HCC-bearing rats, which indicated that some unknown humoral factor secreted by HCC probably stimulated the sodium pump of body organs.

The majority of patients with high erythrocyte sodium pump activity, according to our observations, exhibited signs of cachexia, suggesting that the increase in activity might be related to this disorder. Theologides (1979) proposed that peptides, oligonucleotides, and other small metabolites produced by cancer were responsible for the appearance of cachexia. These products were probably also the material basis affecting sodium pump activity.

Patients with typical cirrhosis have relatively low activity; on the other hand, despite the fact that the majority of HCC patients had concomitant cirrhosis, erythrocyte sodium pump activity increased in most of them. This indicated that these two diseases might have different effects on sodium pump. Concerning the mechanism of sodium pump alteration in noncancerous liver diseases, it might be that energy production of body organs decreased, owing to diffuse pathological changes and damaged metabolic function in the liver, thereby influencing erythrocyte sodium pump activity.

C. Erythrocyte Sodium Pump Activity in SCHCC Patients

Three SCHCC cases were diagnosed; their erythrocyte sodium pump activity was measured to be lower than that for CHCC cases, whereas no statistical distinction could be found from that in cirrhosis patients or healthy subjects. It might be assumed from the above preliminary observation that malignant tumor does not result in an alteration of erythrocyte sodium pump activity in the early period, but becomes the leading influence on sodium pump as the disease progresses. Further intensive investigation is necessary on this point.

D. Potential Significance

1. Action of Cancer on Host

The relationship between sodium pump and cancer was shown not only in tumor tissues but also, according to our investigation, in erythrocytes of cancer-bearing hosts. As far as the erythrocyte sodium pump activity was concerned, HCC had a minor influence on the host in the early period, whereas an obvious response of HCC to the host could be found in the late stage. Therefore, sodium pump activity might indicate the metabolic change both in tumor tissue and in the host. Importance has been attached to the interaction of cancer and the host, which has become an interesting problem (Woodruff 1982). The alteration of erythrocyte sodium pump activity in HCC provided further evidence for the relationship between cancer and the host; nevertheless, the mechanism has yet to be made clear.

2. Evaluation of Therapeutic Effects

It was shown from contrast data before and after treatment that erythrocyte sodium pump activity decreased after resection of the tumor but mostly increased with palliative treatment which left some tumor residue. This indicated that the existence and curative degree of HCC influenced pump activity, thus suggesting that erythrocyte sodium pump activity reflected the biological effect of HCC treatment. The activity might be reduced by radical resection or other effective anticancer treatment; on the other hand, an increase in activity might imply poor therapeutic response.

3. Prediction of Prognosis

According to the measurement and follow-up study, most HCC patients whose erythrocyte sodium pump activity was higher than 0.7 mmol per liter of RBC/h either before or after treatment died within 3 months after measurement, while those with activity lower than 0.7 frequently survived more than 3 months. This preliminary observation indicates that erythrocyte sodium pump activity might be a factor associated with prognosis in HCC patients.

4. Auxiliary Distinction of Cirrhosis and HCC

In view of the variable changes of erythrocyte sodium pump activity in HCC and cirrhosis, it seems that, for the purpose of differentiation, a significant increase in pump activity may mean the existence of HCC.

The measurement of erythrocyte sodium pump activity may contribute to research on the interaction of cancer and the host and to clinical treatment of HCC patients; therefore, the study of the relationship between liver cancer and sodium pump is worth pursuing.

References

Akagawa K, Watanabe M, Tsukada Y (1980) Activity of erythrocyte Na,K-ATPase in manic patients. J Neurochem 35: 258–260

Alam AN, Poston L, Wilkinson SP, et al. (1978) A study in vitro of the sodium pump in fulminant hepatic failure. Clin Sci Mol Med 55: 355–363

Applegarth DA, Davidson AGF, Haworth EM, et al. (1977) Cystic fibrosis: The effect of medium from cultured cystic fibrosis fibroblasts on ATPase activity. Clin Chim Acta 74: 183–185

Balfe JW, Cole CH, Welt LG (1968) Red-cell transport defect in patients with cystic fibrosis and in their parents. Science 162: 689–690

Banbassat J, Keynan A, Adler R, et al. (1980) Sodium transport in red cells of patients with acute hepatitis. Gastroenterology 79: 655–658

Barclay M, Terebus-Kekish O (1973) Enzyme activities and extrinsic proteins in plasma membranes from normal liver and Morris hepatoma 5123tc. J Natl Cancer Inst 51: 1709–1710

Becker D, Viljoen D, Kramer S (1971) The inhibition of red cell and brain ATPase by δ-aminolaevulinic acid. Biochim Biophys Acta 225: 26–34

Blostein R (1970) Sodium-activated adenosine triphosphatase activity of the erythrocyte membrane. J Biol Chem 245: 270–275

Bray GA, Kral JG, Björntorp P (1981) Hepatic sodium-dependent ATPase in obesity. N Engl J Med 304: 1580–1582

Bray GA, York DA, Yukimura Y (1978) Activity of ($Na^+ + K^+$)-ATPase in the liver of animals with experimental obesity. Life Sci 22: 1637–1642

Brody TM, Akera T (1977) Relations among Na^+,K^+-ATPase activity, sodium pump activity, transmembrane sodium movement, and cardiac contractility. Fed Proc 36: 2219–2224

Burk D, Woods M, Hunter J (1967) On the significance of glucolysis for cancer growth, with special reference to Morris rat hepatomas. J Natl Cancer Inst 38: 839–863

Cameron IL, Smith NKR, Pool TB, et al. (1980) Intracellular concentration of sodium and other elements as related to mitogenesis and oncogenesis in vivo. Cancer Res 40: 1493–1500

Cavieres JD (1977) The sodium pump in human red cells. In: Ellory JC, Lew VL (eds) Membrane transport in red cells. Academic, London, pp 1–37

Charney AN, Donowitz M (1978) Functional significance of intestinal Na^+-K^+-ATPase: in vivo ouabain inhibition. Am J Physiol 234: E629–E636

Chiang Chia-mo, Ji Wen-xing, Sun Lan-ying, et al. (1978) Studies on a transplantable rat hepatoma BERH-2. I. The establishment of the tumor line and its morphology, ultrastructure and α-fetoprotein production. Acta Biol Exp Sinica 11: 87–96[1]

Cole CH (1973) Decreased ouabain-sensitive adenosine triphosphatase activity in the erythrocyte membrane of patients with chronic renal disease. Clin Sci Mol Med 45: 775–784

Dahl JL, Hokin LE (1974) The sodium-potassium adenosine triphosphatase. Ann Rev Biochem 43: 327–356

Dau PC (1978) Preparation of plasma membranes from line-10 and line-1 guinea pig hepatoma. J Natl Cancer Inst 61: 935–938

Davis RA, Kern F Jr, Showalter R, et al. (1978) Alterations of hepatic Na^+,K^+-ATPase and bile flow by estrogen: Effects on liver surface membrane lipid structure and function. Proc Natl Acad Sci USA 75: 4130–4134

DeLuise M, Flier JS (1983) Status of the red cell Na,K-pump in hyper- and hypothyroidism. Metabolism 32: 25–30

DeLuise M, Blackburn GL, Flier JS (1980) Reduced activity of the red-cell sodium-potassium pump in human obesity. N Engl J Med 303: 1017–1022

Eckel RE, Rizzo SC, Lodish H, et al. (1966) Potassium transport and control of glycolysis in human erythrocytes. Am J Physiol 210: 737–743

Edmondson RPS, Hilton PJ, Jones NF, et al. (1975) Leucocyte sodium transport in uremia. Clin Sci Mol Med 49: 213–216

Emmelot P, Bos CJ (1969a) Studies on plasma membranes. IX. A survey of enzyme activities displayed by plasma membranes isolated from normal and preneoplastic liver and primary and transplanted hepatomas of the rat. Int J Cancer 4: 705–722

Emmelot P, Bos CJ (1969b) Studies on plasma membranes. X. A survey of enzyme activities displayed by plasma membranes isolated from mouse liver and three mouse hepatoma strains. Int J Cancer 4: 723–734

Erlinger S, Dhumeaux D (1974) Mechanisms and control of secretion of bile water and electrolytes. Gastroenterology 66: 281–304

Fehlmann M, Ereychet P (1981) Insulin and glucagon stimulation of (Na^+-K^+)-ATPase transport activity in isolated rat hepatocytes. J Biol Chem 256: 7449–7453

Foster JH (1982) Cancer and the liver. In: Gitnick GL (ed) Current hepatology, vol 2. John Wiley and Sons, New York, pp 233–272

Gambert SR, Ingbar SH, Hagen TC (1981) Interaction of age and thyroid hormone status on Na^+-K^+-ATPase in rat renal cortex and liver. Endocrinology 108: 27–30

Garay RP, Elghozi J-L, Dagher G, et al. (1980) Laboratory distinction between essential and secondary hypertension by measurement of erythrocyte cation fluxes. N Engl J Med 302: 769–771

Giese AC (1979) Cell physiology, 5th ed. Saunders, Philadelphia, pp 395–409

Glynn IM, Karlish STD (1975) The sodium pump. Ann Rev Physiol 37: 13–55

Gosalvez M, van Rossum GDV, Blanco MF (1979) Inhibition of sodium-potassium-activated adenosine 5′-triphosphatase and ion transport by adriamycin. Cancer Res 39: 257–261

Haljamäe H, Ender E, Sigström L (1975) Cellular potassium transport and ATPase activity in Bartter's syndrome. Scand J Clin Lab Invest 35: 53–58

Hasan J, Vinko V, Hernberg S (1967) Deficient red cell membrane ($Na^+ + K^+$)-ATPase in lead poisoning. Arch Environ Health 14: 313–318

Hesketh JE, Glen AIM, Reading HW (1977) Membrane ATPase activities in depressive illness. J Neurochem 28: 1401–1402

Himms-Hagen J (1976) Cellular thermogenesis. Ann Rev Physiol 38: 315–351

Hull KL, Roses AD (1976) Stoichiometry of sodium and potassium transport in erythrocytes from patients with myotonic muscular dystrophy. J Physiol (Lond) 254: 169–181

Ismail-Beigi F (1977) Thyroidal regulation of active sodium transport. In: Bronner F, Kleinzeller A (eds) Current topics in membranes and transport, vol 9. Academic, New York, pp 367–388

Israel Y, Kalant H, LeBlanc E, et al. (1970) Changes in cation transport and Na,K-ATPase produced by chronic administration of ethanol. J Pharmacol Exp Ther 174: 330–336

Kaji DM, Thakkar U, Kahn T (1981) Glucocorticoid-induced alterations in the sodium-potassium pump of the human erythrocyte. J Clin Invest 68: 422–430

Kashiwamata S, Goto S, Semba RK, et al. (1979) Inhibition by bilirubin of ($Na^+ + K^+$)-activated adenosine triphosphatase and K^+-activated *p*-nitrophenylphosphatase activities of NaI-treated microsomes from young rat cerebrum. J Biol Chem 254: 4577–4584

Knowles AF, Kaplan NO (1981) Variable ATPase composition of human plasma membranes. Biochem Biophys Res Commun 99: 1443–1448

Koizumi K, Ito Y, Kojima K, et al. (1976) Isolation and characterization of the plasma membranes from rat ascites hepatomas and from normal rat livers, including newborn, regenerating, and adult livers. J Biochem 79: 739–748

Kolata GB (1981) Reevaluation of cancer data eagerly awaited. Science 214: 316–318

Kuhnert BR, Kuhnert PM, Murray BA, et al. (1977) Na/K- and Mg-ATPase activity in the placenta and in maternal and cord erythrocytes of pre-eclamptic patients. Am J Obstet Gynecol 127: 56–60

Lin MH, Akera T (1978) Increased (Na^+,K^+)-ATPase concentrations in various tissues of rats caused by thyroid hormone treatment. J Biol Chem 253: 723–726

Lin MH, Romsos DR, Akera T, et al. (1978) Na^+,K^+-ATPase enzyme units in skeletal muscle from lean and obese mice. Biochem Biophys Res Commun 80: 398–404

Losa G, Morell A (1979) Plasma membrane-linked enzymes in lymphoproliferative diseases. Proc Am Assoc Cancer Res 20: 29

Okuda K, Ohnishi K (1982) Hepatic tumors. In: Arias IM, Frenkel M, Wilson JHP (eds) The liver annual 2/1982. Excerpta Medica, Amsterdam, pp 359–396

Parker JC, Welt LG (1972) Pathological alterations of cation movements in red blood cells. Arch Intern Med 129: 320–332

Parker JC, Orringer EP, McManus TJ (1978) Disorders of ion transport in red blood cells. In: Andreoli TE, Hoffman JF, Fanestit DD (eds) Physiology of membrane disorders. Plenum, New York, pp 773–800

Pietrzyk C, Geck P, Heinz E (1978) Regulation of the electrogenic $(Na^+ + K^+)$-pump of Ehrlich cells by intracellular cation levels. Biochim Biophys Acta 513: 89–98

Quarfoth G, Ahmed K, Foster D, et al. (1976) Action of methanethiol on membrane (Na^+,K^+)-ATPase of rat brain. Biochem Pharmacol 89: 697–700

Racker E (1976a) A new look at mechanisms in bioenergetics. Academic, New York, pp 153–175

Racker E (1976b) Why do tumor cells have a high aerobic glycolysis? J Cell Physiol 89: 697–700

Resh MD, Nemenoff RA, Guidotti G (1980) Insulin stimulation of (Na^+,K^+)-adenosine triphosphatase-dependent $^{86}Rb^+$ uptake in rat adipocytes. J Biol Chem 255: 10938–10945

Ricci RL, Crawford SS, Miner PB Jr (1981) The effect of ethanol on hepatic sodium-plus-potassium-activated adenosine triphosphatase activity in the rat. Gastroenterology 80: 1445–1450

Ridderstap AS, Bonting SL (1969) Na-K-activated adenosine triphosphatase and pancreatic secretion in the dog. Am J Physiol 216: 547–553

Robinson JD, Flashner MS (1979) The $(Na^+ + K^+)$-activated ATPase. Enzymatic and transport properties. Biochim Biophys Acta 549: 145–176

Schmoyer IR, Baglia FA (1974) Cystic fibrosis: Effect of media from cultured cystic fibrosis fibroblasts on ATPase activity. Biochem Biophys Res Commun 58: 1066–1070

Scholnick P, Lang D, Racker E (1973) Regulatory mechanism in carbohydrate metabolism. IX. Stimulation of aerobic glycolysis by energy-linked ion transport and inhibition by dextran sulfate. J Biol Chem 248: 5175–5182

Schwartz A, Lindenmayer GB, Allen JC (1975) The sodium-potassium adenosine triphosphatase: pharmacological, physiological and biochemical aspects. Pharmacol Rev 27: 3–134

Schwartz A, Adams RJ, Ball WJ Jr, et al. (1980) Structure, function and regulation of Na-K-ATPase. Int J Biochem 12: 287–293

Sewell RB, Poston L, Wilkinson SP, et al. (1981) Abnormalities in the leukocyte sodium pump in advanced cirrhosis. Gastroenterology 81: 676–680

Shen SS, Hamamoto ST, Bern HA, et al. (1978) Alteration of sodium transport in mouse mammary epithelium associated with neoplastic transformation. Cancer Res 38: 1356–1361

Simon FR, Sutherland E, Accatino L (1977) Stimulation of hepatic sodium-and-potassium-activated adenosine triphosphatase activity by phenobarbital: Its possible role in regulation of bile flow. J Clin Invest 59: 849–861

Skou JC (1957) The influence of some cations on an adenosine triphosphatase from peripheral nerves. Biochim Biophys Acta 23: 394–401

Skou JC (1965) Enzymatic basis for active transport of Na^+ and K^+ across cell membrane. Physiol Rev 45: 596–617

Smith EKM, Samuel P (1970) Abnormalities in the sodium pump of erythrocytes from patients with hyperthyroidism. Clin Sci 38: 49–61

Smith EKM, Welt LG (1970) The red blood cell as a model for the study of uremic toxins. Arch Intern Med 126: 827–830

Smith TJ, Edelman IS (1979) The role of sodium transport in thyroid thermogenesis. Fed Proc 38: 2150–2153

Stekhoven FS, Bonting SL (1981) Transport adenosine triphosphatases: Properties and functions. Physiol Rev 61: 1–76

Sterling K (1979) Thyroid hormone action at the cell level. N Engl J Med 300: 117–123, 173–177

Suolinna E-M, Lang D, Racker E (1974) Quercetin, an artificial regulator of the high aerobic glycolysis of tumor cells. J Natl Cancer Inst 53: 1515–1519

Suolinna E-M, Buchsbaum RN, Racker E (1975) The effect of flavonoids on aerobic glycolysis and growth of tumor cells. Cancer Res 35: 1865–1872

Swarts HGP, Bonting SL, DePont JJHHM, et al. (1981) Cation fluxes and Na^+-K^+-activated ATPase activity in erythrocytes of patients with essential hypertension. Hypertension 3: 641–649

Sweadner KJ, Goldin SM (1980) Active transport of sodium and potassium ions: mechanism, function, and regulation. N Engl J Med 302: 777–783

Tang ZY, Ying YY, GU TJ (1982) Hepatocellular carcinoma: Changing concepts in recent years. In: Popper H, Schaffner F (eds) Progress in liver diseases vol VII. Grune and Stratton, New York, pp 637–647

Tenney SR, Rafter GW (1968) Leukocyte adenosine triphosphatases and the effect of endotoxin on their activity. Arch Biochem Biophys 126: 53–58

Theologides A (1979) Cancer cachexia. Cancer 43: 2004–2012

Van Dyke RW, Keeffe EB, Gollan JL, et al. (1982) Cholestasis, bile flow, and hyperbilirubinemia: Current clinical and pathophysiologic perspectives. In: Gitnick GL (ed) Current Hepatology vol 2. John Wiley and Sons, New York, pp 327–363

Vates TS Jr, Bonting SL, Oppelt WW (1964) Na-K activated adenosine triphosphatase formation of cerebrospinal fluid in the cat. Am J Physiol 206: 1165–1172

Wallick ET, Lindenmayer GE, Lane LK, et al. (1977) Recent advances in cardiac glycoside – Na^+,K^+-ATPase interaction. Fed Proc 36: 2214–2218

Wallick ET, Lane LK, Schwartz A (1979) Biochemical mechanism of the sodium pump. Ann Rev Physiol 41: 391–411

Wambach G, Helber A, Bönner G, et al. (1979) Sodium-potassium-adenosine triphosphatase activity in red cell ghosts of patients with essential hypertension. Klin Wochenschr 57: 169–172

Wambach G, Helber A, Bönner G, et al. (1980) Sodium-potassium-dependent ATPase activity in erythrocyte ghosts of patients with primary and secondary hypertension. Clin Sci 59: 183s–185s

Weiner MW, Maffly RH (1978) The provision of cellular metabolic energy for active ion transport. In: Andreoli TE, Hoffman JF, Fanestil DD (eds) Physiology of membrane disorders. Plenum, New York, pp 287–314

Whittam R, Ager ME (1965) The connexion between active cation transport and metabolism in erythrocytes. Biochem J 97: 214–227

Woodruff M (1982) Interaction of cancer and host. Br J Cancer 46: 313–322

Ye SL, Tang ZY (1983) An experimental observation on red-cell sodium pump activity in BERH-2 hepatoma rats. Tumor 3: 145–147[1]

Ye SL, Tang ZY, Gu TJ (1983) Alteration in red-cell sodium pump activity in patients with primary liver cancer. Acta Acad Med Primae Shanghai 10: 93–98[1]

York DA, Bray GA, Yukimura Y (1978) An enzymatic defect in the obese (ob/ob) mouse: loss of thyroid-induced sodium-and-potassium-dependent adenosinetriphosphatase. Proc Natl Acad Sci USA 75: 477–481

Young VR (1977) Energy metabolism and requirements in the cancer patient. Cancer Res 37: 2336–2347

Yu ZY, Gu TJ (1983) The effect of tumor on erythrocyte sodium pump in the hosts. Acta Acad Med Primae Shanghai 10: 40[1]

Zaheer A, Singh D, Montgomery R (1981) (Na^+ + K^+)-stimulated ATPase of human kidney, normal and adenocarcinoma. Phosphorylation and inhibition by antitumor proteins. Biochem Biophys Res Commun 102: 86–92

[1] Chinese

14 The Role of Unicentric Origin in Subclinical Hepatocellular Carcinoma

Tang Zhao-you

The problem concerning the multicentric or unicentric origin of hepatocellular carcinoma has been in debate for decades (Berman 1958; Higgins 1970). Many pathologists were of the opinion that both modes of origin might occur; as mentioned by Popper in 1957: „Carcinomas developing in cirrhotic livers usually seem to be multicentric, while in noncirrhotic livers they are unicentric" (Popper and Schaffner 1957; Ying 1981). The literature of the 1970s favored the opinion that unicentric origin may play a more important role and that venous invasion seems to be responsible for the multinodular appearance of many liver cancers (Cameron 1976). Even in experimental hepatoma, the number of nodules also varied, with different carcinogens as well as with the regimen used (Farber 1976). Dysplasia has not yet been thoroughly proven to be pre-neoplastic and reflect a multicentric origin (Robin 1976). Peters (1976) was of the opinion that both unicentric and multicentric genesis may occur. Nakashima emphasized the unicentric origin from the viewpoint of vascular alterations. It cannot be denied that even a cirrhotic liver would develop HCC unicentrically (Nakashima 1976). The current literature seems to continue to support indirectly the unicentric origin, from studies of diffuse-type HCC (Okuda et al. 1981) and of the growth pattern of HCC (Nakashima et al. 1982). This problem is of importance both in theoretical and practical aspects, especially in China, where the mortality for HCC was reported to be as high as 10.09/100000 (Li and Li 1980). The grave prognosis for HCC even after tumor resection has long been considered due to its multicentric origin, leading to a pessimistic view as well as inactive therapeutic strategy. Based on operative findings and a long-term follow-up study of 366 HCC cases, we looked for clinical evidence to support the unicentric theory, even in many patients with concomitant cirrhosis, thus supporting more aggressive surgical management in early-stage patients.

I. Methods

Tumor size was measured according to the longest diameter (cm) of the tumor nodule. The number of tumor nodules (single, more than one nodule) and status of the tumor capsule were determined from operative findings. Intrahepatic venous tumor emboli were examined in patients who underwent resection or autopsy. Two types of associated liver cirrhosis were classified: (a) micronodular (nearly all the nodules less than 3 mm in diameter) and (b) macronodular (many nodules more than 3 mm in diameter) (Anthony et al. 1977).

AFP was measured by radioimmunoassay or radiorocket electrophoresis autography (Sun et al. 1979), and by single agar gel immunoelectrophoresis for high levels. Reverse passive hemagglutination assay (RPHA) was employed for initial mass screening. The survival rates were calculated by the life table method (Peto et al. 1977).

Storage, analysis, and statistical treatment of these data were carried out using an APPLE II PLUS microcomputer.

II. General Data

A. Incidence of Single-Nodule HCC with Relation to Tumor Size

As shown in Table 1, negative correlation could be observed between tumor si- and incidence of single-nodule HCC. The bigger the tumor, the smaller the proportion of single-nodule HCC. A significant difference (74.6% versus 46.3%) could be observed in comparing small HCC (⩽5 cm) with huge HCC (>5 cm).

B. Incidence of Well-Encapsulated Tumor with Relation to Tumor Size

As shown in Table 2, the smaller the tumor, the higher the incidence of well-encapsulated tumor, with the break point at 5 cm. Figure 1 shows four surgical specimens with tumors ⩽2.0 cm, all of which revealed single and well-encapsulated small HCC.

Table 1. Relation between incidence of single-nodule HCC and tumor size

Tumor size (cm)	Total cases	Single-nodule HCC		
		No. of cases	%	
⩽3.0	28	21	75.0	74.6
3.1– 5.0	39	29	74.4	
5.1–10.0	135	72	53.3	46.3
>10.0	120	46	38.3	
Total	322	168	52.2	

Table 2. Relation between tumor capsule and tumor size

Tumor size (cm)	Total cases	Well-encapsulated HCC		
		No. of cases	%	
⩽3.0	27	19	70.4	65.6
3.1– 5.0	37	23	62.2	
5.1–10.0	134	36	26.9	17.3
>10.0	120	8	6.7	
Total	318	86	27.0	

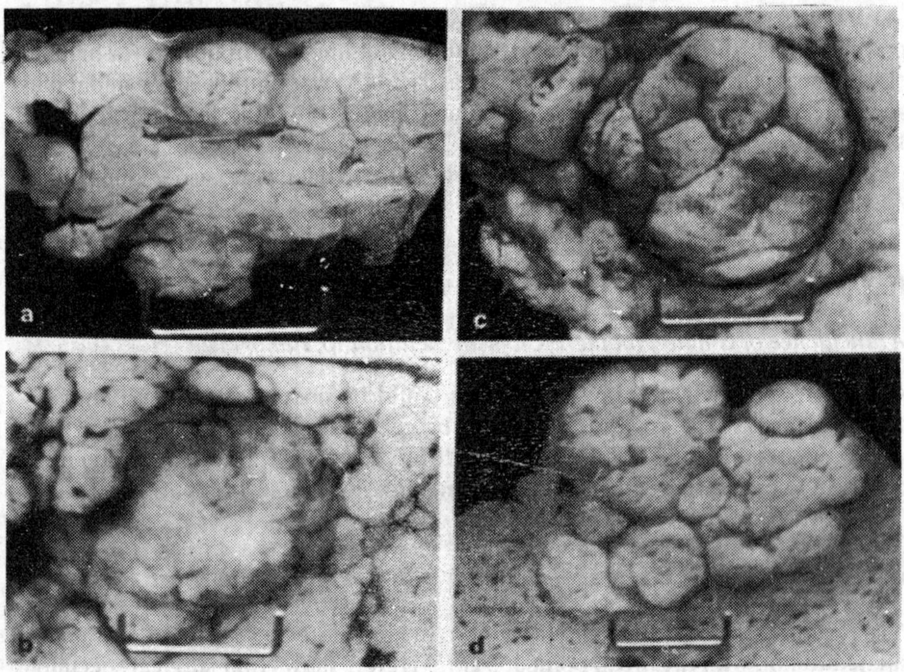

Fig. 1 a–d. Four surgical specimens of single and well-encapsulated small HCC with diameters of **a** 0.7, **b** 1.0, **c** 1.5 and **d** 2.0 cm respectively, showing that the smaller the size, the less the lobulation. AFP declined to ⩽20 ng/ml in all cases after resection. Steel bar = 1 cm

C. Incidence of Intrahepatic Venous Tumor Emboli, with Relation to Tumor Size

It was observed that the larger the tumor, the higher the incidence of intrahepatic venous tumor emboli. Sudden change was also noted when a tumor was larger than 5 cm (Table 3).

D. Relation Between AFP Level and Incidence of Single-Nodule HCC

A higher incidence of single-nodule HCC was noted in patients with lower AFP levels (Table 4).

E. Survival Rate After Resection of Single-Nodule HCC, with Relation to Tumor Size

Negative correlations of tumor size and 1-, 3-, and 5-year survival rates were observed after resection of single-nodule HCC. A dramatically high 5-year survival was noted with HCC ⩽ 5 cm as compared with HCC > 5 cm (Table 5).

Table 3. Relation between intrahepatic venous tumor emboli and tumor size

Tumor size (cm)	Total cases	With tumor emboli		
		No. of cases	%	
⩽3.0	23	2	8.7	9.1
3.1– 5.0	32	3	9.4	
5.1–10.0	81	33	40.7	41.7
>10.0	46	20	43.5	
Total	182	58	31.9	

Table 4. Relation between AFP level and incidence of single-nodule HCC

AFP level (ng/ml)	Total cases	Single-nodule HCC	
		No. of cases	%
51–2000	102	61	59.8
2001–5000	28	15	53.6
>5000	116	53	45.7
Total	246	129	52.4

Table 5. Relation between survival after resection of single-nodule HCC and tumor size

Tumor size (cm)	No. of cases	Survival rate[a]		
		1-year	3-year	5-year
⩽3.0	18	87.5	87.5	87.5
3.1–5.0	24	90.5	65.8	65.8
>5.0	90	71.1	37.8	20.2

[a] Life table method

Table 6. Relation between tumor size and normalization of AFP after resection of single-nodule HCC

Tumor size (cm)	Total cases	AFP ⩽ 20 ng/ml after resection		
		No. of cases	%	
⩽3.0	17	15	88.2	86.8
3.1–5.0	21	18	85.7	
>5.0	50	26	52.0	
Total	88	59	67.0	

F. Normalization of AFP After Resection of Single-Nodule HCC, with Relation to Tumor Size

As shown in Table 6, the smaller the tumor, the higher the percentage of patients whose AFP declined to ⩽20 ng/ml after resection of single-nodule HCC.

G. Incidence of Single-Nodule HCC and Coexisting Liver Cirrhosis

In cases of large HCC, no remarkable correlation could be observed between coexisting cirrhosis and the incidence of single-nodule HCC. Nevertheless, in cases of small HCC, single-nodule HCC was noted less frequently in macronodular cirrhosis than in the micronodular type and in patients without cirrhosis. It should be mentioned that even in patients with associated macronodular cirrhosis, the unicentric pattern still accounted for 68.2% in early-stage HCC (Table 7). Figure 2 shows a typical case of severe macronodular cirrhosis, in which gradually increasing AFP (from 160 to 760 ng/ml) was observed 5 months before the patient died of the cirrhosis; autopsy revealed a solitary small HCC (2.0 cm), and the affected portal trunk as well as its tributaries were filled with tumor emboli.

III. Changing Role of Unicentric Origin in SCHCC

Faced with certain facts established in the past few decades, one would agree to the theory of multicentric origin in human HCC. The multinodular pattern accounted for as much as 82% of HCC (Ervasti 1964), with a low resection rate not exceeding 10% of the overall cases. The extremely low 5-year survival rate after resection of HCC, especially in Asian patients (in 1970 Foster reported 6%), reflected a high incidence of recurrence, up to 90%. Coexisting liver cirrhosis was reported to be up to 90% (Ying 1981).

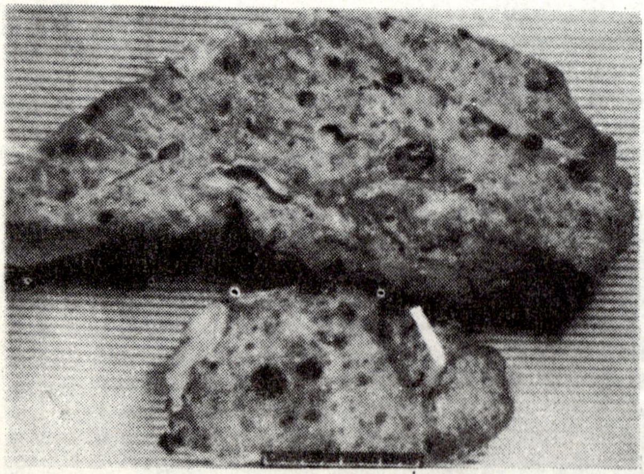

Fig. 2. Autopsy revealed single small HCC (2.0 cm; *arrow*) developed in association with severe macronodular cirrhosis (fibrous tissue amounted to one-fourth of liver parenchyma) and with 760 ng/ml serum AFP. Tumor emboli were filled in the affected portal trunk and its tributaries

However, in view of the changing picture in the 1970s, one might give more consideration to the role of a unicentric origin of human HCC. In contrast to the picture for relatively late-stage patients in the past decades, it is worth noting the great changes in relatively early-stage patients. The percentage of single-nodule HCC was as high as 60% (Okuda et al. 1977) or 76.9% (Chen et al. 1982) in small HCC. A high resectability rate of up to 58.5% was also recorded in SCHCC (Shanghai Coordinating Group, Tang et al. 1979). The relatively low recurrent rate and long survival after resection were noted, although associated with similar rates of coexisting cirrhosis (Tang et al. 1982).

A. Unicentric Origin not Infrequent

A unicentric origin was not infrequently encountered in China in cases of SCHCC or small HCC associated with cirrhosis. The discovery of small HCC by AFP screening in natural population or monitoring in chronic liver disease, and/or angiography as well as ultrasonography, has provided more clues to this problem. On the basis of analysis of 20 cases with minute HCC, Okuda emphasized that HCC arose from a single focus and metastasized throughout the remainder of the liver (Okuda et al. 1977). Tumor nodules were reported to be solitary in the majority of small HCC cases (around 60.0%–83.3%) both in Japan (Okuda et al. 1977; Ishikawa 1976; Shimoyama et al. 1980) and in China (Tang et al. 1979; Huang and Sha 1980; Chen et al. 1982); this was also noted in the West (Mahmood and Schatzki 1976).

More evidence was added in our series. Up to 74.6% of small HCC cases and 66.7% (60/90) of SCHCC cases presented one nodule, thus favoring the theory of unicentric origin, even with associated cirrhosis. After resection of single-nodule small HCC, AFP declined to $\leqslant 20$ ng/ml in 86.8%, indicating that there was no residual HCC nodule after resection. The 5-year survival rate of 65.8%–87.5% after resection of single-nodule small HCC confirmed that no new HCC was formed in the 5-years follow-up study. Even among those patients with recurrence, about one-third had lung metastases, which would exclude the possibility of multicentric origin. The fact that local resection rather than lobectomy achieved substantial success also favored the unicentric hypothesis. The infrequency of single-nodule HCC in the past decades was considered mainly to be a result of relatively late-stage disease.

B. Intrahepatic Spreading

Intrahepatic spreading may be more important than multicentric origin in the majority of cases of large HCC. Evidence of negative correlation between tumor size and incidence of single-nodule HCC, well-encapsulated tumor, and survival rate, and of positive correlation between tumor size and intrahepatic venous tumor emboli, as well as normalization of AFP after resection of single-nodule HCC, indicates that the risk of tumor invasion to the capsule as well as to the portal or hepatic veins is markedly increased with the enlargement of tumor nodule, which results in intrahepatic spreading and finally presents the multinodular pattern. This may be

Table 7. Incidence of single-nodule HCC and coexisting liver cirrhosis

Cirrhosis	Single-nodule HCC (%)	
	Small HCC ($\leq$5 cm)	Large HCC (>5 cm)
None	100.0 (8/8)	45.1 (23/51)
Micronodular	80.0 (12/15)	52.9 (27/51)
Macronodular	68.2 (30/44)	44.9 (62/138)

the reason for the low normalization rate after resection as well as for the low 5-year survival rate. The percentage of well-encapsulated tumors was also reported as high as 61.1% (Ishikawa 1976), 72.7% (Chen et al. 1982), and 90.0% (Okuda et al. 1977). Figure 1 shows that the smaller the tumor size, the less the lobulation, and that once the tumor grows to a certain size, spreading appears. Based on the results in Tables 1–3, 5 and 6, it seems that the break point with marked intrahepatic spreading may occur when the tumor grows to around 5 cm. The excellent description of vasculature in minimal hepatoma by Nakashima – that arterial branches act as afferent vessels and the capillarized sinusoids and portal branches as afferent channels (Nakashima 1976) – and the frequent reversal of portal blood flow in cirrhosis demonstrated by Okuda et al. (1973) may help to explain the intrahepatic spreading along the reverse direction of normal blood flow in the portal system. Figure 2 shows that even in macronodular cirrhosis the very beginning of HCC seems to be a single nodule. However, owing to widespread venous tumor emboli, the multinodular pattern soon appears. Therefore, whether multinodular HCC in cirrhosis is of true multicentric origin, or still a result of spreading owing to the earlier invasion of the intrahepatic venous system in macronodular cirrhosis by HCC remains to be further investigated. Thus, the biological behavior of frequent and early venous invasion by this particular neoplasm, the special vascular pattern of the liver, and the coexisting cirrhosis with portal hypertension may play important roles in the multinodular pattern and in the great difference between HCC and other solid tumors.

C. Aggressive Surgical Intervention

Aggressive surgical intervention remains the policy of choice in the management of early-stage HCC. In contrast to the pessimistic viewpoint and inactive therapeutic strategy based on the hypothesis of multicentric origin, an aggressive surgical approach is suggested, provided the liver function remains at a compensated stage. Our experience has shown that local resection rather than lobectomy provides much higher resectability (76.8%), much lower operative mortality (2.3%), and a similar survival rate for patients with right lobe lesions associated with cirrhosis. The encouraging 5-year survival rates (Table 5) after resection of HCC $\leq$5 cm were remarkably higher than those in HCC>5 cm, strongly attesting to the priority of this policy. The unicentric theory has also led to a more active approach for recurrence as well as for lung metastasis, provided there is a solitary nodule. Reoperation for subclinical recurrence and solitary lung metastasis after an initial radical resection has yielded promising results and prolonged survival.

However, as demonstrated in Table 7, a lower incidence of the unicentric pattern was found in association with macronodular cirrhosis, even in small HCC. Furthermore, with long-term recurrence in the remaining liver the possibility of another new focus cannot be excluded. According to the hypothesis (Anthony 1976) that dysplasia is a precursor lesion of liver cancer in humans, it is logical to conclude that multicentric origin cannot be completely excluded in patients with associated cirrhosis.

Endeavors should be made not only to control the coexisting cirrhosis but also to prevent the early spread of HCC so that the biological behavior of HCC can also be clarified.

References

Anthony PP (1976) Precursor lesions for liver cancer in humans. Cancer Res 36: 2579–2583

Anthony PP, Ishak KG, Nayak NC, et al. (1977) The morphology of cirrhosis – definition, nomenclature and classification. Bull WHO 55: 521–540

Berman C (1958) Primary carcinoma of the liver. Adv Cancer Res 5: 55–96

Cameron HM (1976) The pathology of liver cell cancer. In: Cameron HM, Linsell DA, Warwick GP (eds) Liver cell cancer. Elsevier, Amsterdam, pp 17–43

Chen DS, Sheu JC, Sung JL, et al. (1982) Small hepatocellular carcinoma – a clinicopathological study in thirteen patients. Gastroenterology 83: 1109–1119

Ervasti J (1964) Primary carcinoma of the liver – A pathologic and clinical study of 100 cases. Acta Chir Scand 334: 1s–65s

Farber E (1976) The pathology of experimental liver cell cancer. In: Cameron HM, Linsell DA, Warwick GP (eds) Liver cell cancer. Elsevier, Amsterdam, pp 243–277

Foster JH (1970) Survival after liver resection for cancer. Cancer 26: 493–502

Higgins GK (1970) The pathologic anatomy of primary hepatic tumors. In: Pack GT, Islami AH (eds) Tumors of the liver. Springer, Heidelberg, Berlin, pp 15–37

Huang XY, Sha YW (1980) Diagnosis, surgical resection and prognosis of 38 cases with small hepatocellular carcinoma. Tumor Prevent Treat Study 8: 7–9[1]

Ishikawa K (1976) Follow-up study of patients with primary liver cancer. Report 3. Acta Hepatol Jpn 17: 460–465

Li B, Li JY (1980) National survey of cancer mortality in China. Chin J Oncol 2: 1–10[1]

Mahmood K, Schatzki PK (1976) Solitary small hepatocellular carcinoma. Am J Digest Dis 21: 496–502

Nakashima T (1976) Vascular changes and hemodynamics in hepatocellular carcinoma. In: Okuda K, Peters RL (eds) Hepatocellular carcinoma. John Wiley and Sons, New York, pp 169–230

Nakashima T, Kojiro M, Kawano Y, et al. (1982) Histologic growth pattern of hepatocellular carcinoma – relationship to orcein (hepatitis B surface antigen)-positive cells in cancer tissue. Hum Pathol 13: 563–568

Okuda K, Moriyama M, Yasumoto M, et al. (1973) Roentgenologic demonstration of spontaneous reversal of portal blood flow in cirrhosis and primary carcinoma of the liver. Am J Roentgenol 119: 419–428

Okuda K, Nakashima T, Obata H, et al. (1977) Clinicopathological studies of minute hepatocellular carcinoma – analysis of 20 cases, including four with hepatic resection. Gastroenterology 73: 109–115

Okuda K, Noguchi T, Kubo Y, et al. (1981) A clinical and pathological study of diffuse-type hepatocellular carcinoma. Liver 1: 280–289

Peters RL (1976) Pathology of hepatocellular carcinoma. In: Okuda K, Peters RL (eds) Hepatocellular carcinoma. John Wiley and Sons, New York, pp 107–168

Peto R, Pike MC, Armitage P, et al. (1977) Design and analysis of randomized clinical trials requiring prolonged observation of each patient. II. Analysis and examples. Br J Cancer 35: 1–39

Popper H, Schaffner F (1957) Primary hepatic carcinoma. In: Popper H, Schaffner F (eds) Liver: structure and function. McGraw-Hill, New York, pp 593–612
Robin E (1976) A resume. In: Cameron HM, Linsell DA, Warwick GP (eds) Liver cell cancer. Elsevier, Amsterdam, pp 279–286
Shimoyama T, Kitasato S, Fujitomi Y, et al. (1980) A study of minute hepatocellular carcinoma – clinicopathologic observation on four resected cases. Acta Hepatol Jpn 21: 1009–1015
Sun TT, Wang LC, Chang YL, et al. (1979) Radiorocket electrophoresis autography (RREA) through labelled antigen for AFP assay and its applications in seroepidemiologic investigation of primary hepatocellular carcinoma (PHC). Chin Med J 92: 17–25
Tang ZY, Yu YQ, Lin ZY, et al. (1979) Small hepatocellular carcinoma – clinical analysis of 30 cases. Chin Med J 92: 455–462
Tang ZY, Ying YY, Gu TJ (1982) Hepatocellular carcinoma – changing concepts in recent years. In: Popper H, Schaffner F (eds) Progress in liver diseases. vol VII. Grune and Stratton, New York, pp 637–647
Ying YY (1981) Pathology of hepatocellular carcinoma. In: Tang ZY (ed) Primary liver cancer. Shanghai Scientific and Technical Publisher, Shanghai, pp 115–150[1]

[1] Chinese

15 A New Concept of the Natural History of AFP-positive Hepatocellular Carcinoma

Tang Zhao-you

Survival with hepatocellular carcinoma, from the onset of symptoms or from diagnosis to death, has been frequently reported in the literature; nevertheless, the true natural history of HCC is not clear as yet. In the 1970s, with rapidly growing knowledge about AFP and its application to population screening and long-term monitoring of patients with chronic hepatitis and liver cirrhosis, valuable clues were provided which helped to elucidate the natural history of AFP-positive HCC. This new approach is of great significance in both clinical and theoretical aspects (Tang 1981; Tang et al. 1982).

I. Survival with HCC as Reported in the Literature

Generally, survival from the onset of symptoms or from the establishment of diagnosis to death was reported to be less than 6 months (3–5 months in the majority). For decades, there was little improvement, either in China (Table 1) or in other countries (Table 2). Owing to this relatively short survival, HCC has long been considered an „acute malignancy" and an "incurable disease".

II. A New Concept

Based upon population screening of HCC using AFP as a tumor marker and on long-term follow-up studies, a new concept concerning the natural history of AFP-positive HCC has been developed. Contrary to the previous assumption of a relatively quick development, HCC exists and develops for a relatively long period before symptoms occur.

A. Criteria for Clinical Staging

Clinically, HCC can be arbitrarily divided into four stages: the early subclinical stage (I′), from the onset of HCC to diagnosis of the subclinical stage, represented by low but gradually increasing AFP without associated active liver disease (with normal values for ALT, bilirubin, prothrombin time, etc.); the subclinical stage (I), without obvious HCC symptoms or signs; the moderate stage (II), between criteria for the subclinical and late stages; and the late stage (III), with obvious cachexia, jaundice, ascites, or distant metastases.

Table 1. Survival with HCC in China (Selective data)

Reference	No. of cases	Survival (months)
Yang et al. (1955)	20	4.5
Zhang et al. (1958)	45	2.8
Li et al. (1959)	40	3.5
Jiang (1960)	40	3.8
Wang et al. (1961)	88	4.2
Yan et al. (1964)	150	4.6
Jin et al. (1965).	57	3.8
Shanghai Coordinating Group (Tang et al.) (1974)	3245	5.7
Cao et al. (1979)	224	7.9

Table 2. Survival with HCC in the literature (selective data)

Reference	No. of cases	Survival (months)
Gustafson (1937)	62	3.2
Rosenberg and Oshsner (1948)	55	2.8
Kay (1964)	96	4.4
Ervasti (1964)	100	5.6
Lawrence et al. (1966)	20	5
Chan (1967)	108	5.8
Moseley (1967)	47	3
Alpert et al. (1969)	46	6.7
Geddes and Falkson (1970)	189	4.3
Schreiber et al. (1970)	120	5.0
Sharpstone et al. (1970)	41	5.8
Bengmark et al. (1971)	92	1
Primack et al. (1975)	153	1
Okuda (1976)	134	6.5

B. Material, Methods, and Results

A group of pathologically proven AFP-positive HCC cases receiving nonresectional treatment and follow-up over 2 years were collected for this study, including 15 patients who had complete serial data of AFP from the first appearance of a low (around 50 ng/ml) but increasing level, 32 cases of subclinical HCC, 87 cases of moderate-stage HCC, and 50 cases of late-stage HCC. It is believed that nonresectional treatment seldom results in any marked prolongation of survival; therefore, survival of patients receiving nonresectional treatment may approximate the natural history of the disease.

For initial screening we used RPHA; RREA (Sun et al. 1979) or RIA, CIEP, and AGD were employed for further AFP determination.

AFP-positive SCHCC was diagnosed either by positive CIEP persisting over 3 weeks or by AFP level ⩾200 ng/ml for more than 8 weeks, provided ALT was normal and pregnancy and gonadal teratoma could be excluded. The life table method and median survival were used in assessing the results. A group of 143 patients with HCC who underwent surgical resection were collected for adjunctive study.

The median survival of HCC cases receiving nonresectional treatment was 24 months (7–36) from the first appearance of low (around 50 ng/ml) but increasing AFP, 15 months (3–42) after the diagnosis of SCHCC, 6 months ($1-48^{+}$) for moderate-stage HCC, and 2 months (0.3–6) for late-stage HCC. The overall median survival of clinical HCC including moderate and late stages was 3 months, which mimicked that reported in the literature. The median period from the first appearance of low (around 50 ng/ml) but increasing AFP to the establishment of SCHCC (⩾200 ng/ml) was 10 months (5–21).

The median tumor diameters in subclinical ($n=65$), moderate ($n=74$), and late-stage ($n=4$) HCC measured during operation were 4.0 (0.8–15 cm), 9.0 (3–25 cm), and 10.0 (8–20 cm) cm respectively; the corresponding median AFP levels were 2000 ng/ml, 20000 ng/ml, and 40000 ng/ml.

Of the 36 cases of SCHCC receiving surgical resection, seven had complete serial AFP data. By the time of operation, the median period from the first appearance of low but increasing AFP was 10 (5–21) months. In other words, the median period of the "early subclinical stage (I′)" was around 10 months before the tumor grew to 4.0 cm in diameter.

C. Evolution and Natural History of HCC

The close correlation between HCC and HBV has been adequately reported in the literature (Popper et al. 1982; Okuda et al. 1980). Strong evidence has also been shown in our series, the positive rates of serum HBsAg and anti-HBc being 71.7% and 76.1% respectively, and the overall rate of exposure to HBV (with any one of the HBV markers positive) 93.5%. Furthermore, 85.7% of SCHCC cases had coexistent cirrhosis. In the 63.0% of SCHCC patients who had a history of hepatitis, the median duration was 10 (1–25) years: for 49.2% of them >10 years, for 28.6% 5.1–10 years, and for 22.2% ⩽5 years.

Therefore, from the viewpoint of primary prevention of HCC, it is wise to trace the history back to the first attack of type-B hepatitis. As shown in Fig. 1, HCC will generally appear (of course in only a small proportion of cases) 10 years after the first attack of acute type-B hepatitis. In this period, fluctuation of ALT with correlated low level AFP (<500 ng/ml) was not infrequently (around 20% of the cases) noted. The majority of the patients who eventually developed HCC subsequently progressed through chronic hepatitis to cirrhosis, 75.6% of it the macronodular type.

The natural history of HCC per se might be divided into four periods:

1. The early subclinical stage (I′) is from the onset of disease to the diagnosis of SCHCC, the median period being around 10 months, which is also the time needed for a tumor to grow to 4.0 cm. During this period, nothing could be

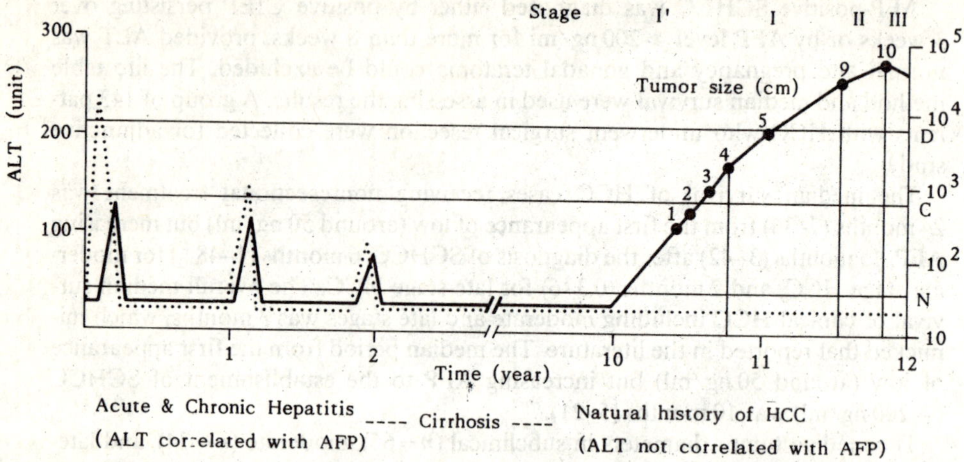

Fig. 1. Evolution and natural history of hepatocellular carcinoma. Stage: *I'*, early subclinical; *I* subclinical; *II* moderate; *III* late. AFP level: *D*, agar gel diffusion; *C*, countercurrent immunoelectrophoresis; *N*, normal. ALT level – *dotted line*

found except slight to moderate AFP elevation (50–200 ng/ml); therefore, early diagnosis and localization are still difficult.

2. The subclinical stage (I) is from the diagnosis of SCHCC to the occurrence of symptoms, lasting 8–9 months, which coincides with our previous report; HCC can be detected by mass screening using AFP on an average of 7.9 months before symptoms occur (Tang et al. 1979). During this period, all of the conventional measurements show positive findings in only 7.8%–32.0% of the patients, and diagnosis is made mainly by combined analysis of absolute value and serial change in AFP and ALT. Angiography may be a valuable aid to the diagnosis. Early tumor resection can be accomplished in 60% of SCHCC patients and 5-year survival achieved by up to 72.9% after resection. These facts indicate that in the majority of cases the disease is still in its curable stage without marked spreading.
3. The moderate stage (II) is from the appearance of symptoms and signs to that of jaundice, ascites, or distant metastasis, and lasts about 4 months. During this period diagnosis is not difficult, since 56.9%–94.2% of patients are positive with enzymology, ultrasound, radionuclide imaging, or angiography. The successful tumor resection rate seldom exceeds 24.7% of these patients and the 5-year survival rate after resection is only 16.1%. This indicates that spreading of tumor has occurred in the majority of cases.
4. The late stage (III) is from the appearance of jaundice (bilirubin >2.0 mg/dl), ascites, or distant metastasis to death, and lasts 2 months. No means can effectively prolong survival. In this stage, tumor emboli in the portal trunk may play an important role in the irreversible course of the disease.

These observations indicate a relatively long natural history of HCC, at least 2 years, because the appearance of AFP in serum usually shows that the tumor has already developed to a certain size, and the true onset might be earlier. The longest record from the first appearance of low but increasing AFP to the establishment of SCHCC ($\geqslant$200 ng/ml) was 21 months, and the longest survival from diagnosis of SCHCC (without resection) was 42 months (it was 57 months in one case of SCHCC which was not proven pathologically). Similarly, it was reported in the literature that the increasing concentration of AFP detectable by RIA might be present up to 18 months before the appearance of symptoms (Johnson and William 1980). Quite recently, Heyward et al. (1982) reported that HBV infection could have occurred as few as 10 years before the recognition of HCC; significant rises of AFP levels occurred as long as 2 years before the clinical onset of HCC.

III. Correlation Between Clinical Performance, AFP Level, Laboratory Findings, Immunostatus, Sodium Pump Activity, and Tumor Size in Different Stages of HCC

As shown in Table 3, alterations in clinical performance, AFP level, laboratory findings, immunostatus, red-cell sodium pump activity, and survival rates were closely correlated to disease stage and tumor size. In the early subclinical and subclinical stages, abnormal clinical or laboratory findings, including those on red cell sodium pump activity and immunostatus, were generally absent in the majority of cases. It should be noted that although the rate of coexisting cirrhosis was similar in different disease stages, clinical or laboratory evidence of cirrhosis (eg. vascular spider, splenomegaly, reverse A/G ratio) was less severe than in the moderate and late stages. This was coincident with our previous pathological findings (Ying and Chai 1978), which suggested that the intensity of cirrhosis usually increases parallel with the enlargement of HCC. Similar results were also observed with ALT levels. When the disease advanced to the moderate stage, marked disturbances represented by a great variety of parameters appeared. Only patients who had undergone radical resection or the few with complete response after nonresectional treatment showed normalization of those disturbances, including those of immunostatus (Lin and Tang 1981) and red cell soidum pump activity (Ye et al. 1983). Severe irreversible disturbances usually appeared in the late stage.

IV. Significance of Studying the Natural History of HCC

A. Change of Pessimistic View

The fact that HCC has a relatively long natural history (around 2 years) indicates that, in many aspects, HCC mimics other solid tumors in their natural evolution. The previous concept of "acute malignancy" and "incurable disease" actually represents the relatively late disease stage. As mentioned, the median HCC in patients with symptoms is as large as 9 cm, which approximates that of other solid tumors in the very late stage, such as those of breast, stomach, or lung. This relatively late disease stage seems responsible for the short survival, as it is in other solid tumors. Of

Table 3. Correlation between clinical performance, AFP level, laboratory findings, immunostatus, sodium pump activity, and tumor size in different stages of HCC

Items compared	Stage			
	Early subclinical	Subclinical	Moderate	Late
Median period (months)	10	8–9	4	2
Median tumor size (cm)	< 4.0	4.0	9.0	10.0
Median AFP (ng/ml)	50–200?	2000	20000	40000
Clinical performance of HCC	None	None	Pain, anorexia weight loss, weakness, epigastric mass, etc	Jaundice, ascites, metastasis, cachexia
With clinical or laboratory evidence of cirrhosis (%)	?	7.0	24.7	
ALT > 40 units (%)	?	10.0	20.7	
γ-GTP > 10 units (%)	?	24.7	77.0	
ALP > 13 units (%)	?	22.5	56.9	
X-ray diaphragm sign (+) (%)	?	7.8	35.7	
Old tuberculin test > 5 mm (%)	?	93.7	65.4	48.9
RBC sodium pump activity[a] mean ± S.E. (mmol/l RBC/h)	?	0.4123 ± 0.0391	0.5215 ± 0.0133	0.7167 ± 0.0506
Survival of whole series (life table method)				
1-year (%)	?	75.5	32.6	1.7
3-year (%)	?	47.7	11.8	0
5-year (%)	?	43.9	5.9	0

[a] Normal value 0.4503 ± 0.0130; cirrhosis 0.3853 ± 0.0125

course, the biological characteristics (such as early invasion of blood sinusoid and intrahepatic veins) as well as the coexistent liver cirrhosis might aggravate the grave prognosis.

B. Change of Therapeutic Attitude

The fact that HCC has a relatively long period (up to around 18 months) without marked impairment suggests that an aggressive therapeutic approach (mainly surgery) might result in radical cure of the disease, as it does with other solid tumors. Our data have demonstrated the priority of aggressive treatment of SCHCC patients: a higher proportion had resections (60.0% versus 24.7%) than did clinical patients, a higher percentage of patients had normal AFP levels after operation (84.2% versus 38.5%), and there was a higher 5-year survival rate after resection (72.9% versus 16.1%). Therefore, it is important to seize the opportunity to treat SCHCC before spreading occurs, and to treat clinical HCC before tumor emboli occur in the portal trunk.

C. Change of Diagnostic Strategy

HCC has a relatively long period with low and moderate AFP levels (50–200 ng/ml), around 10 months before the establishment of SCHCC diagnosis, and the median tumor size even in SCHCC is 3.5 cm (Tang 1981) – 4.5 cm (100 cases of SCHCC in this series), which suggests that a much earlier diagnosis is necessary and feasible, because the AFP level is generally correlated to tumor size in the early stage of AFP-positive HCC (Tang and Yang 1981). This has stimulated the search for HCC markers other than AFP and attempts to detect HCC smaller than 1 cm by radioimmunodetection.

D. Clues to Investigation in Early Evolution of HCC

Materials have accumulated concerning chemically induced liver cell cancer in animals (Craddock 1976; Baldwin and Price 1976: Farber 1976); however, knowledge in regard to the early evolution of human HCC is far from adequate. Despite the fact that a vast amount of work has been done on the pathology, immunology and pathophysiology of human HCC in the past few decades, it has been performed during the relatively late stage of the disease, in the terminal 6 months. The study of the natural history of HCC will provide clues to fill in the gaps concerning the first 18 months or even longer.

References

Alpert ME, Hutt MSR, Davidson CS et al. (1969) Primary hepatoma in Uganda – a prospective clinical and epidemiologic study of forty-six patients. Am J Med 46: 794–802

Baldwin RW, Price MR (1976) Immunology of experimental liver cell cancer. In: Cameron HM, Linsell DA, Warwick GP (eds) Liver cell cancer. Elsevier, Amsterdam, pp 203–242

Bengmark S, Börjesson B, Hafström L, et al. (1971) The natural history of primary carcinoma of the liver. Scand J Gastroenterol 6: 351–355

Cao YZ, Tang ZY, Chai WY, et al. (1979) Factors influencing prognosis of primary liver cancer – clinicopathological analysis of 224 cases. Natl Med J China 59: 35–40[1]

Chan KT (1967) The management of primary liver carcinoma. Ann R Coll Surg Engl 41: 235–282

Craddock VM (1976) Cell proliferation and experimental liver cancer. In: Cameron HM, Linsell DA, Warwick GP (eds) Liver cell cancer. Elsevier, Amsterdam, pp 153–202

Ervasti J (1964) Primary carcinoma of the liver – a pathologic and clinical study of 100 cases. Acta Chir Scand 334: 1s–65s

Farber E (1976) The pathology of experimental liver cell cancer. In: Cameron HM, Linsell DA, Warwick GP (eds) Liver cell cancer. Elsevier, Amsterdam, pp 243–278

Geddes EW, Falkson G (1970) Malignant hepatoma in the Bantu. Cancer 25: 1271–1278

Gustafson EG (1937) An analysis of 62 cases of primary carcinoma of the liver based on 24000 necropsies at Bellevue Hospital. Ann Int Med 11: 889–900

Heyward WL, Bender TR, Lanier AP, et al. (1982) Serological markers of hepatitis B virus and alpha-fetoprotein levels preceding primary hepatocellular carcinoma in Alaskan Eskimos. Lancet 2: 889–890

Jiang ZH (1960) Primary liver cancer – clinical analysis of 40 cases. Natl Med J China 46: 294–298[1]

Jin WT, Li SQ, Ying YY, et al. (1965) Primary liver cancer – clinicopathological study of 57 cases. Acta Acad Med Primae Shanghai 3: 215–224[1]

Johnson PJ, William R (1980) Serum alpha fetoprotein estimation and doubling time in hepatocellular carcinoma – influence of therapy and possible value in early detection. J Natl Cancer Inst 64: 1329–1332

Kay CT (1964) Primary hepatic cancer – review of 96 cases. Arch Int Med 113: 46–53

Lawrence GH, Grauman D, Lasersohn J, et al. (1966) Primary carcinoma of the liver. Am J Surg 112: 200–210

Li RZ, Xia BH, Huang-pu YS, et al. (1959) Primary liver cancer – clinical analysis of 40 cases. Chin J Int Med 7: 358–361[1]

Lin ZY, Tang ZY (1981) Immunostatus and immunotherapy of primary liver cancer. In: Tang ZY (ed) Primary liver cancer. Shanghai Sci and Technical, Shanghai, pp 319–333[1]

Moseley RV (1967) Primary malignant tumors of the liver – a review of the clinical and pathologic characteristics of 47 cases and a discussion of current diagnostic technics and surgical management. Surgery 61: 674–686

Okuda K (1976) Clinical aspects of hepatocellular carcinoma – analysis of 134 cases. In: Okuda K, Peter RL (eds) Hepatocellular carcinoma. John Wiley and Sons, New York, pp 387–436

Okuda K, Nakashima T, Obata H (1980) Hepatitis B virus and primary liver cell carcinoma. In: Bianchi L et al. (eds) Virus and the liver. MTP Press, Lancaster, pp 209–216

Popper H, Gerber MA, Thung SN (1982) The relation of hepatocellular carcinoma to infection with hepatitis B and related viruses in man and animals. Hepatology 2: 1s–9s

Primack A, Vogel CL, Kyalwazi SK, et al. (1975) A staging system for hepatocellular carcinoma – prognostic factors in Ugandan patients. Cancer 35: 1357–1364

Rosenberg DML, Oshsner A (1948) Primary carcinoma of the liver – an analysis of fifty-five autopsied cases, the record of a case with resection, and a review of the recent literature. Surgery 24: 1036–1068

Schreiber WM, Kato H, Robertson JD (1970) Primary carcinoma of the liver in Hiroshima and Nagasaki, Japan. Cancer 26: 69–75

Shanghai Coordinating Group for Research on Liver Cancer, China (Tang ZY, et al.) (1974) Primary liver cancer – Clinical analysis of 3254 cases (from 11 provinces, 21 hospitals in China). Tumor Prevent Treat Study 2: 207–215[1]

Sharpstone P, Fleisher MR, Rake MO, et al. (1970) Diagnosis and prognosis of primary malignant tumors of the liver. Gut 11: 1058

Sun TT, Wan LC, Chang YL, et al. (1979) Radiorocket electrophoresis autography (RREA) through labelled antigen for AFP assay and its application in seroepidemiological investigation on primary hepatocellular carcinoma. Chin Med J 92: 17–22

Tang ZY (1981) A new concept on the natural course of hepatocellular carcinoma Chin Med J 94: 585–588

Tang ZY, Yang BH (1981) Clinical evaluation of alpha fetoprotein as tumor marker for hepatocellular carcinoma. Chin J Oncol 3: 205–209[1]

Tang ZY, Yu YQ, Lin ZY, et al. (1979) Small hepatocellular carcinoma – clinical analysis of 30 cases. Chin Med J 92: 455–462

Tang ZY, Ying YY, Gu TJ (1982) Hepatocellular carcinoma – changing concepts in recent years. In: Popper H, Schaffner F (eds) Progress in liver diseases. vol VII. Grune and Stratton, New York, pp 637–647

Wang CE, Li GC, Li ZC, et al. (1961) Clinical diagnosis of 88 cases of primary liver cancer. Natl Med J China 47: 224–228[1]

Yan ZB, Liu KR, Kuang WF, et al. (1964) Primary liver cancer – clinical analysis of 150 cases. Tientsin Med J 2: 334–336[1]

Yang TY, Zhang XY et al. (1955) Primary liver cancer – analysis of 20 cases. Chin J Int Med 3: 198–203[1]

Ye SL, Tang ZY, Gu TJ (1983) Alteration in red cell sodium pump activity in patients with primary liver cancer. Acta Acad Med Primae Shanghai 10: 93–98[1]

Ying YY, Chai WY (1978) Small hepatocellular carcinoma. III. Pathology of small hepatocellular carcinoma. Acta Acad Med Primae Shanghai 5: 111–118[1]

Zhang ZR, Xu BJ, Chen T (1958) Primary liver cancer – clinical analysis of 45 cases. Chin J Int Med 6: 58–60[1]

[1] Chinese

16 Prognosis of Hepatocellular Carcinoma and Factors Influencing It

Tang Zhao-you

Unquestionable progress has been made in recent years in the etiology, pathology, diagnosis, and treatment of HCC (Okuda and Ohnishi 1982; Foster 1982; Fortner et al. 1981); nevertheless, the overall prognosis has not altered substantially (Okuda et al. 1980). Factors influencing the prognosis of HCC have been analyzed with respect to clinical performance (Primack et al. 1975), clinicopathological findings (Cao et al. 1979), surgery (Tang et al. 1981 a), and small HCC (Tang et al. 1981 b). Encouraging results have been achieved through early detection and early treatment (Sun et al. 1981; Tang et al. 1982 a), which has aroused lively interest in recent years. In this chapter the following questions are answered:

1. Can survival be prolonged if SCHCC is treated early?
2. What is the major factor influencing the prognosis of SCHCC?
3. What should we focus our attention on in the forthcoming years for further improvement of the prognosis of HCC?

I. Prognosis of SCHCC and CHCC

A. Overall Survival with SCHCC and CHCC

The overall survival rates for 566 cases of HCC in this series are listed in Table 1. It should be noted that the survival rates for SCHCC were much higher than those for CHCC. As mentioned in Chap. 15, SCHCC can be diagnosed about 8 months earlier than can CHCC. However, even if 1 year is deducted from SCHCC survival, the 4-year survival (43.9%) is still much higher than that with CHCC (7.2%), and is even higher than the 1-year survival with CHCC (24.5%). Moreover, of the 47 cases with

Table 1. Overall survival of SCHCC and CHCC patients

Survival (Life table method)	SCHCC ($n=100$) %	CHCC ($n=466$) %	Total ($n=566$) %
1-year	75.5 (63)[a]	24.2 (85)	33.3 (148)
2-year	54.5 (39)	11.1 (32)	19.0 (71)
3-year	47.7 (26)	8.4 (21)	16.0 (47)
4-year	43.9 (19)	7.2 (14)	13.9 (33)
5-year	43.9 (10)	4.2 (8)	11.6 (18)

[a] Figures in parenthesis represents number of survivors

3-year survival, 26 cases were from the SCHCC group ($n=100$) and only 21 from the CHCC group ($n=466$). Of the 466 cases of CHCC, only eight patients survived 5 years; however, ten of the 100 patients with SCHCC survived over 5 years during the same follow-up period. It can therefore be concluded that early treatment of SCHCC may prolong survival effectively and markedly, thus improving the overall prognosis. The overall 5-year survival rate for HCC in our selective series (11.6%) was higher than those reported in the current literature.

B. Survival with HCC in Resected and Unresected Groups

As shown in Tables 2 and 3, surgical resection remains the method of choice in treatment of not only CHCC but also SCHCC. No 5-year survival could be obtained in either the SCHCC or the CHCC group with nonresectional treatment. It is worth mentioning that much higher survival was obtained for patients with SCHCC than for those with CHCC receiving similar resectional treatment (72.9% versus 16.1% in 5-year survival). Furthermore, successful resection was achieved in 60.0% of SCHCC patients versus 24.7% of those with CHCC. This indicates that resection of SCHCC plays a major role in the improvement of the overall prognosis of HCC.

Table 2. Survival of HCC patients in resected group

Survival (Life table method)	SCHCC ($n=60$) %	CHCC ($n=115$) %	Total ($n=175$) %
1-year	85.0 (44)[a]	60.1 (51)	69.5 (95)
2-year	76.2 (32)	32.5 (23)	48.5 (55)
3-year	72.9 (23)	26.3 (17)	44.5 (40)
4-year	72.9 (19)	23.0 (12)	41.1 (31)
5-year	72.9 (10)	16.1 (8)	37.3 (18)

[a] Figures in parenthesis represents number of survivors

Table 3. Survival of HCC patients in unresected group

Survival (Life table method)	SCHCC ($n=40$) %	CHCC ($n=351$) %	Total ($n=391$) %
1-year	57.3 (19)[a]	12.1 (34)	17.1 (53)
2-year	19.1 (7)	3.7 (9)	5.6 (16)
3-year	8.0 (3)	2.0 (4)	3.1 (7)
4-year	– (0)	1 (2)	1 (2)
5-year	– (0)	– (0)	– (0)

[a] Figures in parenthesis represents number of survivors

C. Survival with HCC in Different Periods

Owing to the extremely low survival rate for this particular neoplasm, complete data on 1-, 3-, and 5-year survival rates for overall PLC have rarely been reported in the literature. The long-term survival rates reported either from the West (United States – Axtell et al. 1972) or from the East (Japan – Okuda et al. 1980; China – Yang and Tang 1981) covering the period from the 1940s to the 1970s were disappointing. To sum up, the overall 5-year survival rate for PLC from the onset or the diagnosis of disease or after treatment seldom exceeded 4% (Table 4); however, an encouraging improvement of PLC prognosis was observed in our selective series. The close correlation between the increasing proportion of SCHCC in the whole series and the increasing survival rates were particularly notable (Table 5). It is suggested that the "incurable disease" with extremely low 5-year survival actually represents a relatively late disease stage; once the proportion of early-stage patients increases, the "incurable disease" will become curable to a certain extent.

Table 4. Survival rates for PLC patients in the literatures (selective data)

Reference	Country period	No. of cases	Survival rate (%) 1-year	3-year	5-year
Axtell et al. (1972)	U.S.A.				
	1940–49	371	7	4	2
	1950–59	724	5	2	1
	1960–64	505	10	4	4
	1965–69	584	13	6	–
Okuda et al. (1980)	Japan 1968–77	1424 (HCC)	21.5	5.0	2.4
Shanghai Group[a] (Tang et al.) (1974)	China 1967–72	2141	8.6		
Yang and Tang[a] (1981)	China (Zhong Shan Hospital) 1961–70	387	8.7	3.6	2.6
Tang[a] (this series)	China (Zhong Shan Hospital) 1971–82	566	33.3	16.0	11.6

[a] Survival after treatment

Table 5. Survival of PLC patients in different periods (Zhong Shan Hospital, Shanghai)

	1961–1970 ($n=387$)	1971–1976 ($n=250$)	1977–1982 ($n=316$)
Survival (life table method) %			
1-year	8.7	26.5	38.5
3-year	3.6	10.4	21.7
5-year	2.6	6.5	20.6

II. Factors Influencing Survival with SCHCC

Our previous work in regard to factors influencing prognosis of small HCC has shown that early resection of small HCC remains the leading factor, the others being site of the tumor, number of tumors, and state of liver cirrhosis, if any (Tang et al. 1981b). Further investigation of this problem centering on SCHCC is reported herewith.

A. Age

The survival rates in patients younger than the median age with SCHCC (47.5 years) ($n=50$) were mostly higher than those in patients at or older than the median age ($n=50$), being the same (74.2%) for 1-year survival, 55.4% versus 35.3% for 3-year survival, and 51.7% versus 35.3% for 5-year survival. Foster (1970) reviewed the world literature and found that the 5-year survival after resection was 14% in adults, but 33.3% in infants and children. Ishikawa (1976) reported that the 3-year survival after resection in patients below 15 years of age was 24.9%, while it was only 14.8% in adults.

B. Tumor Size, Site, and Number of Tumor Nodules

As shown in Table 6, patients with smaller HCC ($\leqslant$4.5 cm) had a better prognosis than those with tumors $>$4.5 cm, the 5-year survival rate being 69.6% for the former and, so far, 0% for the latter. However, tumors located in the left lobe were not different from those seated in other parts of the liver. Survival with single tumors was significantly longer than it was with multinodular-type carcinomas or massive type with satellites; the longer the follow-up, the greater the difference.

C. Coexisting Liver Cirrhosis

SCHCC patients without cirrhosis or with micronodular cirrhosis ($n=32$) had a higher long-term survival rate than did those with macronodular cirrhosis ($n=59$), being 82.8% versus 74.0% for 1-year survival, 66.5% versus 38.9% for 3-year survival, and 66.5% versus 35.4% for 5-year survival.

D. Original and Postoperative AFP Levels

Table 7 lists the survival rates for SCHCC with relation to original and postoperative AFP levels. It seems that patients with original AFP levels $\leqslant$2000 ng/ml were not significantly different from those with AFP$>$2000 ng/ml. However, SCHCC patients with AFP returning to $\leqslant$20 ng/ml after operation had a much better prognosis, the 5-year survival being 80.4%, but no patient in the group with abnormal AFP surviving 5 years after surgery. This result is coincident with our previous observation that normalization of AFP after resection remains the leading factor for better prognosis (Tang et al. 1981b).

Table 6. Survival rates for SCHCC patients with relation to tumor size, site, and number of tumor nodules

Tumor	No. of cases	Survival %[a]		
		1-year	3-year	5-year
Size ⩽4.5 cm	45	88.2	69.6	69.6
>4.5 cm	42	64.5	28.3	–
Site – left lobe	15	80.0	66.7	50.0
– right, portal, or bilateral lobes	78	73.4	44.9	44.9
Nodule – single	60	88.9	62.9	62.9
– multiple	30	52.4	21.9	–

[a] Life table method

Table 7. Survival rates for SCHCC patients with relation to original and postoperative AFP levels

AFP level (ng/ml)	No. of cases	Survival (life table method) %		
		1-year	3-year	5-year
Original ⩽2000	67	72.9	48.8	45.9
>2000	33	77.0	40.1	40.1
Postoperative ⩽20	52	93.7	80.4	80.4
>20	37	46.9	5.4	–

III. Factors Influencing Survival in Whole Series of PLC

Our previous clinicopathological analysis of 224 cases of PLC indicated that patients with well-encapsulated tumor, with less frequent proliferation, without tumor emboli, without distant metastases, without associated cirrhosis, or with well-differentiated tumor, as well as mass survey patients, had a better prognosis (Cao et al. 1979).

Age, discovery, clinical type and staging, original and postoperative AFP levels, laboratory findings, tumor site, capsule status and number of nodules, treatment modality, and coexisting cirrhosis are here analyzed in relation to survival of a larger series of PLC patients with a higher proportion of SCHCC and longer follow-up study (Table 8).

A. Age

PLC patients ⩽45 years of age had higher long-term survival rates than did those >45 years of age, the 5-year survival being 14.7% in the former and 7.1% in the latter. Single-factor analysis in literature also revealed a better prognosis for young patients (Johnson et al. 1981).

Table 8. Factors influencing survival for entire series of PLC patients

Item	No. of cases	Survival (life table method) %		
		1-year	3-year	5-year
Age ≤45 years	262	36.5	19.8	14.7
>45 years	304	30.0	11.8	7.1
Discovery – AFP survey	145	64.4	40.2	34.7
Clinical	421	22.8	7.3	3.7
Clinical type – Simple	433	37.5	19.1	14.1
Cirrhotic	122	19.2	4.8	2.4
Staging – Subclinical	100	75.5	47.7	43.9
Moderate	335	32.6	11.8	5.9
Late	131	1.7	0	0
Original AFP <5000 ng/ml	301	42.9	20.6	15.2
≥5000 ng/ml	249	21.2	20.6	6.2
Postoperative AFP ≤20 ng/ml	83	94.7	76.1	60.4
>20 ng/ml	200	28.8	4.3	0
γ-GTP <20 units	243	55.0	29.5	21.8
≥20 units	255	10.9	3.3	2.2
OT test ≥5 mm (+)	248	43.1	20.5	15.8
<5 mm (–)	141	24.9	12.0	12.0
Tumor site – left	80	62.3	38.1	30.0
– right, portal, multiple	299	43.3	19.9	13.1
Tumor capsule – good	86	82.3	60.3	49.0
– poor	275	38.4	11.7	5.9
No. of nodules – single	172	68.4	40.5	32.3
– multiple	200	30.0	8.0	5.4
Treatment – resection	175	69.5	44.5	37.3
– nonresection	391	17.1	3.1	0
Resection – radical	64	93.3	69.5	61.5
– palliative	111	55.5	27.0	22.5
Cirrhosis – None or micronodular	142	54.3	30.5	22.2
Macronodular	236	41.5	19.4	16.1

B. Discovery

As mentioned in Chap. 2, patients discovered through AFP serosurvey or monitored because of chronic hepatitis or a cirrhosis background had much higher 5-year survival rates than patients discovered clinically did (34.7% versus 3.7%).

C. Clinical Type and Staging

PLC patients without clinical or laboratory evidence of cirrhosis had a better prognosis in the long run than their counterparts did (14.1% versus 2.4% for 5-year survival).

Clinical staging proved to be one of the most important factors which might influence the overall prognosis of PLC. A significant difference was observed among subclinical, moderate, and late stages, either in 1-year, 3-year, or 5-year survival rates. The literature carries similar reports, that HCC patients in an evidently relatively late stage of disease – serum bilirubin >2 mg/dl, γ-GTP >100 units, GOT $>$ 150 units, occupying lesion $>50\%$ of liver seen by means of scintiscan, etc., would have a poor prognosis (Nishioka et al. 1981).

D. Original and Postoperative AFP Levels

Patients with lower original AFP levels (<5000 ng/ml) had a better prognosis than those with higher AFP levels, their 1-, 3-, and 5-year survivals being two times higher. This is logical, as the AFP level was correlated with the tumor size, and with the disease stage to a certain extent (Tang and Yang 1981). This can also explain the better prognosis for AFP survey patients compared with clinical patients. The median AFP level was lower in the former.

More important results were shown by the analysis of postoperative AFP levels. The data of this series revealed that patients with AFP returning to $\leqslant 20$ ng/ml had a dramatically higher 5-year survival than did their counterparts (60.4% versus 0%). The normalization rates of AFP decreased according to disease stage and mode of treatment: 84.2% in SCHCC after resection, 38.5% in CHCC after resection, 14.8% in SCHCC after nonresectional treatment, and 4.2% in CHCC after nonresectional treatment. These were correlated to the corresponding 3-year survival rates (72.9%), 26.3%, 8.0%, and 2.0% respectively) as well as to the corresponding 5-year survival rates (72.9%, 16.1%, 0%, and 0%). Thus, normalization of AFP after treatment remains the leading prognostic factor in analysis of both SCHCC and small HCC, or in analysis of an entire series of PLC patients.

E. Laboratory Findings

As shown in Table 8, patients with lower serum γ-GTP (<20 units, Orlowski) had a ten times higher 5-year survival rate than those with higher γ-GTP ($\geqslant 20$ units). It has been well documented that the γ-GTP level is correlated to both tumor size and disease stage (Tang et al. 1982b). Similar results were reported by Nishioka et al. (1981).

Theoretically, the immunostatus of PLC patients seems to be of importance in regard to prognosis; however, only a small difference was demonstrated in this series by using the old-tuberculin skin delayed hypersensitivity reaction as an in vivo marker of cell-mediated immunity.

F. Capsule Status, Tumor Site, and Number of Nodules

Data shown in Table 8 reconfirm our previous findings that well-encapsulated tumor is of prime importance for a higher long-term survival. Similar results have been reported in the literature (Kim et al. 1979). Again, a single tumor also provides a better prognosis for PLC, as it does for SCHCC. Different long-term survival rates have also been observed with different tumor sites; left lobe tumors are probably better than those located in the right lobe, the portal area, or bilateral lobes.

G. Treatment

Resection yields a much better prognosis than nonresectional treatment in the long run (37.3% versus 0% in 5-year survival). Moreover, radical resection leads to a nearly three times higher 5-year survival than that after palliative resection (61.5% versus 22.5%).

H. Coexisting Liver Cirrhosis

A minor difference in long-term survival was noted between patients without cirrhosis or with micronodular cirrhosis and those with macronodular cirrhosis (30.5% versus 19.4% in 3-year survival and 22.2% versus 16.1% in 5-year survival). A combined analysis of multiple variations in the literature revealed that cirrhosis does influence prognosis (Johnson et al. 1981).

IV. Approaches to Further Prolongation of Survival in SCHCC and Overall PLC

A. Early and Radical Resection

As shown in Tables 6–8, early and radical resection seems to be the leading approach to further lengthening of survival.

Early resection includes the factors of discovery, clinical staging, original AFP levels, γ-GTP, and tumor size and is indirectly related to tumor capsule and the number of nodules. Radical resection includes the factor of postoperative AFP levels. It is believed that endeavors should be directed toward early detection and radical resection. The comparative study of survey and nonsurvey patients reported in Chap. 2 shows that AFP screening and monitoring of high-risk populations with a background of chronic hepatitis or cirrhosis is the main approach to achieving the purpose. By means of AFP survey we detect a higher proportion of resectable cases and reach a higher percentage of radical resections, owing to the much higher incidence of SCHCC and small HCC. With SCHCC patients, every effort should be focused on earlier diagnosis of smaller tumors.

However, the increase in resectability may be limited because of associated cirrhosis and some biological characteristics of HCC.

B. Investigation of Biological Characteristics of HCC

The biological characteristics of HCC are another important factor influencing prognosis; they include tumor site, tumor capsule, the number of nodules, etc. Our previous study showed that tumor capsule, tumor emboli, metastasis, and differentiation are important factors influencing PLC prognosis (Cao et al. 1979). Apparently, these biological features are also closely related to the major problems in this study, i.e., radical resection and AFP normalization. These characteristics may explain the poor prognosis for HCC to some extent; therefore, elucidation of these special features might provide a new approach to controlling this particular neoplasm. Fortunately, these features are not so advanced in AFP survey patients. Thus, we have found that the earlier the stage, the higher the percentage of well-encapsulated tumor, the higher the incidence of single-nodule tumor, the lower the incidence of tumor emboli, and the better the differentiation (Tang et al. 1980). Meanwhile, it is our conclusion, that early detection and early resection remain the principal approach to a better prognosis until a breakthrough is made in elucidating the biological characteristics of PLC.

C. Research Focused on Coexistent Liver Cirrhosis

In 1970, Foster observed that the prognosis for Asian patients was less favorable than that for non-Asian patients. Even after resection, the 5-year survival was only 11.8% (Okuda et al. 1980), 16.0% (Wu et al. 1980), and 23.6% (Tang et al. 1981 a) for Asian HCC patients, but it was 49% in the United States (Starzl et al. 1980). It was reported that only 20.5% of patients undergoing PLC resection in the United States had associated cirrhosis (Foster and Berman 1977), but in China this was 69.6% (Wu et al. 1980) – 77.1% (Tang et al. 1981 a). Foster and Berman (1977) reported that the 2-year survival for 91 cases without cirrhosis was 72%, but only 25% for ten cases with cirrhosis. Although a minor difference can be seen in our series, considering the high incidence of dysplasia in patients with cirrhosis, it is possible that the disease is of multicentric origin in patients with associated severe macronodular cirrhosis. Our conclusion is that research endeavors should also be focused on coexistent liver cirrhosis.

References

Axtell IM, Cutler SJ, Myers MH (1972) End results in cancer – report nov. 4. US Department of Health, Education and Welfare, Public Health Service, NIH, NCI, Bethesda, pp 72–76

Cao YZ, Tang ZY, Chai WY, et al. (1979) Factors influencing prognosis of primary liver cancer – clinicopathological analysis of 224 cases. Natl Med J China 59: 35–40[1]

Fortner JG, Maclean BJ, Kim DK, et al. (1981) The seventies evolution in liver surgery for cancer. Cancer 47: 2162–2166

Foster JH (1970) Survival after liver resection for cancer. Cancer 26: 493–502

Foster JH (1982) Cancer and the liver. In: Gitnick GL (ed) Current hepatology. vol II. John Wiley and Sons, New York, pp 233–272

Foster JH, Berman MM (1977) Solid liver tumors. Saunders, Philadelphia, pp 62–104

Ishikawa K (1976) Follow-up study of patients with primary liver cancer. Report 3. Acta Hepatol Jpn 17: 460–465
Johnson PT, Melia WM, Palmer MK, et al. (1981) Relationship between serum alpha-fetoprotein, cirrhosis and survival in hepatocellular carcinoma. Br J Cancer 44: 502–505
Kim CI, Takasan H, Arii S, et al. (1979) Clinicopathological study of thirty resectable hepatocellular carcinomas, particularly on prognostic factors. Acta Hepatol Jpn 20: 284–290
Nishioka M, Nawata J, Ando K, et al. (1981) Prognostic factors in patients with hepatocellular carcinoma. Acta Hepatol Jpn 22: 274–279
Okuda K, Ohnishi K (1982) Hepatic tumors. In: Arias IM, Frenkel M, Wilson JHP (eds) The liver annual 2/1982. Excerpta Medica, Amsterdam, pp 359–396
Okuda K, The Liver Cancer Study Group of Japan (1980) Primary liver cancer in Japan. Cancer 45: 2663–2669
Primack A, Vogel CL, Kyalwazi SK, et al. (1975) A staging system for hepatocellular carcinoma – prognostic factors in Ugandan patients. Cancer 35: 1357–1364
Shanghai Coordinating Group for Research on Liver Cancer, China (Tang ZY et al.) (1974) Primary liver cancer – clinical analysis of 3254 cases (from 11 provinces, 21 hospitals in China). Tumor Prevent Treat Study 2: 207–215[1]
Starzl TE, Koep LJ, Weil R III, et al. (1980) Right trisegmentectomy for hepatic neoplasms. Surg Gynecol Obstet 150: 208–214
Sun TT, Tang ZY, Chu YY (1981) Epidemiology, early diagnosis and treatment of liver cell cancer. In: DeCosse JJ, Sherlock P (eds) Gastrointestinal cancer I. Martinus Nijhoff, Hague, pp 387–411
Tang ZY, Yang BH (1981) Clinical evaluation of alpha fetoprotein as tumor marker for hepàtocellular carcinoma. Chin J Oncol 3: 205–209[1]
Tang ZY, Yang BH, Tang CL, et al. (1980) Evaluation of population screening for hepatocellular carcinoma. Chin Med J 93: 795–799
Tang ZY, Yu YQ, Zhou XD, Chen QM (1981 a) Factors influencing primary liver cancer resection rate. Chin Med J 94: 749–754
Tang ZY, Cao YZ, Yu YQ, Lin ZY (1981 b) Small hepatocellular carcinoma. V. Prognosis and factors influencing prognosis of small hepatocellular carcinoma. Acta Acad Med Primae Shanghai 8: 203–207[1]
Tang ZY, Ying YY, Gu TJ (1982 a) Hepatocellular carcinoma – changing concepts in recent years. In: Popper H, Schaffner F (eds) Progress in liver diseases. vol VII. Grune and Stratton, New York, pp 637–647
Tang ZY, Yu YQ, Zhou XD, et al. (1982 b) Research on small hepatocellular carcinoma. China Scientific and Technical Literature Publisher, Beijing, pp 7–11[1]
Wu MC, Chen H, Zhang XH, et al. (1980) Primary hepatic carcinoma – resection over 18 years. Chin Med J 93: 723–728
Yang BH, Tang ZY (1981) Primary liver cancer – a clinical analysis of 1045 cases. In: Tang ZY (ed) Primary liver cancer. Shanghai Scientific and Technical Publisher, Shanghai, pp 366–374[1]

---

[1] Chinese

17 Epidemiology of Primary Liver Cancer

Yu Shun-zhang

Primary liver cancer is a major hazard in China, the number of deaths being 100000 every year. We did a retrospective survey of cancer mortality around 1976, which indicated that the annual rate of death caused by PLC was 14.52/100000 for men and 5.61/100000 for women, the results, standardized with world population, being 19.96 and 8.07 per 100000 respectively. Among men, PLC is the third major cause of cancer deaths, after stomach and esophageal cancers, while among women PLC ranks fourth, after stomach, cervical, and esophageal cancers (Editorial Committee 1979).

The main endemic areas are along the southeast seacoast of China; however, the distribution there is not even. PLC mortality has increased about twofold in the past two decades, with the incidence higher in men than in women. The mortality is dependent on the average age of patients. Wide-range and local studies of PLC show that environmental factors are important, and animal studies show that there may be a common etiology of PLC in man and animals.

Contaminated water, aflatoxin-containing foods, and hepatitis are possible causes. In several areas, liver cancer morbidity or mortality is higher in populations drinking pond and ditch water than in populations drinking well or deep-well water. Case-control studies and cohort studies showed that hepatitis, especially hepatitis B, might play an important role in the disease. Seroepidemiological studies in Shanghai and Qidong County showed that HB_sAg was positive in about 80% of cases but in only 10% of various controls.

The common motto used in the prevention of PLC in Qidong is: "Control of water, control of corn, prevention of hepatitis!" Improving the quality of water and using well water instead of pond water may decrease the incidence of PLC in the endemic area where HB vaccines are to be used.

I. Epidemiology

A. Distribution

According to a retrospective survey done in 1977 involving 2335 counties and cities and 800000000 people, the endemic areas of PLC are near the southeast coast of China (Table 1). The climate is warm and humid, and there is plenty of rainfall because of the monsoon. The main endemic areas for PLC are deltas, valleys, and islands. The counties with the highest mortality (≥30/100000) are Fusui (near Nanning City in the Guangxi Zhuang Autonomous Region), Qidong (near Shanghai

Table 1. Standardized mortality in People's Republic of China (Selected from Atlas of Cancer Mortality in People's Republic of China – Editorial Committee (1979))

Province, municipality, autonomous region	Male (%)		Female (%)		Male/female (%)
	(1)[a]	(2)[b]	(1)	(2)	(2)
Shanghai	26.62	39.09	9.70	15.05	2.60
Fujian	26.04	34.66	8.80	12.58	2.76
Jiangsu	23.81	33.28	9.11	12.95	2.67
Guangxi	26.55	32.51	6.63	8.36	4.90
Zhejiang	22.11	30.52	8.14	11.78	2.59
Jilin	17.03	24.11	6.59	9.57	2.52
Guangdong	16.99	22.70	4.65	6.76	3.40
Heilongjiang	14.61	20.70	4.96	7.35	2.82
Ninxia	13.68	19.48	6.44	9.44	2.06
Tianjin	13.29	19.39	5.54	8.40	2.31
Liaoning	13.12	19.00	6.44	9.44	2.49
Jiangxi	14.22	18.63	5.05	6.88	2.71
Shandong	12.92	18.16	4.65	6.76	2.69
Hebei	12.47	18.03	5.17	7.84	2.30
Beijing	11.87	17.44	4.66	7.29	2.39
Anhui	12.36	17.02	5.06	7.41	2.30
Hunan	12.78	16.51	4.77	6.46	2.56
Hubei	12.79	16.46	4.92	6.94	2.37
Henan	11.39	16.37	5.12	7.70	2.12
Shaanxi	11.47	16.27	6.41	9.57	1.70
Tibet	11.07	15.91	7.25	11.05	1.44
Sichuan	11.73	15.62	4.89	6.88	2.27
Shanxi	9.74	14.22	5.27	8.06	1.76
Inner Mongolia	9.61	13.92	5.12	7.93	1.76
Qinhai	9.11	12.52	5.03	7.04	1.78
Xinjiang	8.07	11.26	4.16	5.90	1.91
Gansu	6.55	9.07	3.97	5.69	1.59
Guizhou	6.62	8.67	2.75	3.83	2.26
Yunnan	6.15	8.26	2.85	3.93	2.10
Overall	14.52	19.96	5.61	8.07	2.47

[a] (1), Standardized according to Chinese population proportion in 1964; [b] (2), standardized according to world population proportion

Municipalty in Jiangsu Province), Zhoushan Prefecture (near Hangzhou City in Zhejiang Province) and Tung'an (near Xiamen City in Fujian Province) (Fig. 1).

The distribution of PLC is uneven from county to county. For example, Qidong is one of the notorious endemic counties; however, the four communes in the north have a lower mortality than those in the south (Fig. 2). The uneven distribution of PLC within endemic areas suggests the possibility of environmental risk factors.

B. Long-term Trend

Since the health of the people has improved in the past 30 years, overall mortality has decreased, but, in Shanghai, for example, cancer mortality moved from 9th place in the 1950s to first or second place in the 1970s. PLC mortality increased

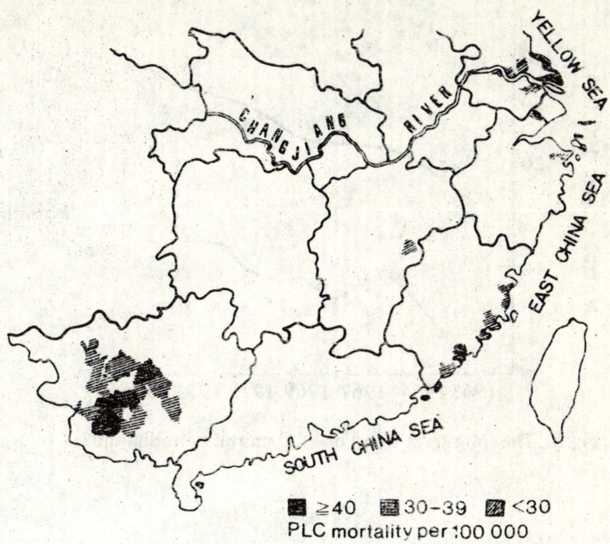

Fig. 1. Hyperendemic areas of PLC in China. (From Editorial Committee 1979)

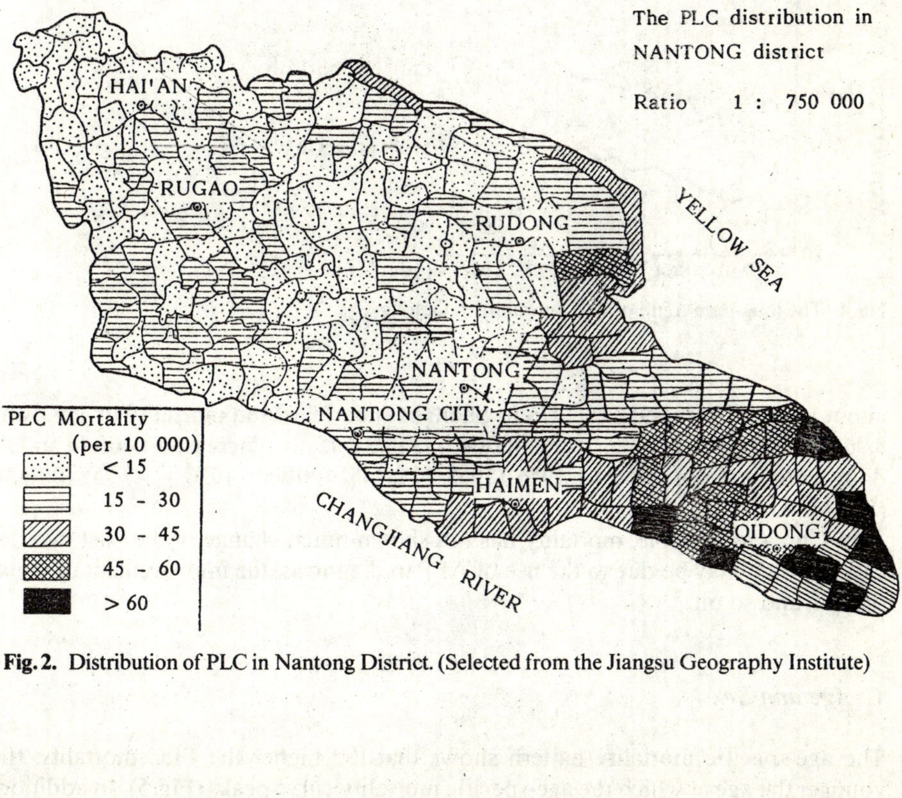

Fig. 2. Distribution of PLC in Nantong District. (Selected from the Jiangsu Geography Institute)

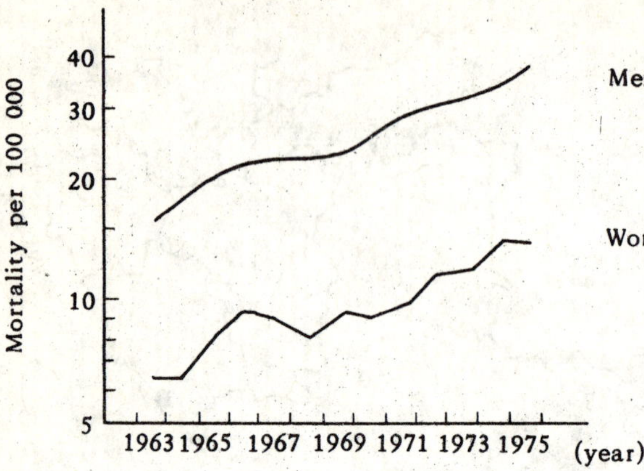

Fig. 3. The long-term trend of PLC mortality in Shanghai

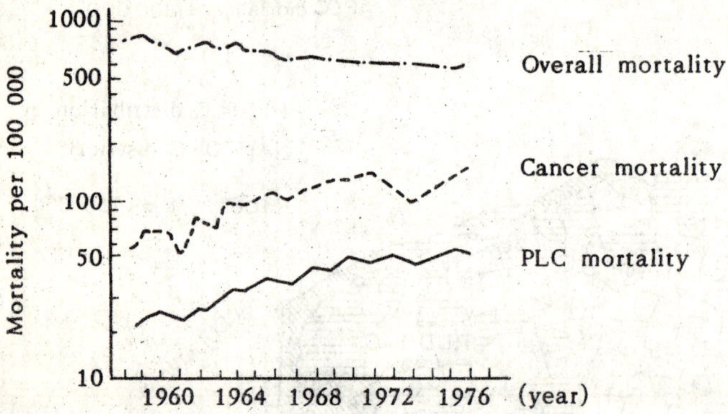

Fig. 4. The long-term trend of PLC mortality in Qidong

about twofold from 1959 to 1976 in Shanghai (standardized mortality in 1959 was 8.96/100000 and in 1976, 16.16/100000) (Fig. 3). It also increased twofold in Qidong county, from 1958 to 1976 (1958 – 20.45/100000; 1976 – 47.71/100000) (Fig. 4).

In China as a whole, mortality has not shown much change in the past two decades, which may be due to the use of AFP in diagnosis, the improvement of registration, and so on.

C. Age and Sex

The age-specific mortality pattern shows that the higher the PLC mortality, the younger the age at which the age-specific mortality curve peaks (Fig. 5). In addition, the higher the mortality, the younger the average age of patients, being only 37.6 years in South Africa, 32 years among Bantu men, 42,5 years in Fusui, China,

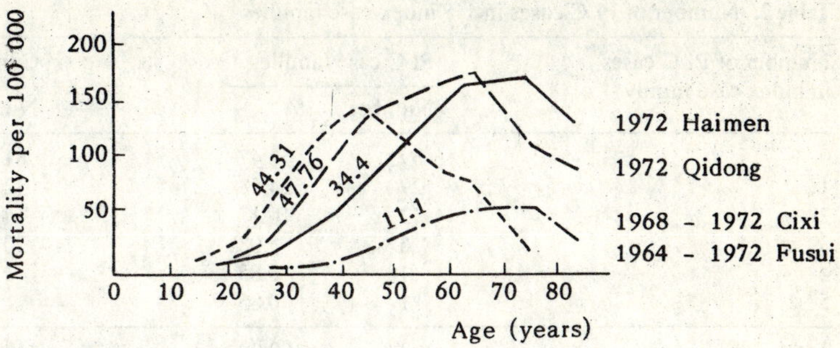

Fig. 5. The age-specific PLC mortality in different counties

48,5 years in Qidong, China, more than 50 years in other places in China, and 64.5 years in Canada. The ratio of men to women with PLC is 3:1 in endemic areas and <2:1 in other nonendemic areas. Most of the patients in China are peasants.

D. Study of Migrants

Wide-ranging studies of migrants were done in the United States and China. The results showed that people among the first migrant generation either from endemic places to nonendemic places or vice versa had the same mortality as those in the places of origin. The second generation, however, showed some changes; e.g., among the first generation of Chinese who migrated to Hong Kong PLC mortality was 12/100000, but it changed to 0.5/100000 for the second generation (Ong and Chan 1976), which indicates that environmental factors are more important than genetic ones.

In both Jiangsu Province and Shanghai, populations migrating from high to low mortality areas and vice versa have also been studied. As shown in Fig. 2 for example, in the Nantong District of Jiangsu Province a low incidence area (the Tongru Ridge) is separated from a high incidence area (the Qihai Plain) by the Daoan-Haijie River. Movement of people from the Tongru ridge to the Qihai Plain has led to a rise in incidence (20.2 to 31.9/100000), while movement in the opposite direction has led to a fall in incidence (36.4 to 29.7/100000) in spite of apparently little change in life style. The total number of migrants in the above-mentioned places was based on some 75000 and 60000 person years respectively.

In Nanhui County, Shanghai, migrants from both high- and low-rate areas to an intermediate-rate area showed changes in mortality toward the intermediate level.

E. Clustering of PLC

There is a tendency for PLC to cluster in families, possibly due to similar diet, mutual infection, or blood relation.

Two case-control studies showed that a history of liver cancer in family members was more common among patients than among controls (12.6% and 16.6% in cases compared with 5.1% and 9.3% in controls). The number of PLC patients in case families was greater than in control families (Table 2).

Table 2. Number of PLC cases in 118 index case families

Number of PLC cases in index case family	PLC case families		Control families	
	Number	%	Number	%
0	69	58.47	81	68.64
1	29	24.58	32	27.12
2	12	10.17	4	3.39
3	6	5.08	0	0
4	1	0.85	1	0.85
5	1	0.85		
Total	118	100.00	118	100.00

Table 3. Relation of relatives to index case

Relation		Male	Female
Blood relation	Often live together with index case	Father's father, father, brother, son, half-blood brother	Father's mother, mother, sister, daughter, half-blood sister
	Seldom live together with index case	Mother's father, uncle, male cousin,	Mother's mother, aunt, female cousin, niece
Non-blood relation	Often live together with index case	Husband, adopted brother, adopted son, "live-in" son-in-law	Wife, adopted sister, adopted daughter, daughter-in-law
	Seldom live together with index case	Brother-in-law, uncle-in-law, nephew-in-law	Sister-in-law, aunt-in-law

Table 4. Prevalence of liver cancer among relatives of index case

Relative		No. of blood relatives	Prevalence (%)	No. of non-blood relatives	Prevalence (%)	x^2	*P*
Male	Often live together	1464	34.84	169	17.75		>0.05
	Seldom live together	3254	16.59	1813	11.03	2.5	>0.05
	X^2		14.65				
	p		<0.01		=0.185		
Female	Often live together	1313	19.80	403	14.86	0.4	>0.05
	Seldom live together	2427	3.29	2071	2.90	0.16	>0.05
	X^2		31.9		10		
	P		<0.001		<0.001		

A history of liver cancer was more common in family members living with the cancer patient than in those living elsewhere, and it was nearly as common in non-consanguineous as in consanguineous relations (Tables 3 and 4). This familial aggregation may, however, be due to environmental rather than genetic factors.

F. Epidemiology of Animals

In Qidong County, PLC was found in ducks, chickens, pigs, and dogs. In September 1973, 1321 duck livers were studied, 43 of which were found to have PLC. The prevalence of duck PLC might be correlated with that of human PLC.

The hypothesis that HBV may be oncogenic is strengthened by recent evidence found in woodchucks (Gerin 1983). These animals contain a virus (WHV) which is morphologically and immunologically related to HBV, and appears to be associated with an extremely high prevalence of chronic hepatitis, cirrhosis, and PLC in these animals. Twenty-nine percent of woodchucks over the age of 4 years have developed PLC. The molecular biological study shows that other factors are involved in woodchuck liver tumorigenesis.

Moreover, the family of hepatitis-B-like viruses now includes HBV, WHV, ground squirrel hepatitis viruses (GSHV), and duck hepatitis B virus (DHBV). Whether a similar pathogenic or oncogenic process occurs in GSHV-infected ground squirrels and in DHBV-infected ducks remains to be seen (Summers 1981).

II. Causes

The causes of PLC are still unclear. According to our data from epidemiological studies, PLC is associated with contaminated water, mycotoxin-containing foods, and hepatitis epidemics.

A. Contaminated Drinking Water

At the turn of the century most concern was centered upon processing water to remove viruses, bacteria, and certain parasites. However, inorganic and organic chemicals have appeared as new, recognizable contaminants as a result of industrial activities (Kraybill 1980).

Comparative studies of a number of environmental factors were made in both high- and low-rate regions. One of the most outstanding factors was that inhabitants drank different types of water. In the high-rate regions, Qidong for instance, most of the inhabitants drank ditch water, whereas people in the low-rate regions, even within the same county, drank river or well (shallow or deep) water (Table 5).

The association of stagnant drinking water with liver cancer hyperendemicity has been noticed not only in Qidong and its three neighboring counties, but also in Nanhui County, a Shanghai suburb, and in the Guangxi-Zhuang Autonomous Region. In Fusui, Guangxi, 35.7% of brigade (rural, farm) people drank pool water, and the PLC mortality was 53.12/100000; however, in another low-mortality coun-

Table 5. Drinking water and number of liver cancer cases and deaths

Type of drinking water	Qidong 1971–1972			Haimen 1968–1972		
	Consumers	Cases of PLC	Incidence per 100000 per year	Consumers	PLC deaths	Death rate per 100000 per year
House ditch	28 614	58	101.35	8 946	28	62.60
Field ditch	37 941	49	64.57	15 246	30	39.35
River	11 727	10	42.64	7 178	13	34.22
Well	5 798	0	0	1 681	1	11.90
Total	84 080	117	69.58	33 051	72	43.57

ty – Ningmin (PLC mortality 8.38/100000) only 5% of brigade people drank pool water. According to a Nanning District survey, PLC mortality was 39.71/100000 among those who drank pool water; 25.77/100000, ditch water; 9.56/100000, river or stream water; 18.74/100000, spring water; 19.10/100000, shallow-well water; and 12.17/100000, deep-well water (more than 20 m deep) (Guangxi Medical College 1973, personal communication).

Beginning in 1972, inhabitants in Qidong County have been consistently encouraged to dig wells. For the assessment of this campaign, the same brigades surveyed in 1973 were surveyed again in the same way in 1978 and 1983. It was found in the second survey that a considerable proportion of the people had changed their habit of drinking ditch water and turned to well water (Table 6). (Su 1979)

B. Eating Mycotoxin-containing Foods

It is well known that there is a positive correlation between aflatoxin quantity and PLC mortality (e.g., Kenya, Swaziland) (Peers and Linsell 1973, Peers et al. 1976). In Guangxi, China, the prevalence of aflatoxin-contaminated foods is positively correlated with liver cancer mortality (Table 7).

Foods most commonly contaminated with aflatoxins are grown in warm, humid areas with plenty of rainfall, places which are also hyperendemic areas of PLC. Corn is the main food in Qidong, and aflatoxin B was detected in up to 72% of samples with an average concentration of 63.5 ppb.

However, PLC mortality is still high in some places with less contaminated water or foods. For example, people in Shanghai drink tap water and eat rice, but the mortality from PLC ist still high (male 26.62/100000, female 9.70/100000). So there may be other, more important factors involved in the cause of PLC.

C. Hepatitis

In the 1950s, in accordance with the correlation of PLC geographical variation with the incidence of viral hepatitis and postnecrotic cirrhosis, Steiner et al. first postulated that a hepatitis virus might play a role in the etiology of PLC (Steiner and Davies 1957).

Table 6. Comparison of source of drinking water and number of liver cancer cases during two periods, 1972–1973 and 1974–1978

Type of drinking water	1972–1973				1974–1978			
	Persons surveyed		Cases	Average number of cases per 100000	Persons surveyed		Cases	Average number of cases per 100000
	No.	%			No.	%		
House ditch	28 614	34.0	58	101.35	13 419	15.2	100	149.04
Field ditch	37 941	45.1	49	64.57	21 816	24.8	116	106.34
River	11 727	14.0	10	42.64	11 121	12.6	30	53.95
Well	5 798	6.9	0	0	41 815	47.4	1	4.78
Total	84 080	100.0	117	69.58	88 171	100.0	247	56.03

Table 7. Aflatoxin detection rate and liver cancer mortality in districts of Guangxi Zhuang autonomous region

District	Number of samples	Aflatoxin B_1 detection rate[a]	Liver cancer mortality/100000
A	226	1.0	8.3
B	87	1.9	9.9
C	61	2.0	15.0
D	147	2.7	15.4
E	200	2.7	16.9
F	197	4.4	23.4
G	499	4.4	25.6

[a] Relative to rate in district A

Four case-control studies in Qidong showed that 39.2% of PLC patients had a previous history of hepatitis, compared with 13.2% of controls. Another cohort study was made of 793 patients with hepatitis or cirrhosis admitted to Qidong County Hospital and 1156 respiratory patients as controls (matched by sex, age, year admitted, year observed, water source, main food, etc.). Based on the PLC incidence among respiratory patients (Table 8) the relative risks of acute hepatitis, chronic hepatitis, and cirrhosis were 2, 7, and 27 respectively. These studies included patients with hepatitis A, which is known to be unrelated to PLC. For example, in 1955–1956 in Delhi, India, a water-born epidemic of hepatitis A was documented, but there was no evidence of elevated PLC mortality when the icteric hepatitis cases were followed up (Chuttani et al. 1966). Such examples were also found in China, where several large epidemics of hepatitis A carried by water and oysters were recorded, but none of them were associated with PLC.

Since Blumberg discovered HB_sAg in 1964, many studies have been done to investigate the frequency of serological markers of HBV infection in the serum of PLC patients and of controls in different parts of the world (Blumberg and London 1981).

Table 8. Standardized incidence ratios of different types of hepatic disease and respiratory disease groups, 1973–1982

Group	Men					Women					Total				
	PY	O	E	SIR	Ratio	PY	O	E	SIR	Ratio	PY	O	E	SIR	Ratio
Respiratory disease	4989.25	5	5.56	0.90	1.0	4275.5	2	1.34	1.49	1.0	9264.75	7	6.90	1.01	1.0
Hepatic disease	4300.75	33	5.12	6.45[b]	7.2	2835.75	8	0.82	9.72[b]	6.5	7136.5	41	5.94	6.90	6.8
Acute hepatitis	2489.75	4	2.28	1.76	2.0	1586.5	1	0.31	3.27[b]	2.2	4076.25	5	2.58	1.94	1.9
Chronic hepatitis	1476.00	15	2.30	6.51[b]	7.2	988.75	3	0.40	7.48[b]	5.0	2464.75	18	2.70	6.65[b]	6.6
Cirrhosis	355.00	14	0.54	26.07[b]	29.0	260.5	4	0.12	34.48[b]	23.1	595.50	18	0.65	27.69[b]	27.4
Respiratory disease and hepatic disease	612.25	4	1.04	3.83[a]	4.2	456.0	2	0.21	9.43[a]	6.3	1068.25	6	1.26	4.78[b]	4.7

PY, Person-year; O, observed PLC cases; E expected PLC cases; SIR, O/E standardized incidence ratio; Ratio, based on respiratory disease as 1

[a] $P<0.05$ [b] $P<0.01$

In Africa, HB_sAg was detected by means of radioimmunoassay in the serum of 63% of 441 PLC patients, as compared with 4.7% of controls. In Asia, HB_sAg was found in the serum of 47% of 801 PLC patients in five studies, as compared with 8% of controls. In the United States and Western Europe, HB_sAg was initially found less frequently in PLC patients; the rate was 12% in two series using radioimmunoassay (Blumberg et al. 1975). However, Tabor et al. (1977) recently reported that 40% of PLC patients in the United States carried HB_sAg as compared with only 1% of white controls and 10% of black controls. Follow-up of PLC patients with HB_sAg revealed that almost all carried this antigen chronically, indicating that PLC was associated with the chronic HBV carrier state.

Beasley et al. (1981) reported a prospective study conducted in Taiwan Province, China, on male civil servants aged 40–59; 3454 were carriers and 19253 were noncarriers. In January 1980, after 3–4 years' follow-up, there were 42 PLC cases in the HB_sAg (+) group and only 1 in the HB_sAg (−) group, the ratio of PLC incidence (relative risk) being about 223 (mortality was 1158/100000 and 5/100000 respectively). Based on this special study, the current population of chronic HB_sAg carriers is estimated to be 200 million worldwide, the mortality from PLC being only 1–10 per 100000.

Obata (1977) in Tokyo reported another prospective study of 30 HB_sAg (+) cirrhosis patients and 85 HB_sAg (−) cirrhosis controls who were followed up and compared with respect to the chance of the development of PLC. During a 3–4 year follow-up, the risk of PLC developing in the HB_sAg (+) patients was four times that in the HB_sAg (−) controls (23.3% and 5.9% attack rate respectively).

We did two seroepidemiological surveys – in Qidong and Shanghai – in 1978, the HB_sAg prevalence being higher in PLC patients (82.9% and 76.9% respectively) and lower in overall controls (12.5% and 10.7% respectively). The prevalence of HB_sAg in other cancer patients, other disease patients, cirrhotic schistosomiasis patients, healthy persons, and blood donors was low, so the increase of HB_sAg prevalence in PLC patients was noticeable (Tables 9, 10). The prevalence of anti-HB_c was 81.8% among PLC patients and 10% among controls.

The possibility was raised that the association between HBV infection and PLC reflected an immunodeficiency in these patients, which made them more likely to develop chronic carrier-type HBV infections. This interpretation was ruled out by several observations: (a) immunological defects were not found in PLC patients; (b) HBV infections in high-prevalence regions in Africa and Asia are almost always acquired early in childhood, or many years before development of PLC; (c) 71.6%

Table 9. Prevalence of HB_sAg and anti-HB_s in PLC patients and controls in Qidong 1978

Persons	No. tested	HB_sAg		Anti-HBs	
		No. positive	%	No. positive	%
PLC	175	145	82.86	2	1.14
Controls other cancers	135	20	14.81	9	6.67
Patients other than cancers	139	21	15.11	9	6.47
Donors	1114	133	11.94	108	9.70

Table 10. Prevalence of HB_sAg and anti-HB_s in PLC patients and controls in Shanghai 1978

Persons	No. tested	HB_sAg		Anti-HB_s	
		No. positive	%	No. positive	%
PLC	143	110	76.92	4	3.64
Controls other cancers	134	17	12.69	24	17.91
Patients other than cancers	112	9	8.04	22	19.64
Cirrhotic schistosomiasis	616	67	10.88	87	14.12
Healthy	26	2	7.69	3	11.51

Table 11. Comparison of two samples of HB_sAg

	HB_sAg (+)	HB_sAg (−)	*P* value
(1973) Number of persons	1472	1478	
Male (%)	50.2	53.99	>0.05
Average age (X±SD)	37.47±1.42	37.52±1.43	>0.05
History of hepatic disease (%)	95.0	95.80	>0.05
(1983) Number of persons			
No. of follow-ups	1328	1294	
Follow-up (%)	90.22	87.55	>0.05
1973–1983 no. of blood samples examined	3.43	3.44	>0.05
1983 samples of 1096 persons			
Corn as staple food (%)	64.17	64.66	>0.05
Smoking (%)	38.57	42.26	>0.05
Drinking (%)	43.09	40.98	>0.05
Spray pesticides in 1982 (%)	23.58	23.86	>0.05

Table 12. 1973–1983 HB_sAg carrier status and PLC in men and women

Status of HB_sAg	Men				Women			
	Py	PLC			Py	PLC		
		Obs.	Exp.	SMR		Obs.	Exp.	SMR
Positive	5631.75	74	8.364	8.85**	4886.75	29	2.323	14.34**
Negative	4701.25	21	7.324	2.87**	5184	7	2.023	3.01*
(−) to (+)	213	2	0.325	6.15*	209.25	1	0.080	12.50
(+) to (−)	1221	6	2.081	2.88*	1242	0	0.592	–

* $P<0.05$ ** $P<0.01$

of mothers with PLC were HBV carriers, as compared with 16.6% of fathers as matched controls, suggesting that most PLC patients acquired this infection during infancy through maternal-fetal or maternal-infant transmission (Blumberg 1980).

We have made a prospective study in Qidong of 1475 discordant pairs of persons; one of each pair was HB_sAg (+), the other (−). They were found in a county-wide screening program (CIEP) and matched by age, sex, and residence (Table 11).

Table 13. 1973–1983 HB_sAg carrier status and age group, sex

Age group (yrs)	HB_sAg (+)			HB_sAg (−)			RR
	Py	PLC cases	MOR ‰	Py	PLC cases	MOR ‰	
Men							
<20	494.5	0	0	407.5	1	2.45	–
20–29	963	6	6.23	706.5	0	0	–
30–39	1447.75	15	10.36	1040	3	2.88	3.60
40–49	1389.5	15	10.80	1147.5	7	6.10	1.77
50–59	874.5	24	27.44	842.5	9	10.68	2.60
60+	462.5	14	30.27	557.25	1	1.79	16.91
	5631.75	74	13.14	4701.25	21	4.47	2.94
Women							
<20	333	0	0	323.5	0	0	–
20–29	660.75	0	0	537.5	1	1.86	–
30–39	1163.5	1	0.86	1083.5	0	0	
40–49	1415.75	11	7.77	1492.75	3	2.01	3.87
50–59	855.5	12	14.03	1158.75	1	8.63	1.63
60+	458.25	5	10.91	588	2	3.40	3.21
	4886.75	29	5.93	5184	7	1.35	4.39

Table 14. 1973–1983 HB_sAg carrier status and PLC in two periods

Period (yrs)	Sex	HB_sAg (+)				HB_sAg (−)				
		Py	PLC	MOR (%)	SMR	Py	PLC	MOR (%)	SMR	RR
1973–1977	M	2790.25	30	5.87	7.79	2230.5	13	2.57	4.03	2.28
	F	2387	5	3.68	16.59	2433.75	2	0.32	2.07	11.50
1978–1983	M	2841.5	44	7.49	7.79	2470.75	8	5.16	1.95	1.45
	F	2499.75	14	2.01	12.50	2750.75	5	1.31	3.72	1.53

Py, Person – year; PLC, PLC cases; MOR, standardized mortality according to chinese population proportion, 1964; SMR, standardized mortality ratio

Table 15. 1973–1983 Hepatitis B antigen status in cohort subjects who developed malignancies, standardized mortality[a] (per 100000)

Cancer sites	HB_sAg (+)		HB_sAg (−)		RR	
	M	F	M	F	M	F
Liver	6.75	2.68	3.11	1.35	2.17	1.98
Stomach	0.28	0.07	0.26	0.12	1.08	0.58
Esophagus	0.20	0	0.17	0.11	1.18	–
Others	0.44	0.24	0.43	0.55	1.02	0.44

[a] Standardized according to Chinese population proportion, 1964

Table 11 shows that there were no significant differences between men and women regarding average age, hepatic disease history, number of blood samples examined, and eating, smoking, and drinking habits (RPHA used to examine blood).

There is a three- to fivefold difference between the standard mortality ratio (SMR) of positive and negative groups (8.85–14.34 to 2.87–3.01) (Table 12). Table 13 shows that the patterns of age-specific mortality for both the HB_sAg (+) and the HB_sAg (−) group are similar, but that the crude relative risks differ by 2.94- to 4.39-fold (Table 13). The HB_sAg carrier status and PLC in two periods, 1973–1977 and 1978–1983, did not show any great difference (Table 14). Table 15 shows that this relation to HB_sAg status is specific for liver cancer but not for other types (Table 15).

Many questions remain to be answered: e.g., in some places the incidence of PLC is reported to be low despite the high HBV carrier rate, and some special geographical distributions cannot be explained by HB_sAg prevalence. However, the present status of our knowledge of the relation between HBV and PLC has practical implications already.

A recent finding from molecular biological research strengthens the hypothesis that HBV may be oncogenic. HBV-DNA was isolated directly from Dane particles obtained from plasma of chronic carriers or from the successful cloning of HBV DNA in *Escherichia coli* by recombinant DNA methods. In 1980, four groups of researchers (Marion et al., Chakraborty et al., Edman et al., Brechot et al.) reported that HBV was integrated into cellular DNA in the PLC/PRF/5 cell line from PLC tissue. Furthermore, integrated HBV DNA was also seen in the DNA isolated from PLC tissue obtained from an HBV carrier who died of PLC (Prince 1981). The conclusion that HBV is an oncogenic virus cannot be drawn at this time for HBV-DNA integration in both tumor and nontumor tissue. The presence of both integrated and episomal forms of HBV-DNA in some carriers with serological markers of active viral replication but without hepatoma suggests that integration may be antecedent to PLC. As in chronic HBV infection, both episomal and integrated forms of WHV-DNA have been detected in tumor and nontumor tissues of the infected woodchuck; in one study, however, the prevalence of WHV-DNA in woodchuck tumors and WHV-DNA integration in nontumor tissue was much lower than that observed in human cases of PLC, suggesting that other factors are also involved in woodchuck liver tumorigenesis (Summers 1981).

D. Others

1. Pesticides

There is no difference between healthy people and tumor patients in Shanghai and Qidong with regard to the levels of DDT and BHC in human fat (Table 16).

According to epidemiological investigations in southeastern China to date, the mortality for PLC in different periods and places did not show any association with the type, quality, and quantity of pesticides.

Table 16. Levels of DDT and BHC in human fat

Region	Subjects	Number of samples	pp'-DDE $\bar{X} \pm SE$	pp'-DDT $\bar{X} \pm SE$	BHC $\bar{X} \pm SE$
Shanghai	Healthy people	47	5.26±0.96	2.39±0.51	1.90±0.32
	Tumor patients	16	1.66±1.16	2.45±0.79	1.83±1.33
	Other patients	44	4.17±0.58	2.48±0.38	1.57±0.44
Qidong	Other patients	47	2.78±0.54	1.52±0.36	0.22±0.08
	Tumor patients	16	3.42±0.71	2.28±0.79	0.51±0.22

2. Trace Elements

It is still unknown what role trace elements play in the etiology of PLC. In some areas the concentrations of Cu, Zn, Ni, and Co in drinking water are high and that of Mo is low; in hair and blood, Cu and Mo content are also high and low respectively. The levels of Se in grain and water do not show any close relationship.

3. Ionizing Radiation

The measurements of ionizing radiation in PLC endemic areas were all below the standard of our country.

4. Parasites

Clonorchis sinensis (the Chinese liver fluke) is found only in a few endemic areas of PLC in the southern part of China. This parasite is associated with cancer of the bile duct rather than with primary hepatocellular cancer.

5. Drinking Alcoholic Beverages

According to retrospective studies, there is no association between drinking habits and PLC.

III. Multivariate Analysis of Causes

There are many factors operating simultaneously in PLC mortality. However, for carcinogenic risk factors the question is even more difficult; it may be that one of them is the *most* important factor. It may be that all contribute to PLC, but none is predominant. The methods of multivariate analysis – trend analysis, stepwise regression, and sequential interaction detection algorithm (SIDA), have been used in trying to establish the relationship among factors and to detect the main factor (Andersen et al. 1971; Department of Health Statistics of Hunan Medical College 1980).

We selected 106 counties randomly, including 19 in Fujian, 15 in Jiangxi, 19 in Zhejiang, 12 in Jiangsu, 40 in Anhui, and one in Shanghai (Fig. 6). Twelve variables

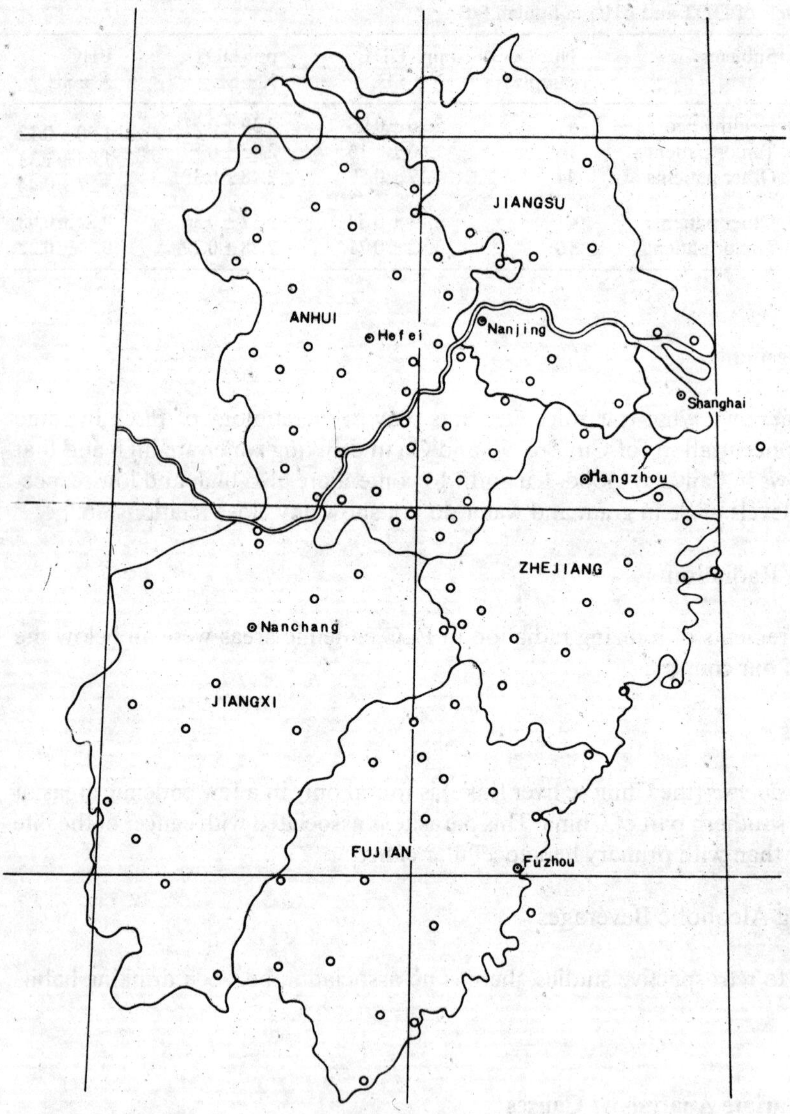

Fig. 6. The location of 106 counties studied

were used, including PLC-standardized mortality, PLC-truncated mortality, cirrhosis-standardized mortality, longitude, latitude, temperature/humidity index (total days of ⩾30 °C and RH⩾80% in 10 years), brackish, island/mainland, or river areas, and the peanut, corn, and sweet potato productions (in 1958).

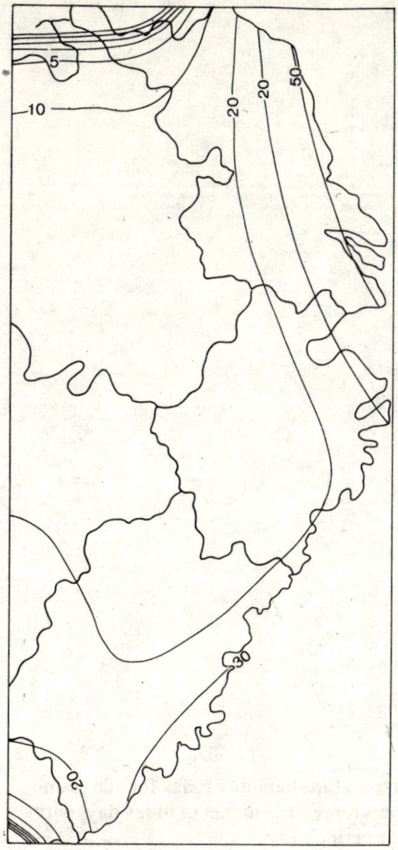

Fig. 7. Standardized mortality of PLC for 106 counties (numbers/100000)

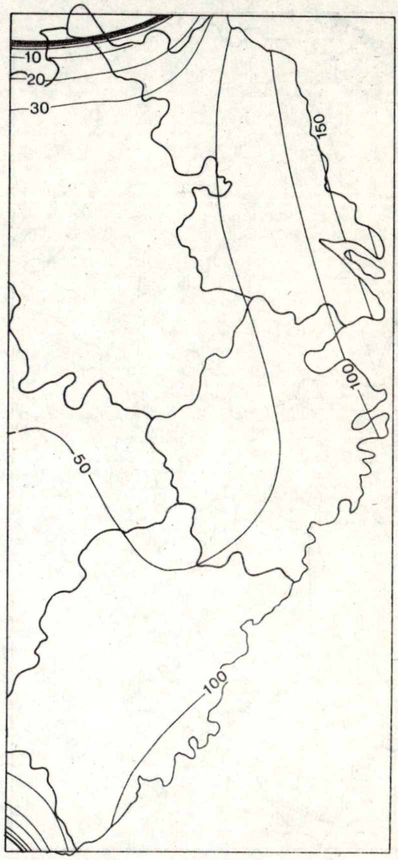

Fig. 8. Truncated mortality of PLC for 106 counties (numbers/100000)

A. Trend Analysis

Latitude and longitude are used as independent variables X_i and Y_i; B_i represents the other, dependent variable. In every county a mathematical model from the data obtained can be acquired as follows:

1st. county $B_1 = a_{11} + a_{12}X_1 + a_{13}Y_1 + a_{14}X_1^2 + a_{15}Y_1^2 + a_{16}X_1Y_1 + a_{17}X_1^3 + \ldots + a_{121}Y_1^5$

2nd. county $B_2 = a_{21} + a_{22}X_2 + a_{23}Y_2 + a_{24}X_2^2 + a_{25}Y_2^2 + a_{26}X_2Y_2 + a_{27}X_2^3 + \ldots + a_{221}Y_2^5$

$\vdots$

106th. county $B_{106} = a_{1061} + a_{1062}X_{106} + a_{1063}Y_{106} + a_{1064}X_{106}^2 + \ldots + a_{10621}Y_{106}^5$

In ordinary cases, the method of least squares can solve this polynomial equation (from $a_1 \ldots a_{21}$); sometimes the single value decomposition (SVD) method is better than that of least squares.

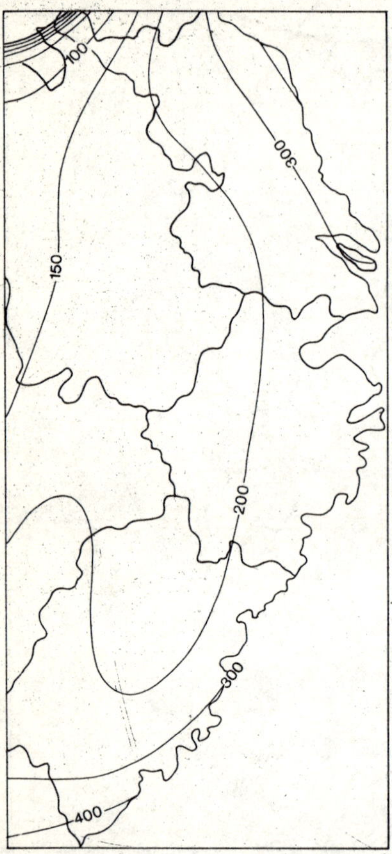

Fig. 9. Temperature-humidity index for 106 counties (numbers represent number of index days within a 10-year period)

All the procedures are done by computer until the geographic figures are drawn. Unfortunately, the results did not show any close association between PLC mortality and variable, other than the temperature/humidity index (degree of fitness =0.355) (Figs. 7–9).

B. Stepwise Techniques

Trend analysis is a kind of mutliple linear regression method. The shortcoming of the method is that the relationship of variables cannot be explained clearly.

Stepwise multiple regression is a statistical technique for analyzing the relationship between dependent variables and a set of independent variables in order of importance. The criterion of importance is based on the reduction of sums of squares, and the independent variables most important in this reduction in a given step are entered in the regression (Table 17). If the longitude and latitude were deleted, the equation would be as follows:

$$
\begin{aligned}
\text{Y (Liver cancer mortality)} = {} & 40.0325 - 5.431\text{Riv}^{***} + 5.57788\text{Brack}^{*} \\
& + 0.0159\text{T–H}^{*} - 0.2498\text{Corn} + 0.0028 \\
& \text{Ele} - 0.0656\text{Cir} - 0.1702\text{Isl} + 0.1159 \\
& \text{Pean} + 0.0117\text{S.Pot}
\end{aligned}
$$

Multiple correlation coefficient = 0.702
(Adjusted for degree of freedom $r = 0.671$)
F = 10.337 (d.f. = 9.96)
* $p < 0.05$ *** $p < 0.001$

C. Sequential Interaction Detection Algorithm

In SIDA analysis, a series of independent variables may be studied simultaneously in relation to one dependent variable to determine which variables enter the analysis and specify the form of the relations between the variables. This is done by successively dividing the original data set into pairs of subgroups, which differ as much as possible from each other with respect to the mean value of the dependent variable. Each of the pairs of subgroups may then be eligible to be further split into a parent group and subdivided at the class of the independent variables, which account for the largest amount of dependent variable variation in the subgroup.

The division ends when two of the subgroups to be formed do not fullfil the desired level of significance. The results of the analysis are presented as follows (Fig. 10):

The entire data set is split initially into brackish and river water (numbers 2, 3, 4 and 5). Thus, an important preventive measure should stress the change of the water sources. Two groups are distinguished within group 4 on the basis of corn, but the quantity does not show the relationship. Group 11 is split into two subgroups of temperature-humidity index. The staple food and the condition in which food is

Table 17. Coefficient correlations of ten variables among 106 counties

	Mor[a]	Ele	T-H	Cir	Isl	Brack	Riv	Pean	Corn	S Pot
Mortality	1.00	−0.07	0.38	−0.21	−0.38	0.62	−0.63	0.11	−0.18	0.21
Elevation		1.00	−0.28	0.02	0.05	−0.15	0.23	−0.06	−0.12	0.19
Temperature-humidity index			1.00	−0.03	−0.24	0.35	−0.24	0.26	−0.04	0.10
Cirrhosis				1.00	0.10	0.18	0.29	0.01	−0.09	−0.00
Island/mainland					1.00	−0.49	0.40	−0.26	0.13	−0.57
Brackish water						1.00	−0.74	−0.74	0.17	0.27
River							1.00	−0.09	0.05	−0.15
Peanuts								1.00	0.13	0.20
Maize									1.00	−0.19
Sweet potatos										1.00

[a] *Mor,* Mortality of PLC (standardized according to Chinese population proportion 1964); *Ele,* elevation; *T-H,* temperature/humidity index; *Cir,* standardized mortality of cirrhosis; *Isl,* island/mainland; *Brack,* brackish water; *Riv,* river water; *Pean,* peanut %; *Corn,* corn %; *S Pot,* sweet potato %

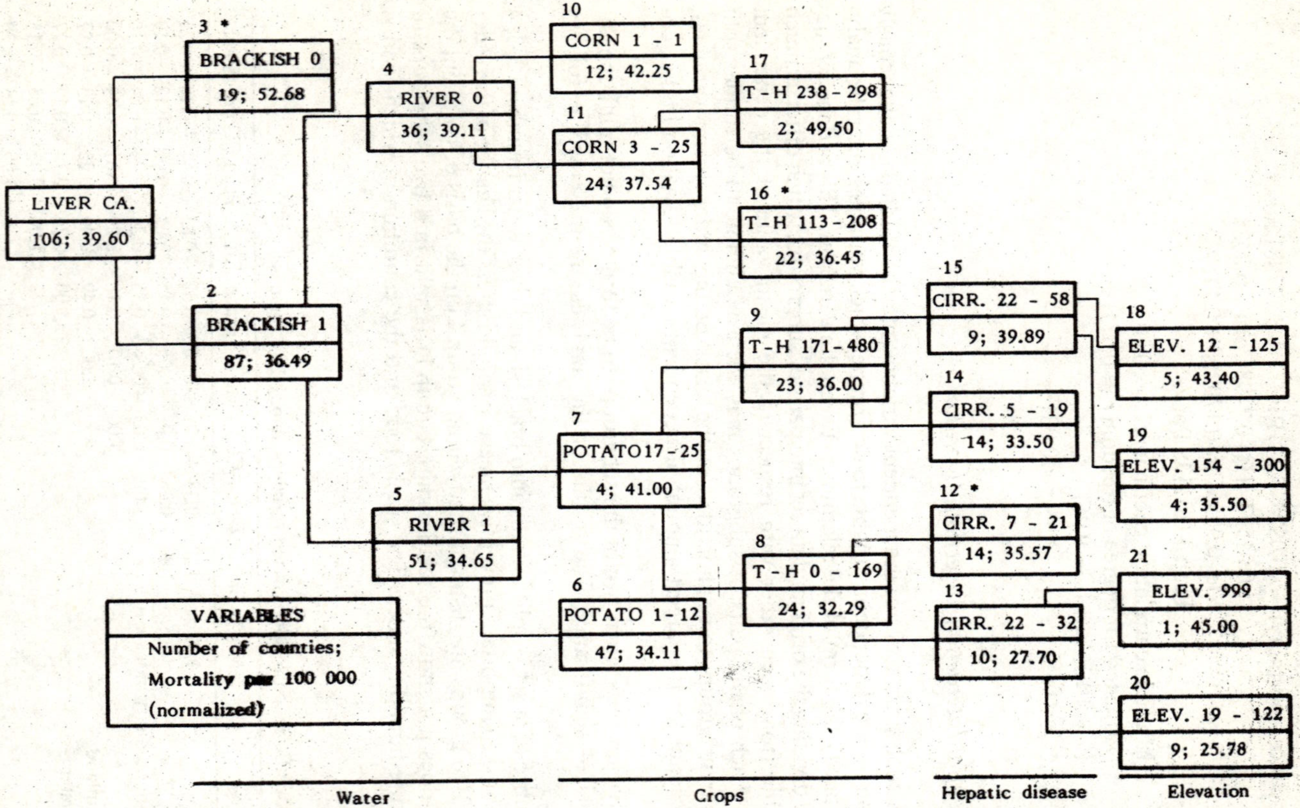

Fig. 10. Epidemiological variables of primary liver cancer in southeastern China (latitudes and longitudes deleted) *Asterisk*, Split end
$R^2 = 0.655$

conserved are also important. The last two sets of the split groups show that hepatic disease (cirrhosis) is associated with PLC.

The stratification model represented by the "tree" (Fig. 10) accounts for 66% of the overall data ($R^2 = 0.665$).

IV. Prevention

Prevention is always being emphasized in China, even though the causes of PLC are still unclear. The common prevention mottoes that have been accepted are "control of water, control of corn, and prevention of hepatitis." Moreover, among high-risk groups we can do PLC screening by AFP for early detection, diagnosis, and treatment.

A. Control of Water

According to the epidemiological investigation, PLC incidence and mortality are high for people who live in hyperendemic areas and drink pond or ditch water. So the government puts stress on improving the quality of drinking water by urging peasants to drink well water and by providing financial aid to them in drilling both shallow and deep wells. For example, in Qidong County, as of 1982 there were hundreds of deep wells supplying tap water for about 11% of local residents and thousands of shallow wells supplying about half of the population.

Hygienic control of drinking water must be supervised periodically by the local antiepidemic station. It is necessary to disinfect shallow-well water, especially in summer. Disinfection not only removes the bacteria, but also resolves nitrates and nitrites and prevents them from forming nitrosamines. However, attention is also paid to organic compounds with mutagenic and carcinogenic properties present in drinking water.

B. Control of Crops

Aflatoxins are detected in certain foods grown in hot and humid areas (corn, peanuts etc.), from which *Aspergillus flavus* can be isolated. These toxins cause disease in animals and fish and are carcinogenic for experimental animals, but adverse effects on man have not been proven. Nevertheless, the presence of aflatoxins in foods presents a serious threat to human health.

Corn and peanuts should be dried as quickly as possible when they are harvested. Before they are stored the water content must be lowered to 12.5%. All storage containers must be disinfected before being filled with corn and peanuts. Should the corn and peanuts be contaminated with aflatoxins, measures such as treatment with alkalis and white kaolin to absorb the aflatoxin in peanut oil are taken to detoxify them.

C. Prevention of Hepatitis

Hepatitis B infection is now shown to be preventable by hepatitis B vaccine. Szmuness et al. (1980) reported a double-blind trial with 1083 homosexual men. The vaccine was found to be safe, with few side effects. Within 2 months, 77% of the vaccinated subjects had high levels of antibody against the HB_sAg. After the booster dose the rate increased to 96%. For the first 18 months of follow-up, hepatitis B or subclinical infection developed in only 1.4%–3.4% of the vaccine recipients as compared with 18%–27% of placebo recipients. According to the experience of Maupas et al. (1981) in Senegal, HB vaccine can also be used in children under 2 years of age. After 12 months of follow-up, the incidence of the HB_sAg carrier state was found to be reduced by 85% among susceptible children ($P<0.0001$). In China we have done a similar trial and the initial anti-HB_s results are encouraging. We are now planning to use vaccine for infants and in PLC hyperendemic areas.

The first pilot trial for infant vaccine shows that about 95% of the 30 infants of HB_sAg (+) mothers injected with HB vaccine when they were born had developed the anti-HB_s within 6 months.

We suggest that all donors be screened regularly for HBV markers, and that the medical instrument which is contaminated with blood be disinfected.

D. Screening

Screening for liver cancer by measuring AFP levels is recommended for people over 30 years of age who have hepatic disease or a family history of it. Mass screening is not recommended, because it is expensive and not easy to organize. So screening is, and should be, limited to high-risk groups and to hyperendemic areas.

Suspected patients with high and persistent AFP titers should be diagnosed, but patients with low and variable titers should also be followed up.

We believe that the implementation of the prevention mottoes will help to control cancer-causing factors, and that the incidence and mortality of PLC will be reduced as time goes on.

References

Andersen R, Smedby B, Eklund G (1971) Approaches and techniques – automatic interaction detector program for analyzing health survey data. Health Serv Res [Summer] 165–83

Beasley RP, Hwang LY, Lin CC, et al. (1981) Hepatocellular carcinoma and hepatitis B virus: a prospective study of 22707 men in Taiwan. Lancet II: 1129–1132

Blumberg BS (1980) The hepatitis B virus. Public Health Rep 95: 427–435

Blumberg BS, London WT (1981) Hepatitis B virus and the prevention of primary hepatocellular carcinoma. N Engl J Med 304: 782–84

Blumberg BS, Larouze B, London WT, et al. (1975) The relation of infection with the hepatitis B agent to primary hepatic carcinoma. Am J Pathol 81: 669–682

Bréchot C, Pourcel C, Louise A, et al. (1980) Presence of integrated hepatitis B virus DNA sequences in cellular DNA of human hepatocellular carcinoma. Nature 286: 533–535

Chakraborty PR, Ruiz-Opazo N, Shouval D, et al. (1980) Identification of integrated hepatitis B virus DNA and expression of viral RNA in an HB_sAg-producing human hepatocellular carcinoma cell line. Nature 286: 531–533

Chuttani HK, Sidhu AS, Wig KL, et al. (1966) Follow-up study of cases from Delhi epidemic of infections hepatitis of 1955–1956. Br Med J 2: 676–679

Editorial Committee (1979) Atlas of cancer mortality in the People's Republic of China. China Map Press, p 41

Department of Health Statitics of Hunan Medical College (1980) Medical multivariate analysis. Human Scientific and Technical Publisher[1]

Edman IC, Gray P, Valenzuela P, et al. (1980) Integration of hepatitis B virus sequences and their expression in a human hepatoma cell. Nature 286: 535–538

Gerin JL (1983) Hepatitis B virus and primary hepatocellular carcinoma. Gastroenterology 84: 869–876

Kraybill HF (1980) Evaluation of public health aspects of carcinogenic/mutagenic biorefractories in drinking water. Prev Med 9: 212–218

Marion PL, Salazar FH, Alexander JJ, et al. (1980) State of hepatitis B viral DNA in a human hepatome cell line. J Virol 33: 795–806

Maupas P, Goudeau A, Coursaget P, et al. (1981) Efficacy of hepatitis B vaccine in prevention of early HB_sAg carrier state in children. Lancet II: 289–292

Obata H (1977) Hepatitis B virus and liver cancer and cirrhosis of the liver. Clinician 24: 63

Ong GB, Chan PKW (1976) Primary carcinoma of the liver. Surg Gynecol Obstet 143: 31–38

Peers FG, Linsell CA (1973) Dietary aflatoxins and liver cancer – a population based study in Kenya. Br J Cancer 27: 473–484

Peers FG, Gilman GA, Linsell CA (1976) Dietary aflatoxins and human liver cancer in Swaziland. Int J Cancer 17: 167

Prince AM (1981) Hepatitis B virus and hepatocellular carcinoma: molecular biology provides further evidence for an etiologic association. Hepatology 1: 73–75

Steiner PE, Davies JNP (1957) Cirrhosis and primary liver carcinoma in Ugandan Africans. Br J Cancer 11: 523–534

Su DL (1979) Drinking water and liver cell cancer: An epidemiological approach to the etiology of this disease in China. Chin Med J 92: 748–756

Summers J (1981) Three recently described animal virus models for human hepatitis B virus. Hepatology 1: 179–183

Szmuness W, Stevens CE, Harley EJ, et al. (1980) Hepatitis B vaccine. N Engl J Med 303: 833–841

Tabor E, Gerety RJ, Vogel CL, et al. (1977) Hepatitis B virus infection and primary hepatocellular carcinoma. J Natl Cancer Inst 58: 1197–1200

18 Hepatitis B Virus and Hepatocellular Carcinoma – Clinical and Serological Aspects

Yang Bing-hui, Tang Zhao-you

Strong evidence of a liver disease background in hepatocellular carcinoma has been noted for decades (Berman 1958). HCC is usually associated with cirrhosis of the liver, which is the case in many areas of the world (Popper 1979). Macronodular, posthepatitic, or postnecrotic cirrhosis rather than micronodular or nutritional cirrhosis have been accepted as HCC-related cirrhosis (Ma and Yang 1965; Mori 1967). The discovery of HBV markers has evoked an increasing interest in the close correlation between HBV infection and HCC. Chronic B-type viral hepatitis has been identified as the main cause of these types of cirrhosis (Blumberg 1975), and a hypothesis of B-type viral heptatitis/macronodular cirrhosis/HCC has been suggested (Vogel et al. 1970; Blumberg 1977). Epidemiological data on the relationship between HBV and HCC have been presented in the preceding chapter, and cellular, molecular, and pathological aspects will be delineated in Chaps. 19 and 20; therefore, only clinical and serological aspects will be discussed in this chapter.

I. Brief Review of Literature Concerning Correlation Between HBV and HCC

The relation of HCC to infection with hepatitis B and related viruses in man and animals had been thoroughly discussed by Popper et al. (1982) and widely discussed in the literature (Zuckerman 1979; Prince 1981). Evidence for the correlation between HBV and HCC in humans stems from (a) epidemiological observations (Szmuness 1978; Prince and Alcabes 1982; Beasley 1982); (b) serological studies of the close association of HBV markers and HCC – both in high-risk areas (Kew et al. 1979; Gibson et al. 1980; Ilardi et al. 1980; Lingao et al. 1981; Chien et al. 1981; Chung et al. 1983) and in low incidence areas (Bassendine et al. 1978; Trichopolo et al. 1978; McCaughan et al. 1979; Yarrish et al. 1980) and found in both noncirrhotic and highly cirrhotic livers (Okuda et al. 1982); (c) the presence of HB_sAg and HB_cAg in hepatocytes of patients with HCC on histopathological observation (Popper et al. 1982; Akagi et al. 1982); (d) the secretion of HB_sAg by HCC cells in culture, detectable in nude mice after transplantation (Shouvel et al. 1981); and (e) signs of integration of HBV-DNA sequences in cellular DNA of human HCC (Bréchot et al. 1980; Shafritz et al. 1981), even in HCC originating in alcoholic liver disease with negative HBV markers in serum (Bréchot et al. 1982). Thus, a virological approach to the prevention of primary liver cancer by either passive or active immunization has been suggested (Zuckerman 1982).

II. Clinical Evidence of Correlation Between HBV and HCC

During the period from May 1978 to April 1983, 138 cases of HCC (HCC group) were collected at the authors' Hospital for the study of the correlation between HBV and HCC. Of the 138 cases, 92 cases were pathologically proven; the rest were diagnosed by means of positive findings of serum AFP, angiography, ultrasonography, scintiscan, and other measurements. A group consisting of 32 cases of secondary liver cancer, hepatic hemangioma, hepatic abscess, adenoma of liver, and diseases other than hepatitis, cirrhosis, and HCC was employed as control.

A. History of Hepatitis and Liver Cirrhosis

In 76 (55.1%) patients of the HCC group there was a history of hepatitis or cirrhosis. The history of hepatitis ranged from 1 to 24 years, averaging 12.1 years. In the control group, however, only six (18.8%) of the 32 patients had a history of hepatitis or cirrhosis, a significant statistical difference ($P < 0.01$) compared with HCC patients.

B. Serological Evidence of HBV Markers

HBV markers were detected in the HCC group and control group using RPHA for HB_sAg, passive hemagglutination (PHA) for anti-HB_s and enzyme-linked immunosorbent assay (ELISA) for anti-HB_c. The results are summarized in Table 1. The positive rates of HBV markers in HCC patients (except for those with anti-HB_s) were significantly higher than those of patients with other liver diseases in the control group ($P < 0.01$), and similar to those in patients with cirrhosis or chronic hepatitis ($P > 0.05$), suggesting that HCC is closely related to HBV infection in China. The positive rates of HBV markers in HCC patients without a history of hepatitis mimicked those of their counterparts (Table 2).

Some investigators demonstrated that the incidence of serum HB_sAg was higher in patients with HCC who were younger and AFP positive (Kew et al. 1979; Vogel et al. 1970; Wu and Lam 1979); however, in the authors' series, sex, age, AFP, and associated cirrhosis were not related to the positive rate of HBV markers in patients with HCC ($P > 0.05$) (Table 3).

C. Other Laboratory and Pathological Findings

Findings of abnormal liver function (ALT and/or ZnTT) in the HCC group were higher than those in the control group: 38.4% (53/138) versus 15.6% (5/32) ($P < 0.05$). Since patients in both groups had local lesions, the higher rate of abnormal liver function indicated the existence of diffuse liver disease in the HCC group.

Pathologically, liver cirrhosis or chronic hepatitis was found in 80 (87.0%) patients of the HCC group who underwent surgery; however, only one (4.5%) case in the control group was associated with mild chronic hepatitis ($P < 0.01$).

Table 1. Serum HBV marker in miscellaneous liver diseases

	No. of cases	HB_sAg *n* (%)	Anti-HB_s *n* (%)	Anti-HB_c *n* (%)	At least one (+) *n* (%)
HCC	138	96 (69.6)	7 (5.1)	105 (76.1)	128 (92.8)
Pathologically proven	92	66 (71.7)	4 (4.4)	70 (76.1)	86 (93.5)
Clinical diagnosis	46	30 (65.2)	3 (6.5)	35 (76.1)	42 (91.3)
Cirrhosis or chronic hepatitis	26	18 (69.2)	1 (3.8)	19 (73.1)	21 (80.8)
Other liver diseases	32	6 (18.8)	8 (25.0)	6 (18.8)	13 (40.6)

Table 2. Serum HBV markers in HCC cases with or without history of hepatitis

	No. of cases	HB_sAg *n* (%)	Anti-HB_s *n* (%)	Anti-HB_c *n* (%)	At least one (+) *n* (%)
History of hepatitis (+)	76	56 (73.7)	4 (5.3)	58 (76.3)	73 (96.1)
History of hepatitis (−)	62	40 (64.5)	3 (4.8)	47 (75.8)	55 (88.7)

Table 3. Factors that may influence positive rate of HBV markers in HCC cases

	No. of cases	HB_sAg *n* (%)	Anti-HB_s *n* (%)	Anti-HB_c *n* (%)	At least one (+) *n* (%)
Sex – Male	126	90 (71.4)	7 (5.6)	97 (76.9)	118 (93.7)
Female	12	6 (50.0)	0	8 (66.6)	10 (83.3)
Age –19	3	2 (66.6)	0	2 (66.6)	2 (66.6)
20–29	11	10 (90.9)	0	6 (54.5)	10 (90.9)
30–39	18	14 (77.8)	1 (5.6)	16 (88.9)	17 (94.4)
40–49	49	31 (65.9)	3 (6.4)	38 (80.9)	45 (95.8)
50–59	50	33 (66.0)	3 (6.0)	36 (72.0)	46 (92.0)
60–	9	6 (66.7)	0	7 (77.8)	8 (86.7)
AFP > 20 ng/ml	115	80 (69.6)	6 (5.2)	86 (74.8)	107 (93.0)
⩽ 20 ng/ml	23	16 (69.6)	1 (4.3)	19 (82.6)	21 (91.3)
Cirrhosis (+)	74	55 (74.3)	4 (5.4)	56 (75.5)	70 (94.6)
(−)	12	6 (50.0)	0	8 (66.7)	10 (83.3)

III. Liver Disease Background of SCHCC

Strong evidence concerning liver disease background has also been found in the study of small HCC (Tang et al. 1979). In 1977, Okuda et al. reported 20 cases with small HCC, 18 (90%) of them associated with cirrhosis (16 cases with severe cirrhosis); mild fibrosis with chronic inflammation was noted in the remaining two cases.

Similar results were observed in our series in 1978. Of the 20 cases of small HCC with complete pathological data, 15 (75%) were associated with chronic hepatitis and 16 (80%) with cirrhosis (Ying and Chai 1978). In 1979, a report from Qidong

Table 4. HBV markers in SCHCC and CHCC patients

	No. of cases	HB_sAg n (%)	Anti-HB_s n (%)	Anti-HB_c n (%)	At least one (+) n (%)
SCHCC	30	21 (70.0)	2 (6.7)	22 (73.3)	28 (93.3)
CHCC	62	45 (72.6)	2 (3.2)	48 (77.4)	58 (95.3)

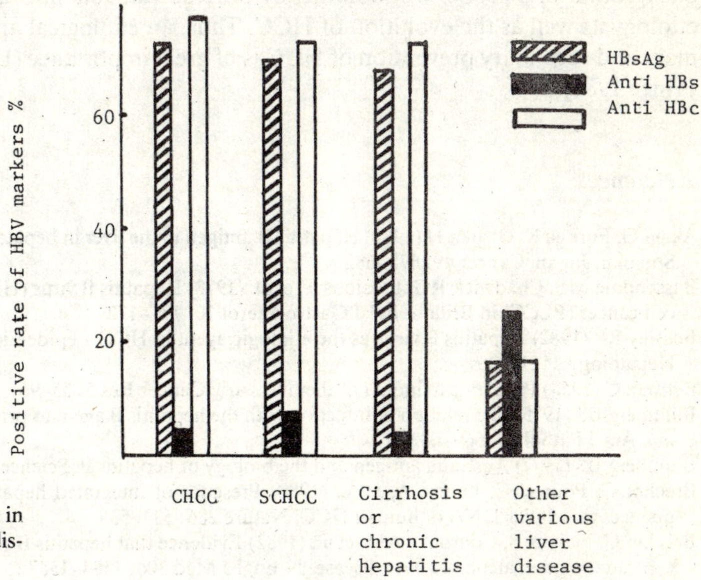

Fig. 1. HBV markers in miscellaneous liver diseases

County, a high-risk area in China, again verified the extremely close association of HBV with hepatitis and cirrhosis. Of the 30 cases with HCC ⩽3 cm, cirrhosis appeared in 28 (91.1%), and hepatitis appeared in the whole series, orcein-positive-stain being found in 90% of the surrounding liver (Sun et al. 1979). Chen et al. (1982) reported 13 cases of HCC ⩽3 cm. The close relation to HBV was also recorded as follows: the positive rate of HB_sAg was 92%, anti-HB_s 8%, HB_eAg 15%, and anti-HB_e 85%; 11 (85%) cases were associated with cirrhosis and the remaining two with fibrosis. Our latest report, comprising 90 cases of SCHCC, revealted that 50 (55.6%) had a history of hepatitis, HB_sAg (RPHA) being positive in 41 of checked 57 (71.9%), and cirrhosis found in 60 of 70 (85.7%) (Tang et al. 1983).

Table 4 lists a comparison of SCHCC and CHCC for positivity of HBV markers, showing similar incidences of HBV infection in both stages. To sum up, akin to large HCC, SCHCC follows a similar pattern in regard to the close relationship with type-B viral hepatitis and cirrhosis.

In accordance with the authors' data, it should be emphasized that the positive rate of anti-HB_s was significantly lower in the HCC group than in the control group. Similar results were found in patients with cirrhosis or chronic hepatitis (Fig. 1).

Blumberg (1977) suggested that a deficiency of anti-HB_s represents an immune deficiency. According to the authors' data, an immune deficiency in HCC patients might begin in the subclinical stage of the disease, or even appear in the stage of cirrhosis and chronic hepatitis. This suggests that an insufficient production of antibody after HBV infection in some patients will lead to persistent infection with HBV, chronic active hepatitis, posthepatitic cirrhosis, and ultimately HCC (Blumberg 1977; Hann et al. 1979; Sung and Chen 1980).

Subclinical HCC is a new concept (Tang et al. 1982); the study of liver disease background in SCHCC will doubtlessly provide valuable information as to the of etiology as well as the evolution of HCC. Thus, an etiological approach to the primary and secondary prevention of HCC is of great importance (Larouze et al. 1979; Prince 1981).

References

Akagi G, Furuga K, Otsuka H (1982) Hepatitis B antigen in the liver in hepatocellular carcinoma in Shikoku, Japan. Cancer 49: 678–682

Bassendine MF, Chadwick RG, Lyssiotis T, et al. (1978) Hepatitis B virus (HBV) and primary liver cell cancer (PLCC) in Britain. Ital J Gastroenterol 10: 171–172

Beasley RP (1982) Hepatitis B virus as the etiologic agent in HCC – epidemiologic considerations. Hepatology 2: 21s–26s

Berman C (1958) Primary carcinoma of the liver. Adv Cancer Res 5: 55–96

Blumberg BS (1975) The relation of infection with the hepatitis B agent to primary hepatic carcinoma. Am J Pathol 81: 669–682

Blumberg BS (1977) Australia antigen and the biology of hepatitis B. Science 197: 17–25

Bréchot C, Pourcel C, Louise A, et al. (1980) Presence of integrated hepatitis B virus DNA sequences in cellular DNA of human HCC. Nature 286: 533–535

Bréchot C, Nalpas B, Courouce AM, et al. (1982) Evidence that hepatitis B virus has a role in liver cell carcinoma in alcoholic liver disease. N Engl J Med 306: 1384–1387

Chen DS, Sheu JC, Sung JL, et al. (1982) Small hepatocellular carcinoma – a clinicopathological study in thirteen patients. Gastroenterology 83: 1109–1119

Chien MC, Tong MJ, Lok J, et al. (1981) Hepatitis B viral markers in patients with primary hepatocellular carcinoma in Taiwan. J Natl Cancer Inst 66: 475–479

Chung WK, Sun HS, Park DH, et al. (1983) Primary hepatocellular carcinoma and hepatitis B virus infection in Korea. J Med Virol 11: 99–104

Gibson JB, Wu PC, Ho JC, Lauder U (1980) Hepatitis B surface antigen in hepatocellular carcinoma and cirrhosis in Hong Kong – a necropsy study 1963–1976. Br J Cancer 42: 370–377

Hann HL, London WT, Whitford P, et al. (1979) Hepatitis B virus and primary hepatocellular carcinoma family studies in Korea. Proc Am Assoc Cancer Res 20: 432

Ilardi CF, Ying YY, Ackerman LV, Elias JM (1980) Hepatitis B surface antigen and hepatocellular carcinoma in the People's Republic of China. Cancer 46: 1612–1616

Kew MC, Desmyter J, Bradburne AF, et al. (1979) Hepatitis B virus infection in Southern African blacks with hepatocellular cancer. J Natl Cancer Inst 62: 517–520

Larouze B, London WT, Werner BG, et al. (1979) Studies on the prevention of primary hepatic carcinoma, parental influences on the transmission of and host responses to hepatitis B virus. Cancer Detect Prev 2: 65–74

Lingao AL, Domingo EO, Nishioka K (1981) Hepatitis B virus profile of hepatocellular carcinoma in the Philippines. Cancer 48: 1590–1595

Ma ZZ, Yang KZ (1965) Relationship between cirrhosis and liver cancer. Acta Acad Med Primae Shanghai 3: 121

McCaughan GW, Parsons C, Gallagher ND (1979) Emerging patterns of hepatitis B chronic liver disease in Australia. Aust NZJ Med 9: 359–364

Mori W (1967) Cirrhosis and primary cancer of the liver. Cancer 20: 627

Okuda K, Nakashima T, Obata H, et al. (1977) Clinicopathological studies of minute hepatocellular carcinoma. Gastroenterology 73: 109–115

Okuda K, Nakashima T, Sakamoto K (1982) Hepatocellular carcinoma arising in noncirrhotic and highly cirrhotic livers – a comparative study of histopathology and frequency of hepatitis B markers. Cancer 49: 450–455

Popper H (1979) Hepatic cancers in man: quantitative perspectives. Environ Res 19: 482–494

Popper H, Gerber MA, Thung SN (1982) The relation of hepatocellular carcinoma to infection with hepatitis B and related viruses in man and animals. Hepatology 2: 1s–9s

Prince AM (1981) Hepatitis B virus and hepatocellular carcinoma. Hepatology 1: 73–75

Prince AM, Alcabes P (1982) The risk of development of hepatocellular carcinoma in hepatitis B virus carriers in New York – a preliminary estimate using death-records matching. Hepatology 2: 15s–20s

Shafritz DA, Shouval D, Sherman HI, et al. (1981) Integration of hepatitis B virus DNA into the genome of liver cells in chronic liver disease and hepatocellular carcinoma – studies in percutaneous liver biopsies and postmortem tissue specimens. N Engl J Med 305: 1067–1073

Shouval D, Reid LM, Chakraborty PR, et al. (1981) Tumorigenicity in nude mice of a human hepatoma cell line containing hepatitis B virus DNA. Cancer Res 41: 1342–1350

Sun ZT, Wang NG, Xia QJ, et al. (1979) Pathological and serological investigation on early primary hepatocellular carcinoma and its liver disease background. Chin J Oncol 1: 13–19[1]

Sung JL, Chen DS (1980) Maternal transmission of hepatitis B surface antigen in patients with hepatocellular carcinoma in Taiwan. Scand J Gastroenterol 15: 321–324

Szmuness W (1978) Hepatocellular carcinoma and hepatitis B virus – evidence for a causal association. Prog Med Virol 24: 40–69

Tang ZY, Yu YQ, Lin ZY, et al. (1979) Small hepatocellular carcinoma – clinical analysis of 30 cases. Chin Med J 92: 455–462

Tang ZY, Ying YY, Gu TJ (1982) Hepatocellular carcinoma – changing concepts in recent years. In: Popper H, Schaffner F (eds) Progress in liver diseases, vol VII. Grune and Stratton, New York, pp 637–647

Tang ZY, Yu YQ, Lin ZY, Yang BH (1983) Subclinical hepatocellular carcinoma. Chin J Oncol 5: 226–228[1]

Trichopolo SD, Gerety RJ, Sparros L, et al. (1978) Hepatitis B and primary hepatocellular carcinoma in European population. Lancet 2: 1257–1219

Vogel CL, Anthony PP, Mody N, et al. (1970) Hepatitis-associated antigen in Ugandan patients with hepatocellular carcinoma. Lancet 2: 621–624

Wu PC, Lam KC (1979) Cytoplasmic hepatitis B surface antigen and the ground-glass appearance in hepatocellular carcinoma. Am J Clin Pathol 71: 229–234

Yarrish RL, Werner BG, Blumberg BS (1980) Association of hepatitis B virus infection with hepatocellular carcinoma in American patients. Int J Cancer 26: 711–715

Ying YY, Chai WY (1978) Small hepatocellular carcinoma. IV. Pathology of small hepatocellular carcinoma. Acta Acad Med Primae Shanghai 5: 111–118[1]

Zuckerman AJ (1979) Role of hepatitis B virus in primary liver cancer. J Toxicol Environ Health 52: 275–280

Zuckerman AJ (1982) Virological approach to the prevention of primary liver cancer. Hepatology 2: 67s–71s

1 Chinese

19 Hepatitis B Virus and Hepatocellular Carcinoma – Cellular and Molecular Aspects

Wen Yu-mei

Epidemiological and histopathological data have provided strong evidence that HBV is one of the major factors in the etiology of primary liver cancer. Studies of HBV viral antigens in PLC tissues or cell lines have been carried out chiefly by means of immunofluorescence or immunoperoxidase staining. Staining of liver sections of HBV seropositive or even seronegative patients usually reveal HB_sAg with or without HB_cAg, and occasionally with HB_eAg. These are located in cells adjacent to tumor cells, whereas HBV viral antigens are rarely found in the latter. Although staining patterns of such sections are suggestive of the association between HBV and PLC, study of the relationship in a cell culture system is preferable. At present, we are handicapped by the fact that HBV has not yet been successfully propagated in cell culture systems; thus, the role of the virus in transforming cells, the transcription, translation, and possible integration of viral DNA in cells, and the regulation and expression of viral antigens in tumor cells, etc. cannot be fully elucidated.

The successful establishment of a number of hepatocellular carcinoma cell lines has provided a useful tool for studying HBV and PLC on a cellular level. Among these cell lines, the PLC/PRF/5 established by Alexander has attracted most attention (Alexander et al. 1976). In the meantime, rapid progress has also been made in the molecular biological studies of HBV and related hepadnaviruses (woodchuck, ground squirrel, and duck hepatitis viruses) (Robinson et al. 1982). Cloning and sequencing of the HBV genome, expression of HBV genome in procaryotic (Charnay et al. 1979; Burrell et al. 1979) and eucaryotic cells (Moriarty et al. 1981), and studies on the replication of hepadna virus DNA have also promoted enthusiastic studies of HBV and PLC on a molecular level. (Summers and Mason 1982). In view of this fascinating and fast-moving field, one can presume that in the near future the role of HBV in carcinogenesis will eventually be clarified.

I. Cellular Expression of HBV Antigens in Hepatoma Cell Lines

A. HBV Markers in Hepatoma Cell Lines

Several hepatoma cell lines have been established by various authors (Chen et al. 1980); however, only the PLC/PRF/5 cell line has been consistently secreting HB_sAg into the supernatant fluid for a number of years. Hep 3B (Aden et al. 1979), another cell line established at the Wistar Institute, can also synthesize HB_sAg, but the concentration detected is far lower than that of PLC/PRF/5. Others (Das and

Nayak 1980) have also claimed to have cell lines secreting HB_sAg, but none has been as reproducible as the two stated above. Since tumor cells from liver sections rarely express HBV antigens, it is not surprising that most of the established hepatocellular carcinoma cell lines fail to synthesize viral antigens.

The production of HB_sAg from the PLC/PRF/5 cell line has stirred up much interest, as this is the first cell culture system available for the study of HBV antigen in vitro. Collection, concentration, and purification of the supernatant fluid from these cells has proved that the particles recovered are similar in size and morphology to the 22-nm spherical form in the serum of persistently infected individuals (Alexander et al. 1978). Polypeptide analysis of the particles produced in vitro has indicated that they are also identical to those from chronic carriers (Skelly et al. 1979). It has been stated, however, that the stability of the particles synthesized in vitro is different from that of the particles present in serum, and that the former tend to become labile during purification by ammonium sulfate precipitation, ultracentrifugation, or concentration by Amicon filter (Alexander et al. 1978). In accordance with these results, we have also detected clumps of particles of aggregated spherical forms in the supernatant of PLC/PRF/5 cells by means of immunoelectron microscopy. In some instances we have observed a few short 20-nm diameter tubular particles entangled with the spherical ones as reported by others, but have never detected Dane particles (Wen et al. 1982a). The kinetic production of HB_sAg by PLC/PRF/5 in different laboratories has had variable results. Serial quantitation of HB_sAg produced by a clone of PLC/PRF/5 (generously provided by Dr. A.J. Zuckerman of the London School of Hygiene and Tropical Medicine), by means of solid-phase RIA, has shown that the production of HB_sAg in the supernatant fluid was usually low in actively dividing cells, but tended to increase at the stage of nutrient depletion and cessation of cell division (Wen et al. 1982a). These findings strongly suggest that HB_sAg production is a terminal event in cultured tumor cells. The maximum titer of HB_sAg from different clones varied. According to our experience, the maximum titer was 707 ng/ml in one series, whereas in another 200 ng/ml was the highest concentration obtained.

For dynamic intracellular studies of HB_sAg production, acetone-fixed coverslips of PLC/PRF/5 cells on different days were stained by indirect immunofluorescence parallel with the quantitation of HB_sAg in supernatant fluid. In spite of a detectable amount of HB_sAg in supernatant fluid, no fluorescent cells could be seen 24 h after the seeding of cells. Immunofluorescence was detected 3 days after subculture, showing very weak staining confined to the cytoplasmic membrane in a few cells. By the 6th day, immunofluorescence developed on the outer membrane of many cells, and cytoplasmic staining could be seen in sparsely distributed cells as well. On the 9th day, correlating with peak production of HB_sAg in the supernatant, bright fluorescent granules could be seen in the cytoplasm. These varied in intensity and size, ranging from fine granules to large coalescent masses. In some cells granule distribution was perinuclear, while in others homogeneous fluorescence partially covering large areas of the cytoplasm could also be seen. After the 9th day, cultures showed increasing numbers of rounded cells which gave bright nonspecific fluorescence, making further detailed immunofluorescent staining impossible (Wen et al. 1981). Although intracellular HB_sAg could be observed by immunofluorescence, its presence was usually too low to be detected by RIA or other serological tests. It may be speculated either that HB_sAg is synthesized in the cytoplasm of PLC/PRF/5 and did not accumulate but was released immediately from the plasma membrane, or that the synthesized HB_sAg is firmly bound to cell organelles, which made its detection by RIA rather difficult. We are inclined to the former possibility, because prior to the detection of intracellular HB_sAg it is already detectable in the culture fluid. The first appearance of HB_sAg confined to the cell membrane is also of interest, as it indicates that HB_sAg expression of integrated viral DNA in tumor cells is first displayed on the membrane of tumor cells.

In spite of the fact that the complete genome of HBV is almost wholly integrated in the PLC/PRF/5, efforts to detect viral antigens aside from HB_sAG, or DNA polymerase in cells or fluid of culture have been so far unsuccessful.

B. Characterization and Immunogenicity of HB_sAg from Hepatoma Cell Line

Skelly et al. (1979) have shown that the purification procedures developed for serum HB_sAg are readily adaptable to that produced by cells, and that HB_sAg derived from both cells and serum contains the two major polypeptides of molecular weights 28000 and 23000 respectively. Since these two polypeptides are of importance in immunogenicity, we studied the antigenicity of the HB_sAg originating from cell culture, as a preliminary step to employing it for diagnostic purposes. Culture media from the PLC/PRF/5 cell line were collected and partially purified by means of an anti-HB_s IgG-linked affinity chromatography column. Purified HB_sAg from serum (designated S-HB_sAg) as well as from PLC/PRF/5 (designated P-HB_sAg) were used together with Freund's adjuvant to immunize different groups of mice intraperitoneally, with 2 μg once a week. After 2 weeks, mice were boosted with HB_sAg without the adjuvant. Serum samples were assayed for anti-HB_s by RIA (Tables 1 and 2).

Table 1. Anti-HB_s response to PLC/PRF/5-derived HB_sAg in mice (SPRIA)

Mouse no.	1	2	3	4	5
P-HB_sAg (P/N)	1.84	17.38	44.89	52.56	48.66
S-HB_sAg (P/N)	143.92	65.91	106.22	163.28	81.42

Table 2. Specificity of anti-HB_s response to PLC/PRF/5-derived HB_sAg in guinea pigs (in cpm)

Guinea pig no.	1[a]	2[a]	3[b]	4[b]
Anti-HBs + HB_sAg-positive serum	5163	4486	5529	5067
Anti-HBs + HB_sAg-negative serum	22357	23137	18584	15748
Inhibition (%)	76.9	80.62	70.3	76.8

[a] P-HB_sAg-immunized guinea pig
[b] S-HB_sAg-immunized guinea pig

Four of the five P-HB_sAg-immunized mice were anti-HB_s positive, whereas all five S-HB_sAg-immunized mice responded with a higher titer of anti-HB_s. In the four immunized guinea pigs, the antibody response against P-HB_sAg versus S-HB_sAg was almost the same. The specificity of the antibody was demonstrated by a blocking test. To study the possible diagnostic use of the antibodies, we isolated IgG from the sera of both groups of guinea pigs and found that the IgG of anti-HB_s against P-HB_sAg can be used to sensitize sheep RBC for RPHA, as well as to coat plates for RIA for detecting HB_sAg (Wen et al. 1982b). Mann et al. (1982) have presented the possibility of using PLC/PRF/5 as an antigen source for HBV vaccine and diagnostic purposes. We believe that employing cell culture antigen source for diagnostic purposes may be a reasonable approach, and may be less tedious during purification than the approach using serum from human carriers.

C. Enhancement and Inhibition of HB_sAg Expression

The availability of PLC/PRF/5-producing HB_sAg has also permitted the investigation of factors involved in the expression of HB_sAg in vitro, i.e., enhancement and inhibition. Even though the in vitro expression is not entirely applicable to the in vivo study, the data obtained might provide information for analysis of viral antigen expressed by integrated HBV genome. In addition, factors increasing production of HB_sAg are necessary for the large scale preparation of such an antigen. On the other hand, substances inhibitory to HB_sAg production might be useful in clinical practice as reference for its possible use in treatment.

Since we observed a correlation between an increase of HB_sAg production and nutrient depletion, the effect of decreasing concentration or omission of calf serum in culture media was studied. Sequential quantitation of supernatants from PLC/PRF/5 cultured in 10% and 2% calf serum were compared. During the first few days after subculture, more HB_sAg appeared to be produced in the cells cultured in those with less calf serum. However, after 9–12 days, the amounts of HB_sAg produced in the two series were almost the same (Wen et al. 1982a). Cells could be maintained in media free of calf serum only up to 4 days, after which sheets of cells would detach. No increase in HB_sAg production was observed while cells were cultured in serum-free medium. Polysaccharides of Radix astragali seu halysari (Astragalus membranaceous [Fisch] Bunge), a Chinese herb which has been shown to extend the life span of the human embryo lung diploid cell strain from around 40 to over 100 passages, was added to the culture media of PLC/PRF/5. No significant enhancement or decrease of HB_sAg production was noted (Wen et al. 1982a). Oefinger et al. (1981) have reported that dexamethasone could increase HB_sAg synthesis in PLC/PRF/5 cells and induce its synthesis in Hep 3B cells. However, our preliminary attempt to increase HB_sAg production by dexamethasone was unsuccessful.

It has been shown that treating confluent cultures of PLC/PRF/5 with 100 units/ml of interferon has no effect. However, a definite decrease of HB_sAg by interferon was shown by treating a semiconfluent cell monolayer. This effect is probably due to the anticellular effect of interferon, rather than to anti-HB_sAg expression. Our experiments showed that on a confluent monolayer of PLC/PRF/5 cells neither leukocyte interferon nor specific immune RNA prepared from HB_sAg immunized sheep spleen had any effect on HB_sAg production, but interferon did inhibit HB_sAg production and cell growth in a semiconfluent culture of PLC/PRF/5.

II. Status of HBV-DNA in Liver Cancer

A. HBV-DNA Hybridization Test

The transfer hybridization technique described by Southern (1975) has been used to detect specific sequences among DNA fragments separated by gel electrophoresis, using a ^{32}P-labeled DNA probe. The successful cloning of HBV-DNA overcame the difficulty of obtaining enough DNA to employ this technique in studies of liver diseases. Studies can be carried out either by a spot test or by Southern blot, combining hybridization with agarose gel electrophoresis. The former is a qualitative test, highly sensitive but less specific, while the latter is more specific and can be used to determine the status of DNA in cells or tissues. We employed a spot test to analyze serum DNA. Samples were digested with proteinase K and extracted with phenol, chloroform, and isoamyl alcohol. The DNA fragments were denatured by sodium hydroxide, neutralized, and then transferred by a special system to a nitrocellulose filter and baked at 80 °C for 2 h. Cloned HBV-DNA was labeled by nick translation, denatured, and hybridized with the sample DNA on filter. After hybridization, the filter was exposed to an X-ray film for autoradiography, and positive sera showed dark spots which were comparable to a positive control (Fig. 1).

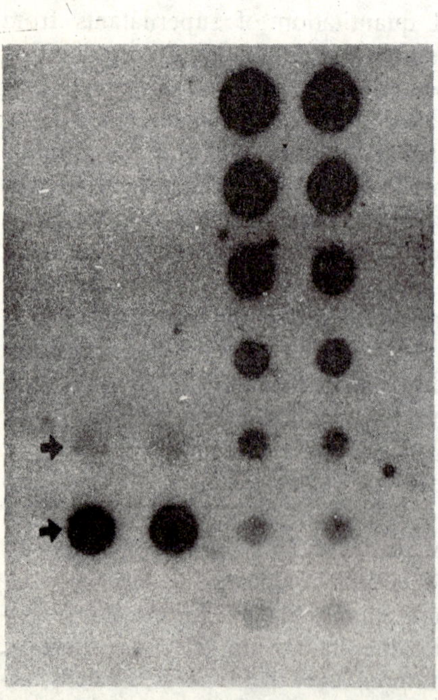

Fig. 1. HBV-DNA spot hybridization. ^{32}P-labeled cloned HBV-DNA, with sera from chronic hepatitis B patients. *Left,* serum samples. *Arrows* indicate strong-positive *(bottom)* and weak-positive results. *Right,* HBV-DNA from top to bottom: 160 pg, 80 pg, 40 pg, 20 pg, 10 pg, 5 pg, 2.5 pg

By this technique we have screened 50 samples of serum from PLC patients. Only two showed traces of HBV-DNA in the serum, whereas sera from many chronic hepatitis B patients were positive, which suggested that there was little demonstrable HBV-DNA in HB_sAg-positive sera of liver cancer patients, despite the possibility that they might have had the viral DNA in their sera prior to the development of liver cancer. It should be mentioned that integrated HBV-DNA in tumor tissues of liver cancer patients has been found by scientists from different laboratories (Koshy et al. 1981; Shafritz 1982). This is an area of great significance.

B. HBV-DNA Integration in Cells

Marion presented data on the integration of HBV-DNA in PLC/PRF/5 cell line (Marion et al. 1980). Koshy et al. (1981) confirmed such findings and demonstrated integration in another hepatocellular carcinoma cell line secreting HB_sAg. Employing endonuclease *Eco*RI and *Bam*HI to cleave PLC/PRF/5 DNA and hybridize it with labeled HBV-DNA, they detected no free DNA whatsoever. Using *Eco*RI and *Hind*III to cleave PLC/PRF/5 DNA, we also detected integrated HBV-DNA.

More interest has been centered on the status of HBV-DNA in tumor and nontumor tissues. Bréchot et al. (1982) analyzed 46 liver tissue samples from hepatocellular carcinoma patients and found the presence of HBV sequences integrated in the host cellular DNA. They claimed that HBV sequences were found not only in the tumor tissues but also in the nontumor part of the liver of PLC patients. They also stated that there was integration of viral DNA at specific cellular sites. However, Schafritz (1982) reported that only 12 of 17 cases of PLC had HBV-DNA integration, and detected no free viral DNA. The patterns of integration varied, but some bands were common in several tumors. Molecular hybridization can now be performed on small pieces of liver tissues obtained by percutaneous biopsies. In situ hybridization is also feasible (Gowans et al. 1981). These improvements will accelerate further studies on the DNA status in various liver diseases, which may eventually be helpful in identyfying carriers or patients who are at the greatest risk of developing hepatocellular carcinoma.

III. HBNA (Hepatitis B Virus-Associated Nuclear Antigen) in Hepatoma Cell Lines

A. Detection of HBNA

Studies on the relationship between HBV and PLC have been pursued along another line, i.e., to study the possible transforming antigen of HBV in hepatome cell lines. Some DNA tumor viruses of animals (e.g., papovaviruses, adenoviruses and herpesviruses) can produce transformation through the action of viral genes that regulate the replication and integration of the viral genome, and usually transformed cells can bear a "T"(tumor) antigen. Since there is direct or indirect evidence of an etiological relationship between HBV and hepatocellular carcinoma, anticomplement immunofluorescence, as employed in studies of EBNA (EB virus-

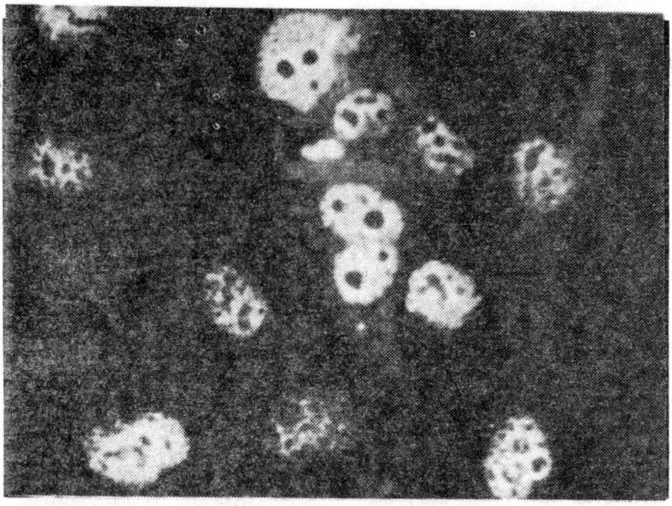

Fig. 2. Anticomplement immunofluorescent staining of PLC/PRF/5 with anti-HBNA, showing nuclear fluorescence that spares nucleoli

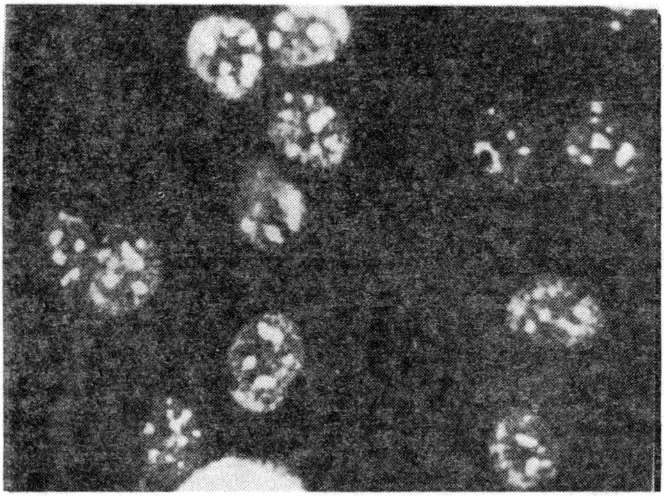

Fig. 3. Anti-complement immunofluorescent staining of PLC/PRF/5 with anti-HBNA, showing nucleolar staining

associated nuclear antigen), was used to search for an antigen analogous to EBNA (Reedman and Klien 1973). Cold-acetone-fixed PLC/PRF/5 cells served as substrates and serum samples from liver cancer patients as antibodies for anticomplement immunofluorescence. Positive sera stained the cells in two patterns. One was homogeneous, showing reticular nuclear fluorescence that sometimes spared the nucleoli, and resembled the T antigen in SV_{40}-transformed cells (Fig. 2); the other showed nucleolar fluorescence that spared the rest of the nucleus (Fig. 3).

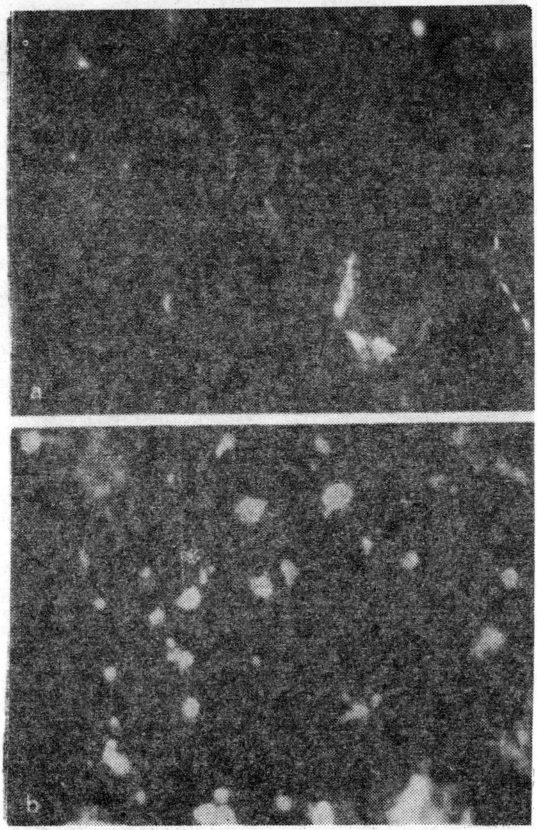

Fig. 4. Sections from tumors of PLC/PRF/5 grown in nude mice, **a** stained with normal serum and **b** stained with anti-HBNA, showing nuclear staining

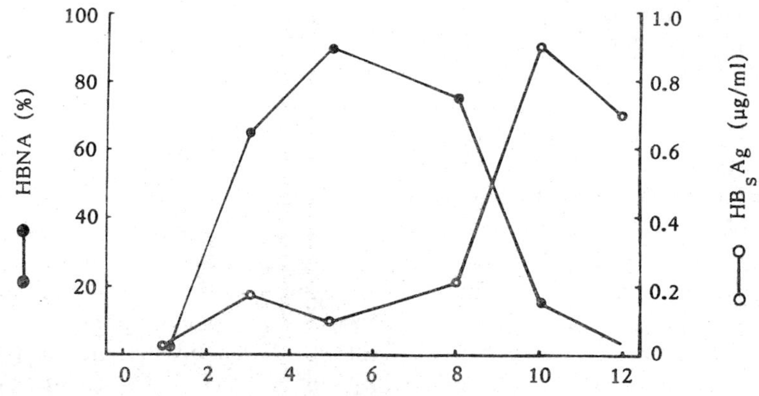

Fig. 5. Expression of HBNA (percentage of cells stained) and HB_sAg in PLC/PRF/5 cells on various days after subculture

Sera from normal controls or non-A, non-B patients failed to stain PLC/PRF/5, whereas sera from a few chronic hepatitis B patients stained the cells with less intensity of immunofluorescence. The specific association of this antigen with HBV was demonstrated by positive staining of hepatom cell lines which contained HBV genome integrated into cellular DNA, while Mahlavu, a cell line without detectable HBV genome, was negative in staining. All sera positive for anti-HBNA were from HB_sAg-positive liver cancer patients. Subcutaneous inoculation of PLC/PRF/5 into nude mice induced tumor formation. Cryostat sections of the tumor from nude mice were processed for anticomplement immunofluorescent staining; the result was mainly in nucleolar staining, and only a few cells had a homogeneous pattern (Fig. 4).

Anti-HBNA-positive serum was around 7%–8% among the liver cancer patients tested, including specimens collected separately from China, Japan, Italy, and Africa (Johnson et al. 1982; Wen et al. 1983).

B. Characterization of HBNA

Expression of HBNA in PLC/PRF/5 and Hep 3B was serially studied in parallel with production of HB_sAg in the supernatant fluid. As shown in Fig. 5, HBNA is expressed in the early stage of cell replication in vitro, which may be related to the synthesis of nucleoprotein in chromosomes.

For characterization of HBNA, fixed coverslips of cells were first incubated with RNase, DNase, or proteinase and then stained by anticomplement immunofluorescence. It was found that the immunofluorescence was abolished, or significantly diminished, by incubation with all three enzymes. It appears that this antigen shares some characteristics with SV40 T antigen, which has been described as a protein bound to DNA as well as to RNA. To assess the influence of antimetabolites on HBNA expression, cycloheximide was added to the cell culture as an inhibitor of protein synthesis; the result was markedly decreased HBNA staining. Blocking of nucleic acid synthesis by iododeoxyuridine or actinomycin D did not show significant differences in HBNA staining. All these findings suggest that HBNA is protein in nature.

C. Immunoprecipitation of HBNA

The presence of HBNA needs to be verified by immunoprecipitation with anti-HBNA-positive serum; however, many attempts have failed to show a reproducible, uniform result. Difficulties lie chiefly in the heat lability of this antigen, which may deteriorate while being processed. Modifications of the immunoprecipitation technique have identified this antigen with an extra band not seen in the controls (Fig. 6). PLC/PRF/5 cells were labeled with ^{35}S-methionine, and preparation of cell lysate was carried out on ice. Incubation of cell lysate with anti-HBNA-positive or control sera was also done at 4 °C. Staphylococcus protein A Sepharose was added to precipitate the antigen-antibody complex, followed by release of adsorbed antigen at 37 °C. SDS-polyacrylamide gel electrophoresis (SDS-PAGE) and subsequent

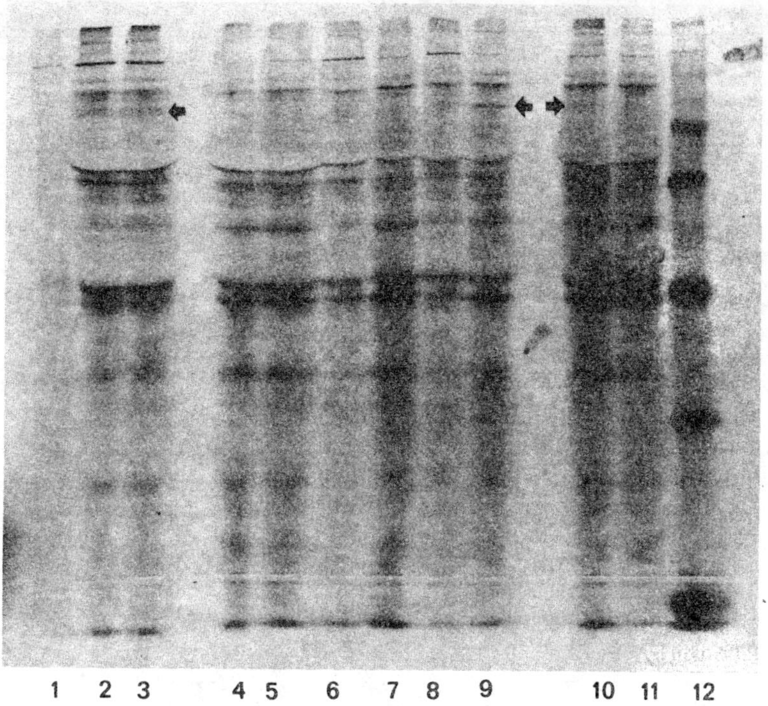

Fig. 6 Immunoprecipitation of HBNA. ^{35}S-methionine-labeled PLC/PRF/5 cell lysates were separately precipitated with different sera and exposed to film after SDS-PAGE.
lane 1 – precipitated with PBS; lanes 2 and 3 – precipitated with anti-HBNA-positive serum; lanes 4 and 5 – precipitated with HB_sAg positive, anti-HBNA-negative serum from liver cancer patients; lane 6 – precipitated with anti-HB_s-positive, anti-HBNA-negative serum; lane 7 – precipitated with normal serum without HBV markers; lane 8 – precipitated with normal serum without HBV markers; lane 9 – precipitated with anti-HBNA strong-positive serum; lane 10 – precipitated with anti-HBNA weak-positive serum; lane 11 – precipitated with HB_sAg-positive, anti-HBNA-negative serum from liver cancer patient; lane 12 – protein markers; 93000; 65000; 46000; 30000. *Arrows* indicate extra band of 10000, which may be a polymer of nuclear antigen

autoradiography revealed an extra band in the lane of cell lysate precipitated by anti-HBNA. The molecular weight of this band which may be a polymer of this nuclear antigen, was approximately 100000.

D. Possible Association of HBNA with Transformation

Transforming antigens have been demonstrated in different viruses, and their major properties are compared with those of HBNA in Table 3. From the data summarized it is obvious that to define HBNA as a transforming antigen, actual transformation by HBV in vitro is necessary. Unfortunately, numerous attempts to propagate this virus in a tissue culture system have been so far unrewarding. The successful cloning of HBV genome and its transfection and expression in eucaryotic

Table 3. Transforming antigens from DNA viruses

	HBNA	EBNA	SV40 (T)	Adeno (T)
Presence	HBV genome positive hepatoma cell lines	EBV genome positive tumor cells; cells transformed by EBV	SV40-induced tumor cells; SV40-transformed cells; permissively or nonpermissively infected cells	Adenoviral tumor; adenovirus-transformed cells; cells lytically infected
Virus specificity	+	+	+	+
Localization	Nucleus	Nucleus	Nucleus, cell surface	Nucleus; cytoplasm
Methods of detection	ACIF	ACIF, CFR	ACIF, CFR, indirect IF	IF, CFR
Kinetics of appearance	36 h after seeding cells	Within 24 h after infection	18 h after seeding cells	4 h after infection
Heat lability	Labile	Stable (at 80 °C)	Labile	Labile
Treatment of:				
– DNase	Abolished	Abolished	Abolished	
– RNase	Abolished	–	Abolished (IF)	
– Proteinase	Abolished	Abolished	Abolished	
Inhibition by:				
– Ara-A	–		–	–
– IDU	–		–	–
– Gyclohexi-mide	+		+	
– Interferon	–		+	
Binding to:				
– DNA	?	+	+	+
– RNA	?	?	+	?
Nature	Protein	Protein	Proteins (T, t)	Proteins
Molecular wt.	100000±	150000–200000 (tetramer) 28000–50000 (monomer)	90000	53000–58000 (major)
Association with transformation	?	+	+	+

ACIF, anti-complement immunofluorescence;
CFR, complement fixation test;
IF, immunofluorescence

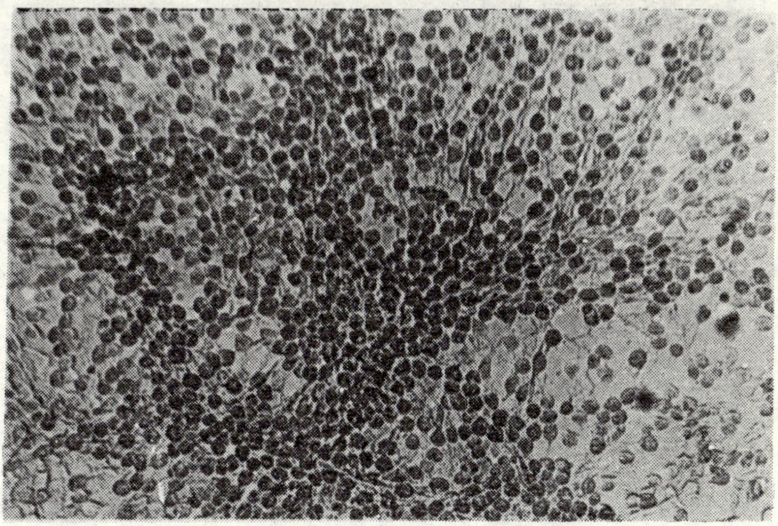

Fig. 7. Round and refractile NIH/3T3 cells transformed by PLC/PRF/5 DNA

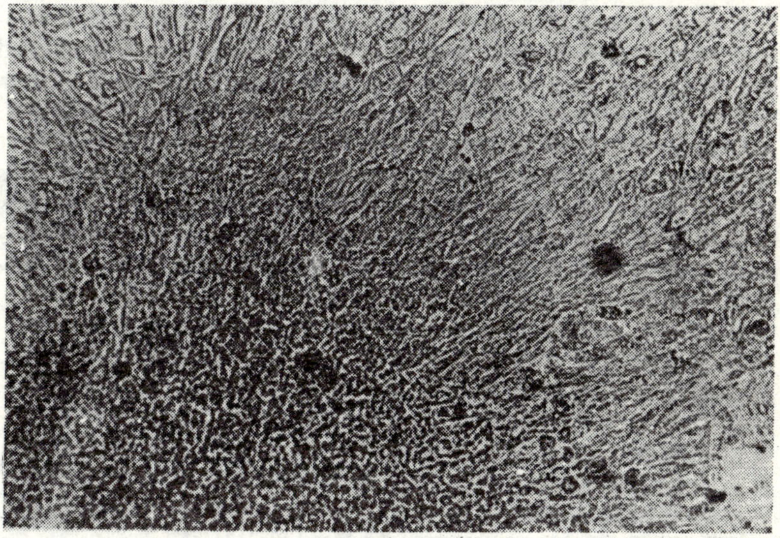

Fig. 8. Spindle-shaped NIH/3T3 cells transformed by PLC/PRF/5 DNA, showing marked disorientation in growth

cells have made in vitro transformation feasible. However, attempts to transform various cells with HBV-DNA were not promising; despite the fact that a few transformed foci did appear, they failed to be passaged. We have attempted to transfect NIH/3T3 cells with DNA extracted from PLC/PRF/5 cell lines. Foci of transformed cells were cloned using a cloning cylinder and cultured in flasks. Preliminary studies revealed two distinct morphological types of transformed cells, one be-

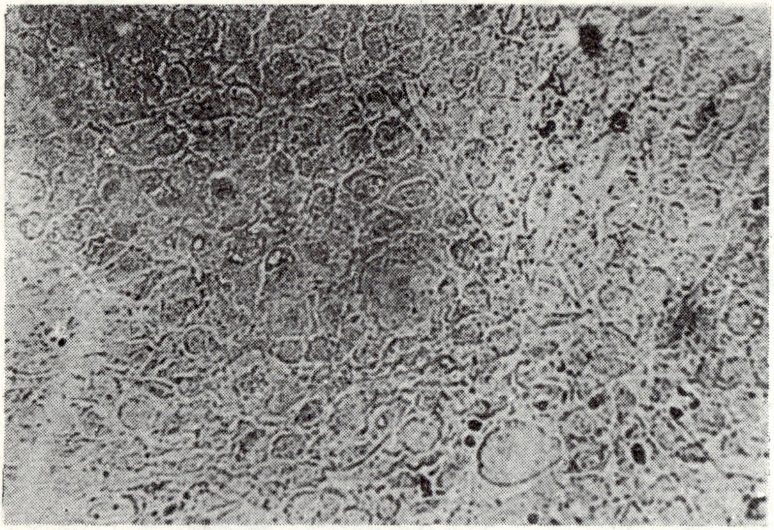

Fig. 9. NIH/3T3 cells transfected with NIH/3T3 DNA. No transformation was detected

ing round and refractile (Fig. 7), the other spindle-shaped with marked disorientation in growth (Fig. 5, 8 and 9). Both types require less serum in the growth media and are able to grow in soft agar. Staining these cells with anti-HBNA produced weak, dotted immunofluorescence in the nucleus which was absent in the controls. The intensity of the staining was far inferior to that in PLC/PRF/5 cells. Therefore, it seems necessary to study the different cells transformed by HBV-DNA, or hepatoma DNA with integrated HBV-DNA, and to make clear the role of HBNA in transformation. There are the possibilities that HBNA is a virus-coded protein or that it might be a cellular protein turned on by the viral genome.

References

Aden DP, Fogel A, Plotkin S, et al. (1979) Controlled synthesis of HB_sAg in a differentiated human liver carcinoma-derived cell line. Nature 282: 615–616

Alexander JJ, Bey EM, Geddes EW, et al. (1976) Establishment of a continuously growing cell line from primary carcinoma of the liver. S Afr Med J 50: 2124–2128

Alexander JJ, Macnab G, Saunders R (1978) Studies on in vitro production of hepatitis B surface antigen by a human hepatoma cell line. Perspect Virol 10: 103–120

Burrell CJ, Mackay P, Greenway PJ, et al. (1979) Expression in *E. coli* of hepatitis B virus DNA sequences cloned in plasmid PBR322. Nature 279: 43–47

Bréchot G, Pourcel C, Hadchouel M, et al. (1982) State of hepatitis B virus DNA in liver diseases. Hepatology 2: 27S–34S

Charnay P, Pourcel C, Louise A, et al. (1979) Cloning in *E. coli* and physical structure of hepatitis B virion DNA. Proc Natl Acad Sci USA 76: 2222–2226

Chen R, Zhu D, Ye X, et al. (1980) Establishment of three human liver carcinoma cell lines, and some of their biological characteristics in vitro. Scientia Sinica 23: 236–247[1]

Das PK, Nayak NC (1980) Ultrastructure of cultured human hepatocellular carcinoma cells releasing hepatitis B virus surface antigen. Indian J Exp Biol 18: 1511–1514

Gowans EJ, Burrell CJ, Jilbert AR, et al. (1981) Detection of hepatitis B virus DNA sequences in infected hepatocytes by in situ cytohybridization. J Med Virol 8: 67–78

Johnson RA, Mitamura K, Kew MC, et al. (1982) A "new" antigen associated with possible hepatitis B virus-induced malignancy. Viral Hepatitis 1981 International Symposium. Franklin Institute Press, Philadelphia, pp 713–714

Koshy R, Maupas P, Muller R, et al. (1981) Detection of hepatitis B virus-specific DNA in the genome of human hepatocellular carcinogens and liver cirrhosis tissue. J Gen Virol 57: 95–102

Mann GF, Copeland JA, Skelly J, et al. (1982) In vitro study on the PLC/PRF/5 hepatoma cell line. Viral Hepatitis 1981 International Symposium. Franklin Institute Press, Philadelphia, pp 67–79

Marion RL, Salazas FH, Alexander JJ, et al. (1980) State of hepatitis B viral DNA in a human hepatoma cell line. J Virol 33: 795–806

Moriarty AM, Hoyer BH, Shih JW-K, et al. (1981) Expression of the hepatitis B virus surface antigen gene in cell culture by using a simian virus vector. Proc Natl Acad Sci USA 78: 2606–2610

Oefinger PE, Bronson DL, Dreesman GR (1981) Induction of hepatitis B surface antigen in human hepatoma-derived cell line. J Gen Virol 53: 105–113

Reedman BM, Klien G (1973) Cellular localization of an Epstein-Barr virus (EBV)-associated complement-fixing antigen in producer and nonproducer lymphoblastoid cell line. Int J Cancer 11: 499–520

Robinson WS, Marion P, Feitalson M, et al. (1982) The hepadna virus group: Hepatitis B and related viruses. Viral Hepatitis 1981 International Symposium. Franklin Institute Press, Philadelphia, pp 57–68

Shafritz DA (1982) Hepatitis B virus DNA molecules in the liver of HB_sAg carriers: mechanistic considerations in the pathogenesis of hepatocellular carcinoma. Hepatology 2: 35s–41s

Skelly J, Copeland JA, Howard CR, et al. (1979) Hepatitis B surface antigen produced by a human hepatoma cell line. Nature 282: 617–618

Southern EM (1975) Detection of specific sequences among DNA fragments separated by gel electrophoresis. J Mol Biol 98: 503–517

Summers J, Mason WS (1982) Replication of the genome of a hepatitis B-like virus by reverse transcriptase of an RNA intermediate. Cell 29: 403–415

Wen YM, Copeland JA, Mann GF, et al. (1981) Detection of HB_sAg in a clone derived from the PLC/PRF/5 human hepatoma cell line. Arch Virol 68: 157–163

Wen YM, Zhang W, Lou HZ, et al. (1982a) Studies on hepatitis B surface antigen production in PLC/PRF/5 hepatoma cell line. Acta Acad Med Primae Shanghai 9: 1–6[1]

Wen YM, Feng TH, Zhang W, et al. (1982b) Studies on immunogenecity of HB_sAg produced by PLC/PRF/5 cell line. Shanghai Med J 5: 514–517[1]

Wen YM, Mitamura K, Merchant B, et al. (1983) A nuclear antigen detected in hepatoma cell line containing integrated hepatitis B virus DNA. Infect Immun 39: 1361–1367

1 Chinese

20 Hepatitis B Virus and Hepatocellular Carcinoma – Viral Antigens HB_sAg and HB_cAg In Primary Hepatocellular Carcinoma Tissue

Cao Yun-zhen

Epidemiological, clinicopathological, and virological data suggest an etiological relationship between persistent infection with HBV and PLC (Szmuness 1978; Popper 1978; London 1981). The evidence for this relationship includes the following: (a) the high prevalence of HBV serum markers in patients with PLC (Szmuness 1978; Cao and Lin 1980); (b) the strong geographical correlation between HB_sAg prevalence and PLC incidence (Yu 1981; Popper et al. 1982); (c) the high prevalence of HB_sAg in families of patients with PLC (Szmuness et al. 1975; Larouze et al. 1976; Tong et al. 1979; Hann et al. 1979; Cao and Lin 1980); (d) in prospective studies, the high relative risk of PLC among patients with chronic liver diseases and among HBV carriers (Tang et al. 1980; Beasley et al. 1981; Beasley 1982); (e) the observation that several cell lines derived from human PLC secrete HB_sAg into culture medium and, when implanted into nude athymic mice, secrete AFP and HB_sAg into the murine serum (Alexander et al. 1976; Desmyter et al. 1978; Aden et al. 1979; Bassendine et al. 1980; Sattler et al. 1982); (f) persistent infection with the woodchuck hepatitis virus (WHV), an HBV-like virus which causes chronic hepatitis and PLC in woodchucks *(Marmota monax)*, and with two other HBV-like viruses, ground squirrel hepatitis virus (GSHV) and duck hepatitis B virus (DHBV), which are similar to HBV in the structure of their DNA genomes, function of endogenous DNA polymerase, and morphology. WHV, GSHV, and HBV have antigenically similar core and surface antigens and about 70% nucleic acid homology (Summers et al. 1978b; Marion et al. 1980; Mason et al. 1980); (g) the finding, using molecular hybridization methods, of HBV-DNA sequences integrated into hepatocytes and tumor cells in human beings and woodchucks (Summers et al. 1978a; Shafritz and Kew 1981; Shafritz et al. 1981; Ogston et al. 1982); (h) the presence of HBV antigen in cytoplasm or nuclei of hepatocytes and tumor cells, demonstrated by electronmicroscopy (Goudeau et al. 1979; Michalak et al. 1980), orcein staining, immunofluorescence, and peroxidase immunohistochemical methods (Nayak et al. 1977; Huang and Neurath 1979; Goudeau et al. 1979; Ilardi et al. (1980); Ying et al. 1982). Detailed data on electron-microscopic findings and immunohistochemical staining results in PLC tissue are presented in this chapter.

I. Electron-microscopic Findings – Virus-like Particles

Australia antigen was discovered by Blumberg et al. (1965), and was associated with hepatitis in 1967 (Blumberg et al. 1967). Shortly thereafter, Bayer et al. described 19- to 22-nm spherical and rod-shaped particles in density gradient fractions containing

Australia antigen (Bayer et al. 1968). In 1970, Dane et al. observed 40- to 45-nm particles in the serum of patients with Australia antigen (now called HB_sAg). Dane particles are thought to be the complete infectious virions of HBV. These particles have HB_sAg as their outer lipoprotein coat and contain an internal 27-nm core particle (Gerin and Shin 1978).

Three types of virus-like particles associated with HBV have been detected in infected liver cells by means of electron-microscopy. Spherical particles 20–27-nm in diameter are seen mainly in the nucleus and sometimes in the cytoplasm (Ahmed et al. 1971; Michalak et al. 1980), and tubular particles 20–30 nm in diameter are noted in the cisternae of smooth endoplasmic reticulum (SER) and rough endoplasmic reticulum (RER) (Ma and Blackburn 1973; Tanikawa 1979). Larger round, coated particles of 35–40 nm have been seen in the cytoplasm (Huang 1971). These particles are similar to those reported in the serum of hepatitis patients (Bayer et al. 1968; Dane et al. 1970). Immunofluorescent-microscopic (Ray et al. 1976) and immunoelectron-microscopic studies of such particles with ferritin-labeled antibodies (Huang et al. 1972) and peroxidase-labeled antibodies (Gerber et al. 1974; Yamada and Nakane 1977) revealed that HB_sAg is associated with the larger tubular cytoplasmic particles in the SER and the membranes of the liver cells and that HB_cAg is associated with the smaller nuclear particles.

Recently, 20 cases of PLC were studied with electron microscopy (Cao et al. 1983b). A variety of particles resembling virions were found in tumor cells and surrounding non-neoplastic cells in the livers of two of the patients.

Case 1. A 34-year-old man, previously diagnosed as having had acute hepatitis in December 1976, was admitted to the hospital on March 21, 1981 with complaints of loss of appetite, bloating, coughing, and weight loss. For the 5 years between 1976 and 1981 his ALT level fluctuated between normal and 152 units, and his direct serum bilirubin/total serum bilirubin was 0.5–3.8/1.2–7.2 mg%. Prior to hospitalization his serum AFP, tested monthly by countercurrent immunoelectrophoresis, showed elevated values only once, in January 1978. Serum HB_sAg and anti-HB_c were positive continuously from the time of first testing for the antigen and antibody (July 1979). Supporting treatment, including vitamins and glucose in combination with Chinese medicinal herbs, was given every day for 5 years. In March 1981 the patient's AFP rose to 700 ng/ml and he was admitted to the hospital. On May 28, 1981, 2 months after entering the hospital, he died of liver failure. Liver samples were taken at autopsy, which was performed 24 h post mortem.

Light microscopy showed grade IV hepatocellular carcinoma with associated active cirrhosis and chronic active hepatitis. Electron microscopy revealed numerous spherical virus-like particles measuring 23 nm in diameter in many nuclei of the non-neoplastic tissue. The particles occupied almost all of the chromatin areas (Fig. 1a). The cores of some of the particles were electron dense, while others were electron lucent. In addition, particles of 16–18 nm in diameter were seen in the cytoplasm (Fig. 2); also the peroxidase-antiperoxidase staining (PAP) showed strongly HB_sAg-negative and HB_cAg-positive in the non-neoplastic cells.

Case 2. In a mass screening project, a 40-year-old woman who was completely asymptomatic with regard to the liver was found to have a positive AFP level by means of countercurrent immunoelectrophoresis; her serum was also positive for

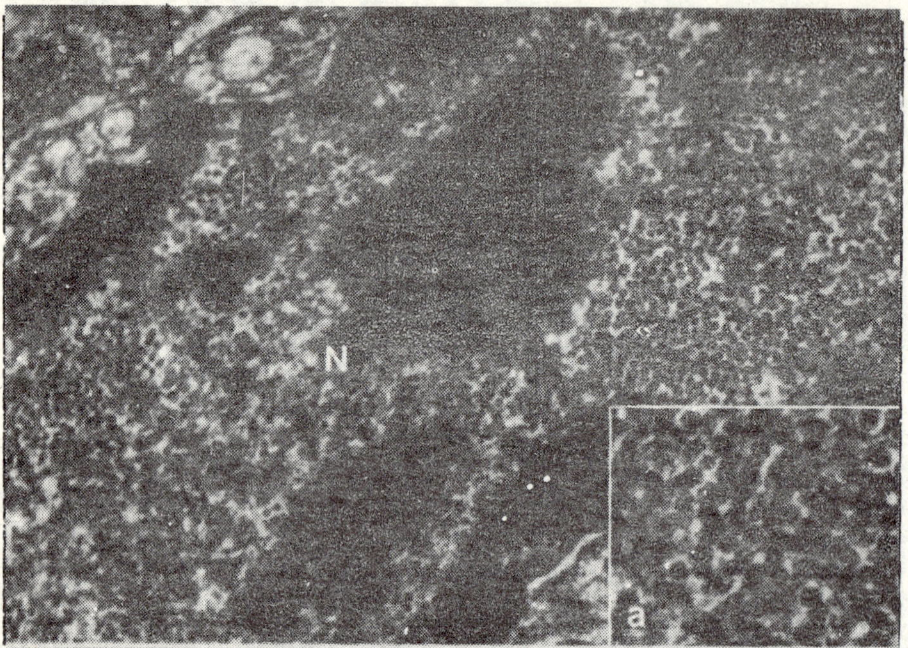

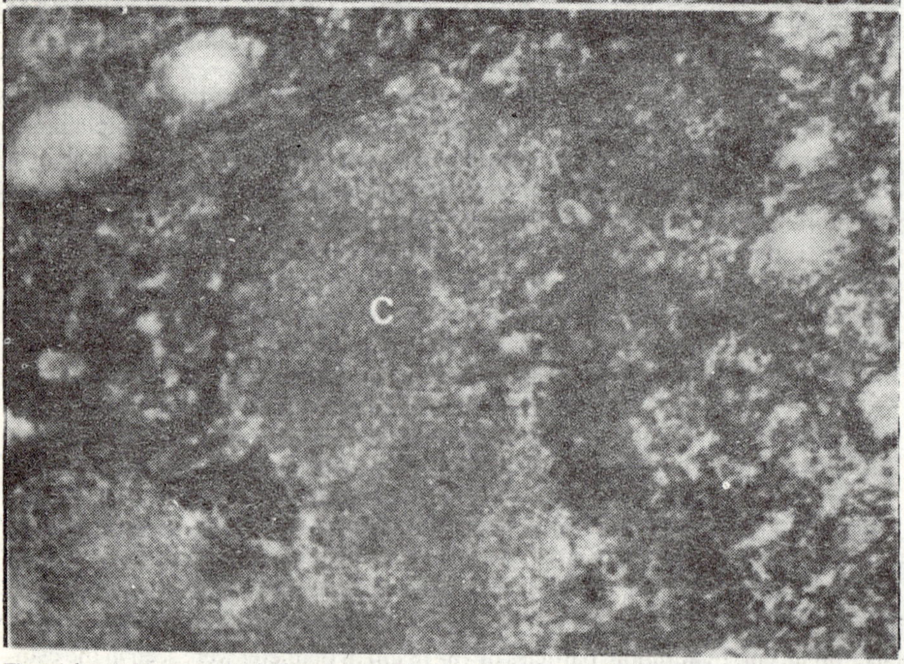

Fig. 1 *(above)*. Non-neoplastic liver tissue with virus-like particles, 23 nm in diameter, in the nucleus *(N)*. × 80 000 *Insert:* high magnification of nuclear virus-like particles. × 135 000. (Reproduction by 25%)

Fig. 2 *(below)*. Virus-like particles, 16–18 nm in diameter, in cytoplasm *(C)* of non-neoplastic cells. × 100 000. (Reproduction by 25%)

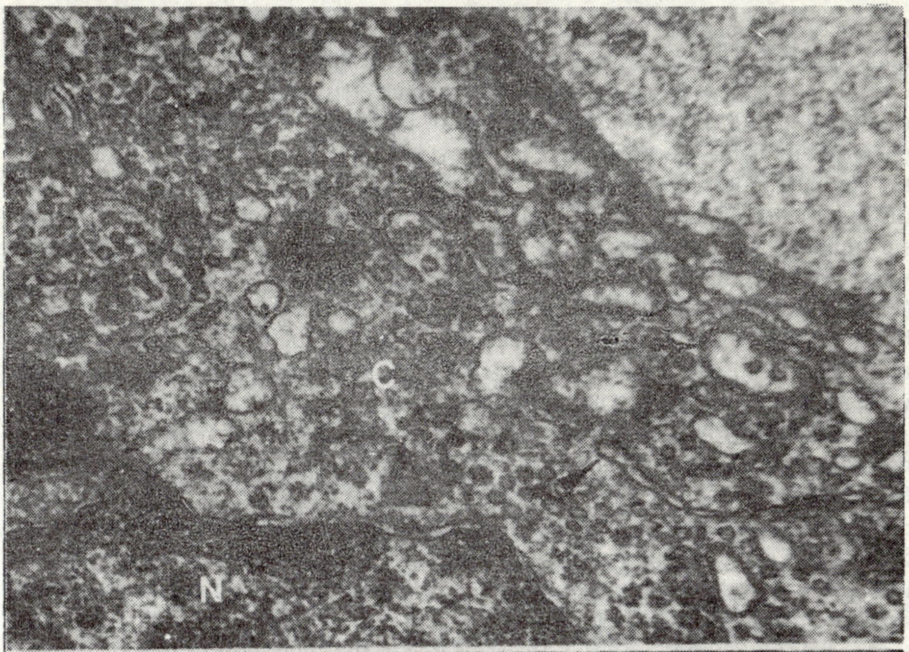

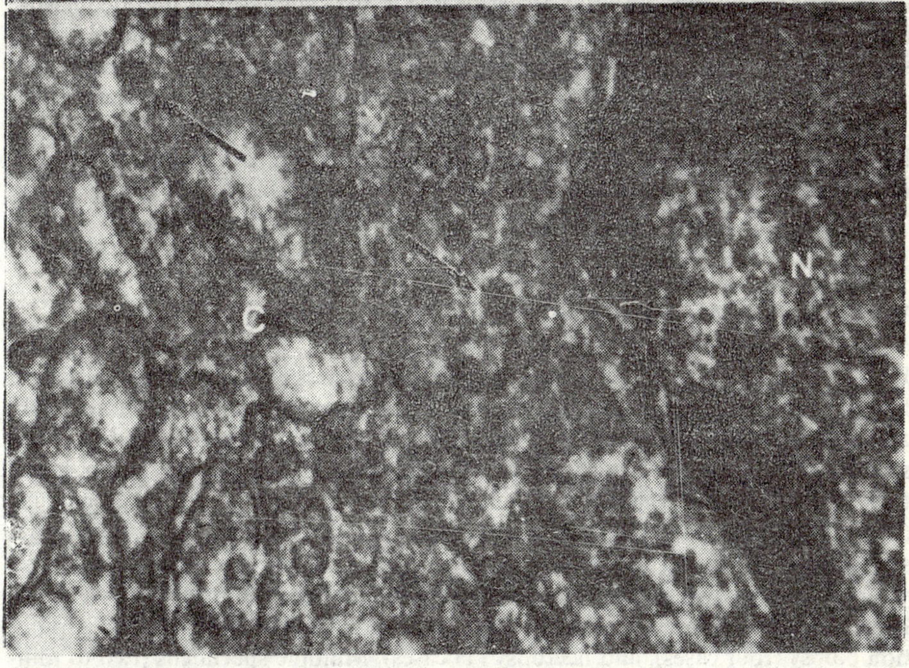

Fig. 3 *(above)*. Hepatoma tissue with spherical virus-like particles, 40–60 nm in diameter, in the cytoplasm *(C)*. Some particles are enclosed in membranes *(short arrows)*. Tubular particles are also noted *(triangle)*. *N*, nucleus; ×50000 (Reproduction by 25%)

Fig. 4 *(below)*. High magnification of spherical virus-like particles *(long arrows)* and tubular particles *(triangle)*. *C*, cytoplasm; *N*, nucleus; ×100000 (Reproduction by 25%)

HB_sAg. A left hemihepatectomy was performed on December 14, 1981. Light-microscopic examination of the surgical specimen showed grade III hepatocellular carcinoma with associated cirrhosis and chronic persistent hepatitis. The tissue was classified as well differentiated by means of electron microscopy; many particles 40–60 nm in diameter were present in the cytoplasm of tumor cells (Fig. 3). Some of the particles appeared in groups inside double membranes. Higher magnification of the tissue revealed that some spherical particles had an outer membrane, 5 nm thick, surrounding a central particle 30–50 nm in diameter (Fig. 4). Tubular structures were also discernible, as they were interspersed between the spherical particles (Figs. 3 and 4). The tubules had an average diameter of 36 nm, with an outer membrane 5 nm thick; the longest tube measured 500 nm. Particles were not seen in nontumorous cells. PAP staining showed HB_sAg positive in both tumor and nontumor cells and HB_cAg positive in nontumor cells.

Our study of virus-like particles would support the view that each case should be considered on an individual basis, as a unifying concept between the cases was not found. A comparison between our findings concerning the virus-like particles and results of previous studies reveals both similarities and discrepancies. With case 1, hepatocytes surrounding the tumor – numerous uniform spherical particles 23 nm in diameter – were found not only in the nuclei but also in the cytoplasm, and not associated with the SER. In terms of the relation of particle morphology and location (primarily nuclear, and to a lesser degree in the cytoplasm of non-neoplastic liver tissue), these particles might represent HB_cAg. In case 2, such particles had similarities to Dane particles, described in association with hepatitis: they consisted of a central portion (core), 25–27 nm in diameter and surrounded by a membrane. The tubules were similar in structure to those noted in serum containing HB_sAg. Particles suspected to be Dane particles have been described in both tumor and nontumor tissue of patients with liver carcinoma (Ma and Blackburn 1973).

II. Immunohistochemical Studies – Antigen-Positive Pattern

HB_sAg and HB_cAg have been detected in the hepatocytes of infected liver cells, and less frequently in tumor cells, by means of PAP staining (Sternberger et al. 1970) and orcein staining (Shikata et al. 1974), using conventional formalin-fixed paraffin sections. The frequency of positive orcein staining for HB_sAg was reported as 50% to 90% in infected liver tissue containing PLC and as 1.6% to 12.5% in tumor cells (Ying 1981; Ying et al. 1982). The results of PAP staining for HB_sAg and HB_cAg are summarized in Table 1.

Thirty patients with PLC were studied by the author. The diagnosis was confirmed by light microscopy of tissue obtained at surgical resection (15 cases), aspiration biopsy (four cases), and necropsy (11 cases). Multiple specimens (two to four blocks) including both tumor and uninvolved liver, were obtained in 25 cases; in the remaining five single samples including tumor and adjacent liver were collected. For immunohistochemistry, the tissues were fixed in 10% neutral formalin, embedded in paraffin, sectioned at 5 μm, and stained with appropriate PAP for viral antigen components. In staining for HB_sAg and HB_cAg the PAP method of Sternberger

Table 1. Frequency of positivity for HB_sAg and HB_cAg in PLC patients

Reference	No. of patients	HB_sAg (+) Nontumor tissue	(%)	Tumor cells	(%)	HB_cAG (+) Nontumor tissue	(%)	Tumor cells
Nayak and Sachdeva (1975)	13	10/11	(90.9)	4/12	(33.3)			
Nayak et al. (1977)	50	47	(94)	4	(8)	9/41	(22)	0
Omata et al. (1978)	20	11	(55)	0		10	(50)	0
Kew (1978)	44	13	(29.5)	8	(18.2)			0
Thung et al. (1979)	9			7	(77.8)	0		0
Ilardi et al. (1980)	18	15	(83.3)	3	(16.7)			–
Cao et al. (1984a)	30	28	(93.3)	15	(50)	16	(53.3)	0

(Sternberger et al. 1970) was used, as well as the commercial DAK PAP KIT (Accurate Chemical & Scientific Corp., Westbury, NY). Sections were deparaffinized and hydrated, and endogenous peroxidase activity quenched with a 0.6% solution of hydrogen peroxide in absolute methanol, then placed in 0.05 *M* Tris-buffer at pH 7.6. Staining procedures were performed according to the manufacturer's instructions. Tissues were counterstained with hematoxylin. Control sections were treated with normal swine serum or normal rabbit serum instead of the antibody.

HB_sAg is limited mainly to non-neoplastic hepatocytes with several distribution patterns: (a) inclusion pattern – the PAP-positive material occupies the cytoplasm in round or oval inclusion bodies (Fig. 5); (b) spotty pattern – the PAP-positive material is irregular and unevenly distributed; sometimes it is located in one pole of the cytoplasm, in other cells it is perinuclear (Fig. 6); (c) membrane-expression pattern – the HB_sAg is partially to completely distributed along the cell membrane (Fig. 7), occasionally occupying intercellular spaces. The distribution varied from whole lobular involvement to small foci in otherwise negative lobules, or occasionally to isolated positive cells in negative lobules. HB_sAg was detected in non-neoplastic hepatocytes as frequently in the serum HB_sAg (−) group as in the HB_sAg (+) patients, but the expression of HB_sAg was different. In 14 of 16 patients who were positive for HB_sAg in their serum and liver, HB_sAg was present in clumps of cells or in lobules or pseudonodules; in nine of 12 patients who were negative for HB_sAg in their serum but had HB_sAg in liver cells, the HB_sAg-positive cells were few and isolated. HB_sAg was found in the cytoplasm of a few carcinoma cells. Sometimes positive-staining cells blended into tumor cells and could have been misclassified as such (Cao et al. 1983 a).

The proportion of HB_cAg positivity in liver tissue appears to be much lower than that of HB_sAg. However, the validity of these results is questionable because of an inadequate sampling method (aspiration biopsy). We believe that the true frequency of HB_cAg positivity will prove to be higher than reported. HB_cAg is usually detected in nuclei, less commonly in cytoplasm of hepatocytes (Fig. 8), and rarely in cell membranes (Cao et al. 1983 a), suggesting that it is synthesized on cytoplasmic ribosomes and migrates through nuclear pores to the nucleus, forms core particles, and is then released together with other HB_sAg-positive forms into the intercellular space (Yamada and Nakane 1977). The stain is usually found in isolated cells, occa-

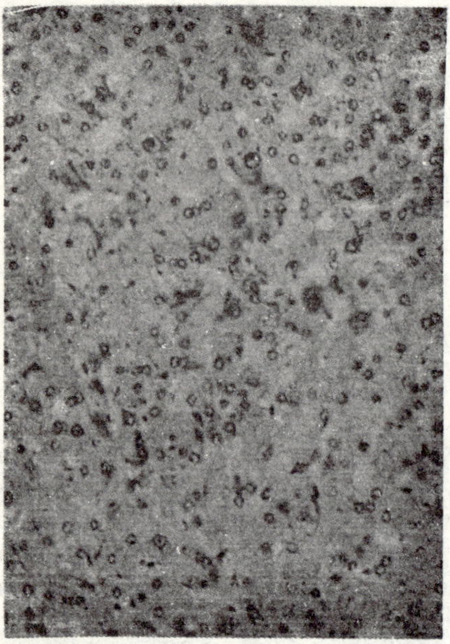

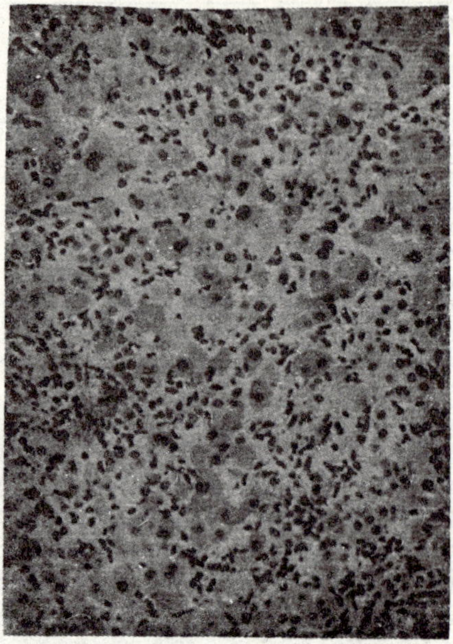

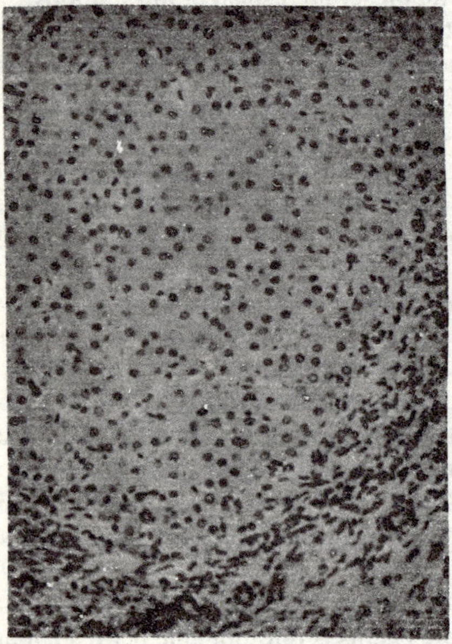

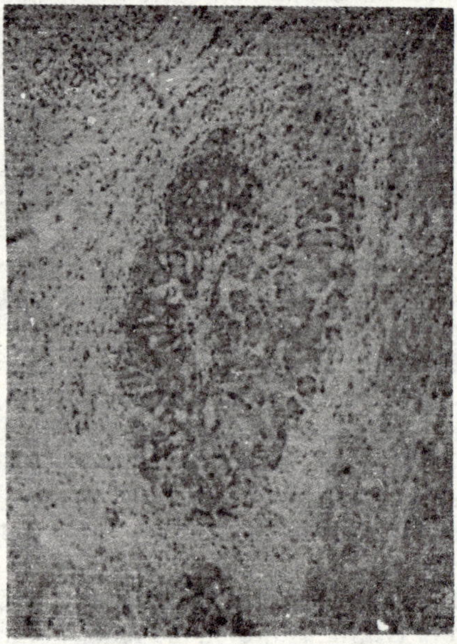

Fig. 5 *(upper left).* Inclusion pattern of HB_sAg expression in infected liver cells. PAP; ×340. (Reproduction by 25%)

Fig. 6 *(upper right).* Spotty pattern of HB_sAg expression. PAP; ×340. (Reproduction by 25%)

Fig. 7 *(lower left).* Membranous expression pattern of HB_sAG. PAP; ×340. (Reproduction by 25%)

Fig. 8 *(lower right).* Positive HB_cAg in nucleus. PAP; ×340. (Reproduction by 25%)

sionally clumped or limited to regenerative lobules. HB_cAg is always absent in tumor cells (Table 1), suggesting defective replication of HBV in the tumor cells (Nayak et al. 1977; Trubitt et al. 1977; Wu 1979; Ilardi et al. 1980; Popper et al. 1982).

Some authors emphasize that the patterns of HB_sAg and HB_cAg PAP staining can be used to estimate the chronicity and severity of liver disease, and that certain qualitative and quantitative expressions of HB_sAg and HB_cAg may have diagnostic and prognostic implications (Ray et al. 1976; Yamada and Nakane 1977; Huang and Neurath 1979). There are different patterns of HB_sAg expression – especially a peculiarly heavy membranous staining in severe active cirrhosis and chronic active hepatitis – in which we also observed HB_cAg in nuclei. With chronic persistent hepatitis and inactive cirrhosis or cirrhosis with little activity HB_cAg is in the cytoplasm, and membrane-localized HB_sAg is sometimes present, albeit in weak or moderate intensity (Ray et al. 1976; Huang and Neurath 1979; Cao et al. 1983a). We consider the pattern and quantity of HBV antigens in liver cells to reflect changes in the dynamics of HBV replication and the interrelationships between HBV and host cells.

For the most part, dysplastic hepatocytes failed to stain for HB_sAg. In two cases, dysplastic epithelial lining of proliferating bile ducts stained positively for HB_sAg. To our knowledge, this finding has not been reported previously.

The information reviewed at the beginning of the chapter, together with the data cited above, strongly associates HBV with PLC and supports the hypothesis that HBV is the major etiological agent of PLC in humans. The electron-microscopic observations and histochemical studies appear to permit discernment of HBV proteins in the infected liver tissue, but direct evidence for HBV oncogenicity is still far from satisfactory. Unless HBV can be proven to transform cells in culture, or to cause tumors experimentally in animals, or unless HBV vaccination reduces the frequency of PLC in high risk areas, the role of HBV in the pathogenesis of PLC will remain in doubt.

Acknowledgments. The work reported in this chapter was done under the guidance of Dr. W. T. London in Dr. B. S. Blumberg's laboratory and supported by the International Agency for Research on Cancer and the Reimann Fellowship from the Institute for Cancer Research, For Chase Cancer Center, Philadelphia, PA, USA.

I am very grateful to Dr. M. E. Bayer and Dr. R. P. Custer for their advice and constant encouragement. I also wish to thank S. Shepardson for her excellent technical assistance.

References

Aden DP, Fogel A, Plotkin S, et al. (1979) Controlled synthesis of HB_sAg in a differentiated human liver carcinoma-derived cell line. Nature 282: 615–616

Ahmed MN, Huang SN, Spence L (1971) Australia antigen and hepatitis. Arch Path 92: 66–72

Alexander JJ, Bay EM, Geddes EW, et al. (1976) Establishment of a continuously growing cell line from a primary carcinoma of the liver. S Afr Med J 50: 2124–2128

Bassendine MF, Arborgh BAM, Shipton U (1980) Hepatitis B surface antigen- and alpha-fetoprotein-secreting human primary liver cell cancer in athymic mice. Gastroenterology 79: 528–532

Bayer ME, Blumberg BS, Werner B (1968) Particles associated with Australia antigen in the sera of patients with leukemia, Down's syndrome and hepatitis. Nature 281: 1057–1059

Beasley RP (1982) Hepatitis B virus as the etiologic agent – hepatocellular carcinoma – epidemiologic considerations. Hepatology 2: 21S–26S
Beasley RP, HWang LY, Lin CC, et al. (1981) Hepatocellular carcinoma and hepatitis B virus. A prospective study of 22707 men in Taiwan. Lancet 2: 29–33
Blumberg BS, Alter HJ, Visnich S (1965) A "new" antigen in leukemia sera. JAMA 191: 541–546
Blumberg BS, Gerstley BJS, Hungerford DA, et al. (1967) A serum antigen (Australia antigen) – Down's syndrome, leukemia and hepatitis. Ann Intern Med 46: 924–927
Cao YZ, Lin ZY (1980) Detection of serum HB_sAg, anti-HB_s and anti-HB_c in 100 cases of primary liver cancer. Acta Acad Med Primae Shanghai 7: 125–130[1]
Cao YZ, Custer RP, London WT (1984a) primary hepatocellular carcinoma liver cell dysplasia and hepatitis B virus: pathology and histochemical studies in 30 cases from Shanghai, China. Am J Pathol (in press)
Cao YZ, Shepardson S, Bayer ME (1984b) Ultrastructure of primary hepatocellular carcinoma – analysis of 20 cases. Am J Pathol (to be published)
Dane DS, Cameron CH, Briggs M (1970) Virus-like particles in serum of patients with Australia antigen-associated hepatitis. Lancet 1: 695–698
Desmyter J, Ray MB, Bradburne AF, et al. (1978) Human HB_sAg-positive hepatoma in nude athymic mice. In: Vyas GN, Cohen SN, Schmid R (eds) Viral hepatitis. Franklin Institute Press, Philadelphia, pp 459–463
Gerber MA,Hadziyannis S, Vissoulis C, et al. (1974) Electron microscopy and immunoelectron microscopy of cytoplasmic hepatitis B antigen in hepatocytes. Am J Pathol 75: 489–495
Gerin JL, Shin JWK (1978) Structure of HB_sAg and HB_cAg. In: Vyas GN, Cohen SN, Schmid R (eds) Viral hepatitis. Franklin Institute Press, Philadelphia, pp 147–153
Goudeau A, Maupas P, Coursaget P, et al. (1979) Hepatitis B virus antigens in human primary hepatocellular carcinoma tissue. Int J Cancer 24: 421–429
Hann HL, London WT, Blumberg BS (1979) Hepatitis B virus and primary hepatocellular carcinoma: Family studies in Korea. Proc Am Soc Clin Oncol 20: 584–588
Huang SN (1971) Hepatitis-associated antigen hepatitis: An electron-microscopic study of virus-like particles in liver cells. Am J Pathol 64: 483–500
Huang SN, Neurath AR (1979) Immunohistologic demonstration of hepatitis B viral antigen in liver with relation to its significance in liver injury. Lab Invest 40: 1–17
Huang SN, Millman I, O'Connell A, et al. (1972) Virus-like particles in Australia antigen-associated hepatitis: An immunoelectron-microscopic study of human liver. Am J Pathol 67: 453–460
Ilardi CF, Ying YY, Ackerman LV, et al. (1980) Hepatitis B surface antigen and hepatocellular carcinoma in the People's Republic of China. Cancer 46: 1612–1616
Kew MC (1978) Hepatoma and the HBV. In: Vyas GN, Cohen SN, Schmid R (eds) Viral hepatitis. Franklin Institute Press, Philadelphia, pp 436–450
Larouze B, London WT, Blumberg BS (1976) Host responses to hepatitis infection in patients with primary hepatic carcinoma and their families. A case/control study in Senegal, West Africa. Lancet 2: 534–538
London WT (1981) Primary hepatocellular carcinoma – etiology, pathogenesis, and prevention. Hum Pathol 12: 1085–1097
Ma MH, Blackburn CRB (1973) Fine structure of primary liver tumors and tumor-bearing liver in man. Cancer Res 33: 1766–1774
Marion P, Oshiro LS, Regnery DC, et al. (1980) A virus of Beechey ground squirrels that is related to hepatitis B virus of humans. Proc Natl Acad Sci USA 77: 2941–2945
Mason WS, Seal G, Summers J (1980) Virus of Pekin ducks with structural and biological relatedness to human hepatitis B virus. J Virol 36: 829–836
Michalak T, Krancywski K, Ostrowski J, et al. (1980) Hepatitis B surface antigen and albumin in human hepatocytes. Gastroenterology 79: 1151–1158
Nayak NC, Sachdeva R (1975) Localization of hepatitis B surface antigen in conventional paraffin sections of the liver. Am J Pathol 81: 481–492
Nayak NC, Dhan A, Sachdeva R, et al. (1977) Association of human hepatocellular carcinoma and cirrhosis with hepatitis B virus surface and core antigens in the liver. Int J Cancer 20: 643–654
Ogston CW, Jonak GJ, Rogler CE, et al. (1982) Cloning and structural analysis of integrated woodchuck hepatitis virus sequences from hepatocellular carcinoma of woodchucks. Cell 29: 385–395

Omata M, Asheawai M, Liew CT, et al. (1978) Hepatocellular carcinoma in the USA. Etiologic considerations. Gastroenterology 76: 279–287

Popper H (1978) Considerations on an association between hepatocellular carcinoma and hepatitis B. In: Vyas GN, Cohen SN, Schmid R (eds) Viral hepatitis. Franklin Institute Press, Philadelphia, pp 451–454

Popper H, Gerber MA, Thung SN (1982) The relation of hepatocellular carcinoma to infection with hepatitis B and related viruses in man and animals. Hepatology 2: 1S–9S

Ray MB, Desmet Y, Bradburne AF, et al. (1976) Differential distribution of hepatitis B surface antigen and hepatitis B core antigen in the livers of hepatitis B patients. Gastroenterology 71: 462–467

Sattler FR, Paolucci S, Kreiden JW, et al. (1982) A human hepatoma cell line (PLC/PRF/5) produces lung metastases and secretes HB_sAg in nude mice. Eur J Cancer Clin Oncol 18: 381–389

Shafritz DA, Kew MC (1981) Identification of integrated hepatitis B virus DNA sequences in human hepatocellular carcinomas. Hepatology 1: 1–8

Shafritz DA, Shouval D, Sherman HI, et al. (1981) Integration of hepatitis B virus DNA into the genome of liver cells in chronic liver disease and hepatocellular carcinoma. Studies in percutaneous liver biopsies and postmortem tissue specimes. N Engl J Med 305: 1067–1073

Shikata T, Uszw T, Yoshiwara N (1974) Staining methods of Australia antigen in paraffin section – detection of cytoplasmic inclusion bodies. Jap J Exp Med 44: 25–36

Sternberger LA, Hard PH, Cuculis JJ, et al. (1970) The unlabeled antibody-enzyme method of immunohistochemistry preparation and properties of soluble antigen-antibody complex (horseradish peroxidase-antiperoxidase) and its use in identification of spirochetes. J Histochem Cytochem 18: 315–319

Summers J, O'Connell A, Maupas P, et al. (1978a) Hepatitis B virus DNA in primary hepatocellular carcinoma tissue. J Med Virol 2: 207–214

Summers J, Smolec JM, Snyder R (1978b) A virus similar to hepatitis B virus associated with hepatitis and hepatoma in woodchucks. Proc Natl Acad Sci USA 75: 4533–4537

Szmuness W (1978) Hepatocellular carcinoma and hepatitis B virus – evidence for a causal association. Prog Med Virol 24: 40–69

Szmuness W, Harley EJ, Prince AM (1975) Intrafamilial spread of asymptomatic hepatitis B. Am J Med Sci 270: 293–304

Tanikawa K (1979) Ultrastructural aspects of the liver and its disorders, 2nd edn. Igaku-Shoin, Tokyo, pp 338–348

Tang ZY, Yang BH, Tang CL, et al. (1980) Evaluation of population screening for hepatocellular carcinoma. Chin Med J 93: 795–799

Thung SN, Gerber MA, Sarno E (1979) Distribution of five antigens in hepatocellular carcinoma. Lab Invest 11: 101–105

Tong JM, Weiner JM, Ashcavai MW, et al. (1979) Evidence for clustering of hepatitis B virus infection in families of patients with primary hepatocellular carcinoma. Cancer 44: 2338–2342

Trubitt ML, Patrick RS, Gaudis PB, et al. (1977) Incidence in southwest Scotland of hepatitis B surface antigen in the livers of patients with hepatocellular carcinoma. J Clin Pathol 30: 1124–1128

Wu PC (1979) Patterns of hepatitis B surface antigen. Arch Pathol Lab Med 103: 165–168

Yamada G, Nakane PK (1977) Hepatitis B core and surface antigen in liver tissue. Light and microscopic localization by the peroxidase-labeled antibody method. Lab Invest 36: 649–659

Ying YY (1981) Pathology of hepatocellular carcinoma. In: Tang ZY (ed) Primary liver cancer. Shanghai Scientific and Technical Publisher, Shanghai, pp 55–84[1]

Ying YY, Yan R, Xu B, et al. (1982) Relationship between hepatocellular carcinoma, liver cirrhosis and hepatitis B – a pathological study. Natl Med J China 62: 257–261[1]

Yu SZ (1981) Epidemiology of primary liver cancer. In: Tang ZY (ed) Primary liver cancer. Shanghai Scientific and Technical Publisher, Shanghai, pp 55–80[1]

1 Chinese

21 Duck Hepatitis Virus: A Member of the Human Hepatitis B-like Family of Viruses

Zhou Yi-zhong

A great amount of epidemiological data has shown that there is a close correlation between HBV and primary HCC (Blumberg et al. 1975; Szmuness 1978; Tabor et al. 1977; Trichopolous et al. 1978; Beasley et al. 1981). In recent years integration of HBV-DNA in human liver cancer lines, in liver cancer tissues and in the cells surrounding liver cancer nodules has been detected (Brechot et al. 1980, 1981; Chakraborty et al. 1980; Edman et al. 1980; Marion et al. 1980a; Chen et al. 1982), and assumptions of HBV carcinogenesis have been presented by some researchers. However, it is still unclear what role HBV plays in chronic active hepatitis and hepatocarcinogenesis, because HBV has not been successfully propagated in vitro and there is no satisfactory animal model available. Some progress has been made in searching for animal hepatitis viruses which have properties similar to those of HBV. Summers et al. (1978) and Marion et al. (1980b) have found woodchuck hepatitis virus (WHV) in woodchuck serum and ground squirrel hepatitis virus (GSHV) in ground squirrel serum. It has been shown that these viruses possess some properties identical to those of HBV – for example, the morphology under the electron microscope, the presence of endogenous DNA polymerase, an immunochemically weak cross-reaction between the animal viruses and HBV antigen-antibody systems (Werner et al. 1979; Gerlich et al. 1980), the genome composed of circular double-stranded DNA with a partially single-stranded region (Siddiqui et al. 1981; Summers 1981). In particular, the evidence of the integration of WHV-DNA into woodchuck liver cancer cells (Mitamura et al. 1982) and the correlation between WHV and chronic active hepatitis and hepatocellular carcinoma have shown that the woodchuck is a useful model in studies on the pathogenetic mechanism of chronic hepatitis and hepatocarcinogenesis (Popper et al. 1981).

In China, a high incidence of liver cancer has been found in ducks over 2 years of age in Qidong County of Jiangsu Province, a district with a high incidence of liver cancer in the human population as well. Gross pathological changes have been observed frequently in ducks in this district. Consequently, many scientists have shown much interest in whether these changes are caused by duck viruses. In 1980 we isolated a strain of duck hepatitis virus (DHBV) from duck sera (Zhou et al. 1980, 1982), and found the livers of all ducks with DHBV in serum had pathological changes. DHBV showed close resemblance to HBV and WHV in shape, gene composition, and pathogenic and other structural characteristics. Identical results were also obtained by Mason et al. (1980). The purpose of this chapter is to outline the studies on DHBV structural characteristics, distribution, and the possible correlation between DHBV and hepatopathogenesis of the duck.

I. Structure and Characterization of DHBV

Human HBV is known to be a spherical particle, termed a Dane particle, with a diameter of about 40 nm (Dane et al. 1970), composed of a bilayer coat and an inner core with a diameter 28 nm (Almeida et al. 1971). The HBV genome is a double-stranded DNA circle containing about 3200 base pairs (Robinson et al. 1974) and a region of single strands of heterogeneous lengths (Summers et al. 1975; Lander et al. 1977). The viral inner core contains DNA polymerase (Kaplan et al. 1973), which is capable in vitro of converting single-stranded DNA into intact double-stranded DNA.

DHBV in duck serum displays two forms. One is a 40–45 nm spherical particle with an approximately 27-nm core, similar to a Dane particle. The other is a fuller spherical particle with a diameter of 35–55 nm and an irregular surface; some of these do not show any inner core, and some of them seem to have been disrupted (Fig. 1).

Employing the method to test for HBV-DNA polymerase (Zhou et al. 1979), we found that the isolated DHBV from duck serum also revealed DNA polymerase activity (Table 1). CsCl gradient ultracentrifugation of DHBV yielded two portions (see Fig. 2). DNA polymerase activity was detected only in the fractions between 1.20 and 1.21 g/ml, near the first protein peak. Under electron microscopy, two forms of particles were concentrated in this portion. A 35–55 nm particle was also found in the second protein peak with densities of 1.14–1.15 g/ml; in this region most particles seemed to have a disrupted protein coat. Neither spherical nor tubular particles of 22 nm in diameter were found in these fractions.

Nine specimens showing DHBV-DNA polymerase activity, obtained in the suburbs of Shanghai, were determined in an HB_sAg RIA system for comparing the antigenicity of DHBV with that of HB_sAg. A weak cross-reaction in all the specimens

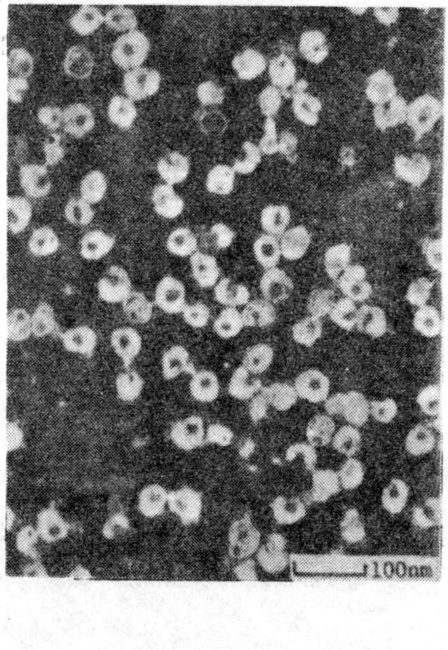

Fig. 1. DHBV particles in duck serum

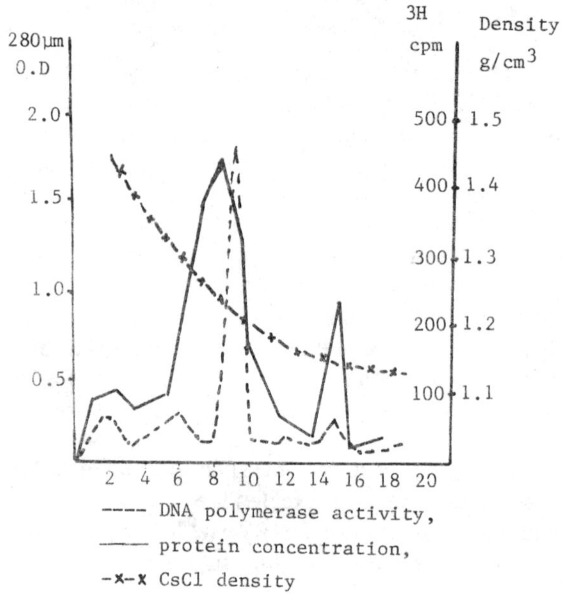

Fig. 2. Isolation of DHBV from duck serum by CsCl gradient centrifugation

Table 1. DNA polymerase activity in duck serum

Specimens	^{3}H (cpm)
DHBV (−), Act. D (−)	−9
DHBV (+), Act D (−)	497
DHBV (+), Act. D (+)	−11
Dane particles	1725
Purified HB_sAg	−2

Act. D, actinomycin D

Table 2. Endogenous DNA polymerase activity in DHBV (+) specimens and HB_sAg antigenicity

No.	Endogenous DNA polymerase activity (cpm)	RIA for HB_sAg (P/N)	Inhibition after adding anti-HB_s (%)
D- 1	848	1.68	37
D-23	51	4.30	33
D-15	358	1.88	37
D- 8	4768	5.00	67
D-11	496	1.91	53
D-19	2471	4.00	88
D-21	836	1.88	53
D-25	381	2.78	74
D-34	286	3.31	71

$$P/N = \frac{\text{cpm of specimen}}{\text{cpm of negative control}}$$

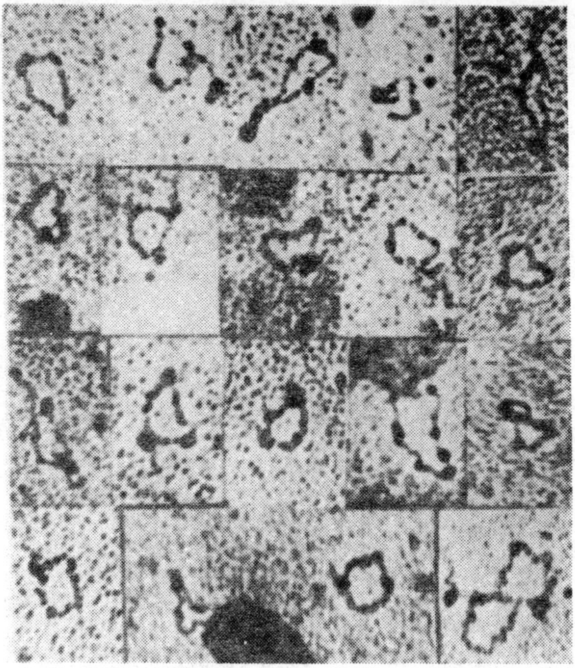

Fig. 3. DHBV-DNA

1 μ

resulted from the competition of DHBV to anti-HB_s with HB_sAg (Table 2). This experiment suggests that both HBV and DHBV possess some common polypeptide chains or common determinant(s), or that there are some similarities in their antigenicity.

After being treated with SDS, porteinase K, phenol extraction, and ethanol precipitation, DHBV was observed under electron microscopy to release a double-stranded DNA circle of DHBV (Fig. 3). Analyses of DHBV-DNA using agarose gel electrophoresis and autoradiography showed a region of single strands of heterogeneous lengths; the single-stranded DNA could be converted into a more complete, double-stranded circle of about 3000 base pairs (Fig. 4). Using the Southern blot method, Mason et al. (1982) reported that the DHBV-DNA isolated from seven ducks was mainly of more complete, double-stranded circles, with smaller single-stranded regions.

II. Transmission of DHBV

DHBV exists not only in ducks from high-incidence liver cancer districts but also in various species of ducks from different sources. Of 138 specimens of older ducks 2–4 years of age from districts other than Qidong County, 44 were also DHBV positive. A detailed analysis showed that the ducks fed on collective farms had a much higher frequency of DHBV (ca. 50%) than the ones fed by individuals (10%–20%).

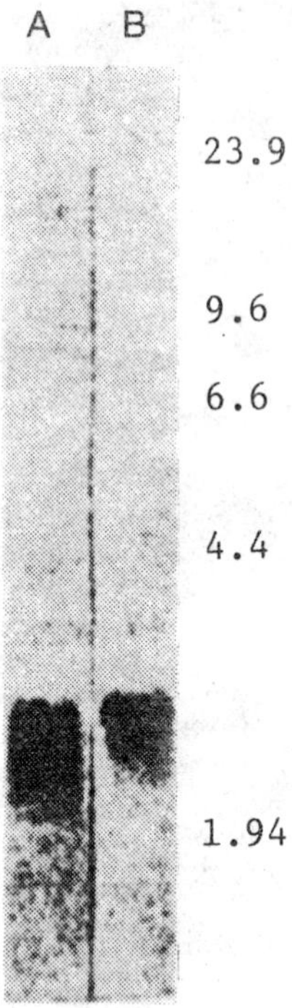

Fig. 4. Electrophoretic pattern of DHBV-DNA after DNA polymerase reaction. *A*, 0.5 h; *B*, 4 h

The higher frequency of DHBV in the collective farms group might be associated with the close contact among the ducks raised with collective feeding methods.

Young ducks, 1 month in age, were experimentally infected with purified DHBV by peritoneal infection. Five infected ducks were killed every 2 weeks up to the 6th month for sequential observation of DHBV proliferation. DHBV could be seen in the sera of two-thirds of the ducks under electron microscopy. These results suggest that at least one route of transmission is horizontal.

We have also found that 10%–20% of young ducks just after birth – aged 1, 3, 5 and 7 days – harbored DHBV in their sera. O'Connell et al. (1983) reported that 14% of serum samples from duck embryos were found to be positive for endogenous DNA polymerase activity characteristic of hepatitis B-related viruses. DHBV-DNA was also found by hybridization with cloned DHBV-DNA in the livers of embryos incubated for 12 or 18 days. These findings suggest that the vertical route is possibly a major pathway of DHBV transmission.

III. Correlation Between DHBV and Duck Liver Histopathology

In a series of ducks with DHBV in the serum, the liver tissue of all 18 ducks showed pathological changes of varying degrees, there being generalized parenchymal damage with disruption of normal liver cell cord arrangement. The hepatic cells were swollen and had distinct margins and pale granular cytoplasm. Focal necrosis was

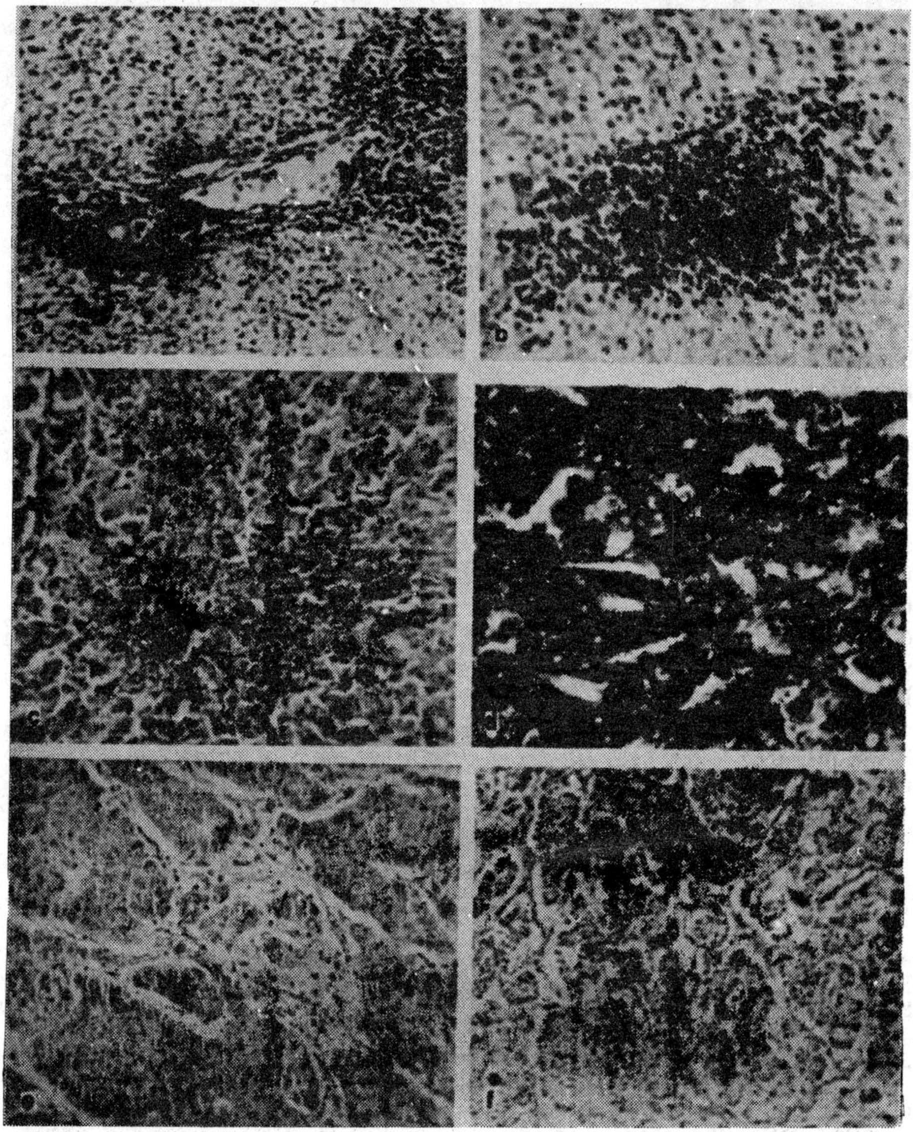

Fig. 5 a–f. Histopathological observation of livers from DHBV (+) ducks. **a** Portal space infiltrated by inflammatory cells. **b** Local necrosis of liver cells. **c** Biliary epithelial cell proliferation in the liver lobules. **d** Immature cell proliferation in the liver lobules. **e** Cancer cells of HCC arranged as coarse trabeculae. **f** Cancer cells of HCC arranged as nests

present, with lymphocytes infiltrating the portal areas and sinusoids throughout the lobules. Variable degrees of fatty change were observed. Smaller bile ducts showed proliferative change. Fibrous tissue extended from the portal zones into lobules, occasionally separating cells or clumps of cells in a star-like fashion. Perilobular necrosis was associated with fibrosis and infiltration by lymphocytes. The periportal zones showed some proliferation of a kind of primitive cell which broke through the limiting plate and extended further into the parenchyma. These round or oval cells showed sparse, basophilic cytoplasm and relatively uniform nuclei with sparse chromatin and one to two prominent nucleoli. Two of these 18 cases were primary HCC. In one case the trabecular pattern of liver-cell carcinoma was recognizably liver-like, but the trabeculae were misshapen and up to many cells thick; in the other, the arrangement of carcinoma cells was nest-like (Fig. 5).

In controls without DHBV in the serum the lobules of liver tissue were histologically normal; no inflammatory cell infiltration or necrosis of cells was found, but varying degrees of fatty change were present. Sometimes the infiltration of a few inflammatory cells in the periportal zones could be seen. The morphological investigation described above seems to provide evidence that there is a close correlation between the pathological changes in duck liver tissue and the presence of DHBV infection.

Five years ago HBV was thought to be a unique virus, not included in any known family of viruses. Following the discoveries of WHV, GSHV, and DHBV, scientists have confirmed the existence of an HBV-like family of viruses in birds and mammals classified as hepadnaviruses. In addition to those stated above, scientists have also predicted the existence of this family of viruses in other animal species. The similarities and differences among HBV, WHV, GSHV, and DHBV in structure, genome, antigenicity, and endogenous DNA polymerase may result from the evolution of their hosts. The fact that there are pathological changes in the livers of ducks with DHBV (+) in serum samples indicates that there is a close correlation among DHBV, hepatitis, and liver cancer, though there is no direct evidence. Ducks, duck eggs, and DHBV are no doubt much easier to obtain than WHV, GSHV, and their hosts. Therefore, it may be presumed that DHBV and its host will become a useful model for the investigation of DHBV proliferation and pathogenesis in vivo, as well as for further understanding of HBV in human beings.

References

Almeida JD, Rubenstein D, Scott EJ (1971) New antigen-antibody system in Australia antigen-positive hepatitis. Lancet 2: 1225–1227

Beasley RP, Lin CC, Hwang LY, et al. (1981) Hepatocellular carcinoma and hepatitis B virus. Lancet 2: 1129–1132

Blumberg BS, Larouze B, London WT, et al. (1975) The relation of infection with the hepatitis B agent to primary hepatic carcinoma. Am J Pathol 81: 669–682

Bréchot C, Pourcel C, Louise A, et al. (1980) Presence of integrated hepatitis B virus DNA sequence in cellular DNA of human hepatocellular carcinoma. Nature 286: 533–535

Bréchot C, Hadchouel M, Scotto J, et al. (1981) State of hepatitis B virus DNA in hepatocytes of patient with hepatitis B surface antigen-positive and -negative liver diseases. Proc Natl Acad Sci USA 78: 3906–3910

Chakraborty PR, Ruiz-Opazo N, Shouval D, et al. (1980) Identification of integrated hepatitis B virus DNA and expression of viral RNA in an HB_sAg-producing human hepatocellular carcinoma cell line. Nature 286: 531–533

Chen DS, Hoyer BH, Nelson J, et al. (1982) Detection and properties of hepatitis B viral DNA in liver tissue from patient with hepatocellular carcinoma. Hepatology 2: 42S–46S

Dane DS, Cameron CH, Briggs M (1970) Virus-like particles in serum of patients with Australia antigen-associated hepatitis. Lancet 2: 695–698

Edman JC, Gray P, Valenzuela P, et al. (1980) Integration of hepatitis B virus sequences and their expression in a human hepatoma cell line. Nature 286: 535–538

Gerlich WH, Feitelson MA, Marion PL, et al. (1980) Structure relationships between the surface antigen of ground squirrel hepatitis virus and human hepatitis B virus. J Virol 36: 787–795
Kaplan PM, Greenman RL, Gerin JL, et al. (1973) DNA polymerase associated with human hepatitis B antigen. J Virol 12: 995–1005
Lander TA, Greenberg HD, Robinson WS (1977) Structure of hepatitis B Dane particle DNA and nature of the endogenous DNA polymerase reaction. J Virol 23: 368–376
Marion PL, Salazar FH, Alexander JJ, et al. (1980a) State of hepatitis B viral DNA in a human cell line. J Virol 33: 795–806
Marion PL, Oshire LS, Regnery DC, et al. (1980b) A virus of Beechey ground squirrel that is related to hepatitis B virus of human. Proc Natl Acad Sci USA 77: 2941–2945
Mason WS, Seal G, Summers J (1980) Virus of Pekin ducks with structural and biological relatedness to human hepatitis B virus. J Virol 36: 829–836
Mason WS, Yaylor JM, Seal G, et al. (1982) An HBV-like virus of domestic ducks. In: Szmuness W, Alter HJ, Maynard JE (eds) Viral hepatitis. 1981 International Symposium. Franklin Institute Press, Philadelphia, pp 107–116
Mitamura K, Hoyer BH, Ponzetto A, et al. (1982) Woodchuck hepatitis virus DNA in woodchuck liver tissues. Hepatology 2: 47S–50S
O'Connell AP, Urban MK, London WT (1983) Naturally occurring infection of Pekin duck embryos by duck hepatitis B virus. Proc Natl Acad Sci USA 80: 1703–1706
Popper H, Shih JWK, Gerin JL et al. (1981) Woodchuck hepatitis and hepatocellular carcinoma – correlation of histologic observations. Hepatology 1: 91–98
Robinson WS, Clayton DA, Greenman RL (1974) DNA of a human hepatitis B virus candidate. J Virol 14: 384–388
Siddiqui A, Marion PL, Robinson WS (1981) Ground squirrel hepatitis virus DNA: Molecular cloning and comparison with hepatitis B virus DNA. J Virol 38: 393–397
Summers J (1981) Three recently described animal virus models for human hepatitis B virus. Hepatology 1: 179–183
Summers J, O'Connell A, Millman I, et al. (1975) Genome of hepatitis B virus: Restriction of enzyme cleavage and structure of DNA extracted from Dane particles. Proc Natl Acad Sci USA 72: 4597–4601
Summers J, Smolec JM, Synder R (1978) A virus similar to hepatitis B virus associated with hepatitis and hepatoma in woodchucks. Proc Natl Acad Sci USA 75: 4533–4537
Szmuness W (1978) Hepatocellular carcinoma and hepatitis B virus – evidence for a causal association. Prog Med Virol 24: 40–69
Tabor E, Gerety RJ, Vogel CL, et al. (1977) Hepatitis B virus infections and primary hepatocellular carcinoma. J Natl Cancer Inst 58: 1197–1200
Trichopolous D, Tabor E, Gerety RJ, et al. (1978) Hepatitis B and primary hepatocellular carcinoma in a European population. Lancet 2: 1217–1219
Werner BG, Smolec JM, Synder R, et al. (1979) Serological relationship of woodchuck hepatitis virus to human hepatitis B virus. J Virol 32: 314–322
Zhou YZ, Tao QM, Wang JQ, et al. (1979) DNA polymerase activity in patients with primary liver cancer and hepatitis B carriers. Natl Med J China 59: 298–301[1]
Zhou YZ, Kou PY, Shao LQ (1980) A virus possibly associated with hepatitis and hepatoma in ducks. Shanghai Med J 3: 1–3[1]
Zhou YZ, Ding HZ, Dai PH, et al. (1982) A virus in ducks similar to human hepatitis B virus. Shanghai Med J 5: 1–4[1]

---

1 Chinese

22 Hepatitis B Vaccine

Zhou Yi-zhong

The epidemiology of HBV, worldwide distribtuion of HB_sAg, and correlation between this virus and primary hepatocellular carcinoma have been described and commented on by many scientists (Blumberg and London 1981; Maupas and Melnick 1981; Prince 1981). Prevention and control of HBV are becoming more and more important in eliminating infection; for this reason many laboratories have paid great attention to the development of a hepatitis B vaccine.

Several years ago, the discovery of Australia antigen by Blumberg (1964) and the identification of strains MS-1 and MS-2 by Krugman et al. (Krugman and Giles 1970; Krugman et al. 1971) laid the groundwork for studies on hepatitis B, HBV biological characterization, and a hepatitis B vaccine. Further studies showed that three forms of particles might exist in the serum of hepatitis B patients and of HBV carriers: spherical particles 22 nm in diameter, tubular particles 22 nm in diameter, and Dane particles 42 nm in diameter (Dane et al. 1970). The first two have a protein coat and neither DNA nor infectious activity, while the third is regarded as intact HBV. All these particles possess common antigenicity of HB_sAg and can be immunologically precipitated and coagulated by antiserum to HB_sAg (anti-HB_s). Dane particles are composed of a protein coat and a core (Almeida et al. 1971), the core being 27 nm in diameter HB_cAg and consisting of DNA and DNA polymerase (Kaplan et al. 1973; Robinson et al. 1974). To date, in vitro proliferation of HBV has not been successful; therefore, extensive studies on hepatitis B vaccine have concentrated on how to obtain a large amount of HB_sAg material with HB_sAg antigenicity and on how to strengthen their immunogenicity.

I. Purified Serum HB_sAg as Vaccine

Hilleman et al. (1975) and Purcell and Gerin (1975) purified 22 nm HB_sAg particles from the sera of HB_sAg carriers as a vaccine to immunize the chimpanzee challenged by infectious material. Both groups found their vaccines were efficacious and had no harmful effects. Since then, a great number of more sophisticated vaccines have been developed in the United States, France, and Japan. Very encouraging evaluations of the safety and efficacy of these vaccines have resulted from large-scale field trials among high-risk populations, susceptible populations, natural populations, and infants whose mothers were HB_sAg carriers (Hilleman et al. 1978; Purcell and Gerin 1978; Maupas et al. 1978, 1981; Prince et al. 1978; Szmuness 1979; Szmuness et al. 1980, 1981).

In China since 1975, Tao et al. in the Shanghai Institute of Biological Products, Zhou et al., and the Beijing Institute of Biological Products have also purified 22-nm HB_sAg particles from the sera of HB_sAg carriers as a vaccine to inoculate human volunteers. Twenty-two healthy subjects were injected subcutaneously over the deltoid muscle with 1.0 ml of adjuvant vaccine prepared by Tao et al., the immunization being carried out three times, once a month. Eleven of them were found to be anti-HB_s positive 1 month after inoculation, 13 to be positive 2 months after, and 16 3 months after (positive rate 72.7%); all of them had neither detectable HB_sAg and anti-HB_c nor elevation of ALT activity (Tao et al. 1980).

To determine the safety and efficacy of the vaccine prepared by the Shanghai Institute of Biological Products, 33 healthy subjects were vaccinated. They received three injections of vaccine (protein concentration 273 µg/ml, 1.0 ml subcutaneously). The interval between the first and second injections was 1 month, that between the second and third injections 4–6 months. Of the vaccinated subjects 90.9%, were anti-HB_s positive 3 months after the first injection and none revealed HB_sAg or a rise of ALT (Liu et al. unpublished). The safety and efficacy of the HB_sAg vaccine purified by Zhou et al. were also observed by Kang et al. (unpublished). Nine volunteers, who were HB_sAg, anti-HB_s, and anti-HB_c negative, were injected subcutaneously three times at 1-month intervals with 1.0 ml vaccine which contained 50 µg/ml purified formalin-treated HB_sAg. Seven of nine were anti-HB_s positive by RIA 2 months after the first injection, and eight were positive 4, 6, or 9 months after. The P/N average value[1] at 2, 4, 6, and 9 months was 23, 81.8, 36.5, and 23.1 respectively. None of the vaccinated subjects was HB_sAg positive, and none had elevation of ALT. Characterization of serum 22-nm HB_sAg vaccines now available is listed in Table 1.

Table 1. Characterization of reported vaccines

Reference	HB_sAg subtype	Composition
Hilleman et al. (USA) (1978)	adw	Subunit (22-nm particles)
Purcell et al. (USA) (1978)	adw	Subunit (22-nm particles
Maupas et al. (France) (1978)	ad + ay	Subunit (Mixed)
Prince et al. (USA) (1978)	adw	Subunit (5–20-nm particles)
Shikata et al. (Japan)	adr	Subunit (22-nm particles)
Tao et al. (1980, China)	ad	Subunit (spherical particles)
Peking Institute of Biological Products (China)	ad	Subunit (spherical particles)
Shanghai Institute of Biological Products (China) (1982)	ad	Subunit (22-nm particles)
Zhou et al. (China) (1980)	ad	Subunit (22-nm particles)

[1] $P/N - \frac{\text{cpm of specimen}}{\text{cpm of negative control}}$

II. Polypeptides of HB_sAg as Vaccine

Although 22-nm HB_sAg as vaccine has not been found unsafe, controversy still exists among some scientists as to its contaminated host-components, including even some infectious materials (Neurath et al. 1974; Zuckerman 1975). An HB_sAg polypeptide vaccine has been developed to substitute for 22-nm HB_sAg particles. Two main polypeptides, one with a mol. wt. of 22000–26000 (P1) and a polysaccharide-containing polypeptide with a mol. wt. of 28000–30000 (P2), were isolated from different subtypes of HB_sAg using various methods (Gerin et al. 1975; Dreesman et al. 1975; Robinson 1977; Cabral et al. 1978; Skelly et al. 1979; Zhou et al. 1980). P1 and P2 were extremely similar in their amino acids compositions and amino acids sequences of N-, C-terminals (Shih and Gerin 1977; Peterson et al. 1977), which suggested that P2 might be a derivative of P1 after polysaccharification. Both of them possessed immunogenicity identical to that of HB_sAg; chimpanzees immunized with P1 or P2 were capable of preventing HBV attack (Hollinger et al. 1978; Dreesman et al. 1981). P1 and P2 obtained in our laboratory by SDS-urea-mercaptoethanol treatments and SDS-polyacrylamide gel electrophoresis were able to raise specific antibody response to HB_sAg in guinea pigs immunized with dosages of 1, 5, and 20 μg (Table 2, Fig. 1). Eight of the 12 volunteers who received a single injection of 200 μg P1–P2 mixture had raised specific anti-HB_s response, while placebo controls had no anti-HB_s response (Table 3). During 4 years of follow-up none of the 12 vaccine recipients developed side effects or suffered from HBV, though the polypeptide vaccine had raised antibody in lower titer with a longer lag phase and shorter in vivo maintenance as compared with 22-nm HB_sAg vaccine.

Table 2. Immunization of guinea pigs with various doses of HB_sAg and HB_sAg polypeptide

Day after first injection	1 μg/time		5 μg/time		20 μg/times		Control
	P	HB_sAg	P	HB_sAg	P	HB_sAg	
14	0/5	4/4	0/5	5/5	0/5	4/4	0/5
33	2/5	4/4	0/4	5/5	0/5	4/4	0/5
47	4/5	4/4	3/4	5/5	4/5	4/4	0/4
76	3/3	3/3	3/3	5/5	3/4	1/2	0/3
103	0/3	2/2	2/3	5/5	2/4	1/2	0/3

P, polypeptide; denominator: total number of animals; numerator: anti-HB_s(+) number
Each animal was immunized 3 times, every 2nd week

Table 3. Immunization of human beings with HB_sAg polypeptides

Days after 1st injection	Experimental group (12 persons)			Placebo controls (9 persons)		
	HB_sAg	Anti-HB_s	Anti-HB_c	HB_sAg	Anti-HB_s	HB_c
66	0	0	0	0	0	0
637	0	0	0	0	0	0
673	0	3	0	0	0	0
729	0	8	0	0	0	0

200 μg per injection, 4 times; immunizations were carried out on 1st, 19th, 37th, and 637th days.

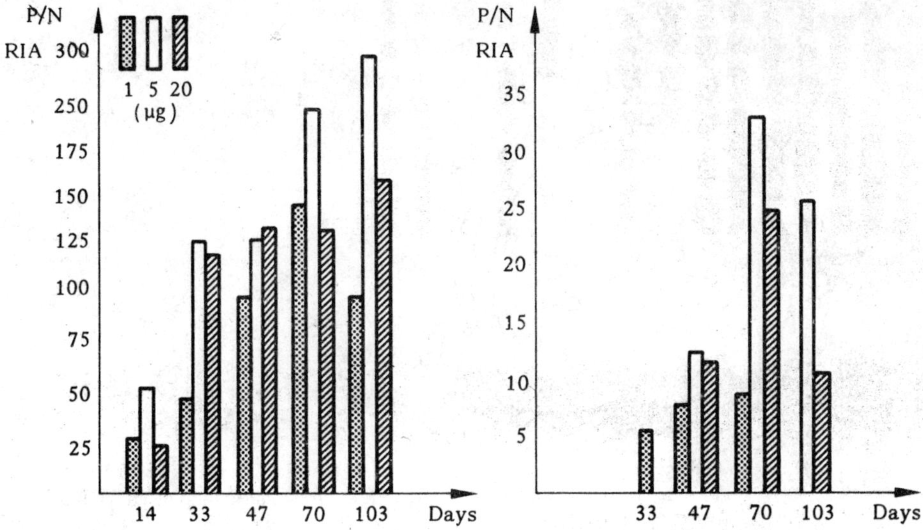

Fig. 1. Anti-HB_s titer maintenance in guinea pigs after *(left)* HB_sAg or *(right)* HB_sAg polypeptide immunization

After triton x-100 treatment, affinity chromatography, and gradient ultracentrifugation, HB_sAg might first be relaxed to form polypeptides and then form clusters, commonly known as polypeptide micelles, which could reveal much stronger immunogenicity than the above-mentioned P1 and P2 vaccines, stronger even than 22-nm HB_sAg (Skelly et al. 1979, 1981). However, controversial results have also been obtained. Antibody titer raised by micelles was only some 50%–80% of that raised by 22-nm HB_sAg in mice (Young et al. 1982), but in chimpanzees it was markedly stronger than that raised by water-soluble polypeptides (Tabor et al. 1982). If the immunogenicity of polypeptide micelles could be further strenthened, they would possibly constitute a safe and efficacious vaccine to substitute for 22-nm HB_sAg in man.

III. Studies on Genetic Engineering of HB Vaccine

To overcome the difficulties of the raw material source, genetic engineering of HBV vaccine was begun in the mid 1980s. Since Summers et al. (1975) found that HBV-DNA consisted of double-stranded DNA containing a single-stranded region, and Landers et al. (1977) found that HBV-DNA with a single-stranded region might be converted in vitro into an intact double-stranded DNA by endogenous DNA polymerase, HBV genetic engineering has been developing very quickly. Scientists in France, the United States, the United Kingdom, and West Germany have succeeded in cloning ayw, adw, and adyw HBV genomes (Charnay et al. 1979a; Valenzuela et al. 1979; Burrell et al. 1979; Sninsky et al. 1979), in making their restriction maps, in sequencing 3200 b.p. of HBV, and in localizing HB_sAg genes and HB_cAg genes in HBV genome as well (Galibert et al. 1979; Charnay et al. 1979b; Valenzue-

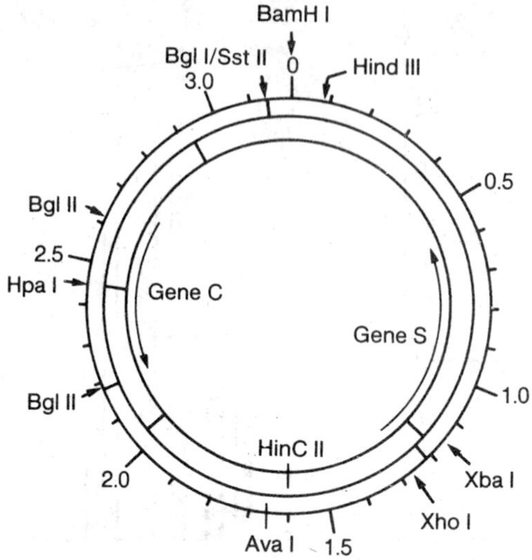

Fig. 2. Restriction map of HBVadr-DNA

Table 4. Comparison of restriction endonuclease action on HBV subtype genomes

Subtype	No. of action sites										
	*Ava*I	*Ava*II	*Bgl*II	*Bam*HI	*Eco*RI	*Hae*III	*Hin*CII	*Hind*III	*Hpa*I	*Pst*I	*Sma*I
adw	2	7	2	2	1	10	5	0	1	1	0
adr	4		2	1	0		3	1	0	0	0
ayw	3	7	3	3	1	13	4	0	0	0	0
adyw		4	2	2		13					
	*Sst*II	*Xba*I	*Xho*I	*Kpn*I	*Sal*I	*Sst*I					
adw	1	1									
adr	1	1	1	0	0	0					
ayw		3	1	0	0	0					
adyw		3	1								

la et al. 1979). In 1982 we succeeded in cloning the adr subtype genome (Wu et al. 1983) and in making its restriction map. The adr genome is clearly distinguishable from ayw, adw, and adyw genomes in its restriction map and nucleotide sequence (Fig. 2, Table 4).

HBV genetic engineering has enabled *Escherichia coli* to express HB_sAg (Charnay et al. 1980; Edman et al. 1981; Mackay et al. 1981). Our adr plasmid, under the control of Lac operon initiation gene, is able to synthesize a β-galactosidase-HB_sAg complex, which possesses HB_sAg antigenicity (Figs. 3 and 4). As is known from the literature, expression of HB_sAg plasmid seems to be very weak and expressed materials are fused components consisting of HB_sAg and bacterial proteins. More recently, we have reconstituted a novel plasmid containing an HB_sAg gene and a bacterial initiation gene, which expresses HB_sAg material much more strongly than the

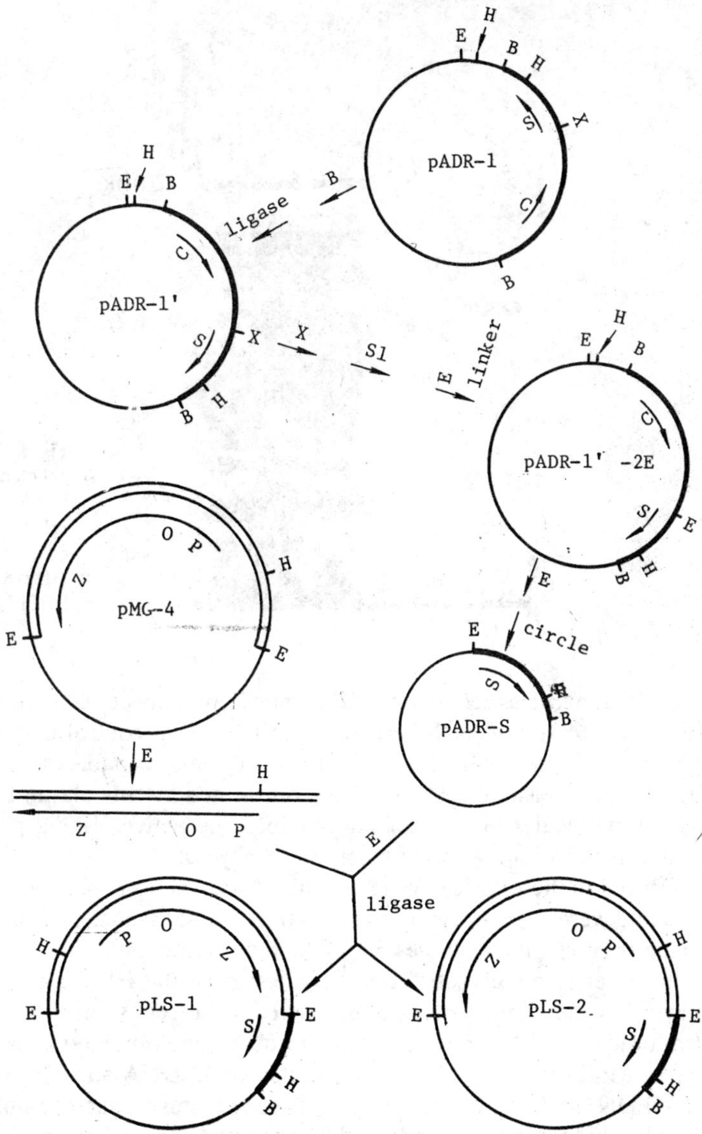

Fig. 3. Construction of recombinant plasmid. *B, Bam*I; *E, Eco,*RI; *H, Hin,*dIII; *X, Xho*I

first one. However, whether HB_sAg fused bacterial proteins could be utilized as a hepatitis B vaccine remains to be studied.

The expression of HB_sAg gene in yeast was much more successful. Valenzuela et al. (1982) reported the synthesis of HB_sAg in the yeast *Saccharomyces cerevisiae* by using an expression vector that employs the 5-flanking region of yeast alcohol dehydrogenase I as a promoter to transcribe surface antigen coding sequences. The protein synthesized in yeast was assembled into particles having properties similar to

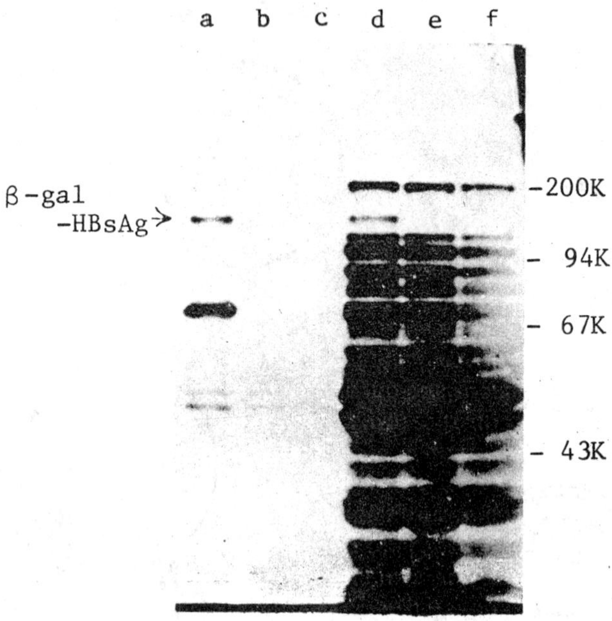

Fig. 4. SDS polyacrylamide gel electrophoresis of bacterial proteins. **a** pLS-1 + anti-HB_s; **b** pADR-S + anti-HB_s; **c** MC106 + anti-HB_s; **d** pLS-1; **e** pADR-S; **f** MC106

the 22-nm particles secreted by the human hepatoma cell line. Recently, Miyanohara et al. (1983) placed the HB_sAg gene under the control of the repressible acid phosphatase promoter of *S. cerevisiae* in a plasmid capable of autonomous replication in both yeast and *E. coli.* Yeast transfomed by this plasmid synthesized up to 5×10^5 molecules per cell of immunologically active HB_sAg polypetide in phosphate-free medium (approximately 3 μg/ml yeast extract). The HB_sAg polypeptides produced in the yeast cell were assembled into 20- to 22-nm spherical or oval particles and were immunogenic in guinea pigs. These results, no doubt, represent heartening progress in the studies on fermented production of hepatitis B vaccine.

In order to obtain satisfactory expression of the HB_sAg gene, a series of trials have also been done in cell culture systems in recent years. Dubois et al. (1980) introduced the HBV gene into mouse fibroblast and obtained 22-nm HB_sAg-like particles. Moriarty et al. (1981) reconstituted SV40 DNA and HB_sAg gene to form an SV40 DNA-HB_sAg DNA complex. The recombinant gene complex proliferated in monkey kidney cells and released 22-nm HB_sAg in culture medium. Stratowa et al. (1982) introduced a recombinant gene of HB_sAg DNA with MSV-DNA into 3T3 mouse fibroblast and obtained HB_sAg at a yield of 4.5 μg/10^7 cells/day. Wang et al. (1983) introduced a recombinant gene of HB_sAg DNA with bovine papilloma virus DNA into mouse fibloblast and obtained a higher yield of HB_sAg. HB_sAg particles produced by means of transformed cells have an elevated efficacy in chimpanzees. However, the cell systems adopted here are all tumor cells, which frightens the vaccine recipients.

More recently, Smith et al. (1983) reported a potential live vaccine against HBV. The HB_sAg gene was linked to a vaccinia control region, which contains information to "turn on" or express the gene. Then the engineered gene was inserted into a

Table 5. Chemicopolypeptides containing HB_sAg antigenicity

Position	Amino acid sequence
2–16[a]	Glu-Asn-Ile-Thr-Ser-Gly-Phe-Leu-Gly-Pro-Leu-Leu-Val-Leu-Gln-Cys
22–35[a]	Leu-Thr-Arg-Ile-Leu-Thr-Ile-Pro-Gln-Ser-Leu-Asp-Ser-Try-Cys
48–81[a]	Cys-Leu-Gly-Gln-Asn-Ser-Gln-Ser-Pro-Thr-Ser-Asn-His-Ser-Pro-Thr-Ser-Cys-Pro-Pro-Thr-Cys-Pro-Gly-Tyr-Arg-Trp-Met-Cys-Leu-Arg-Arg-Phe-Ile
95–109[a]	Leu-Val-Leu-Leu-Asp-Tyr-Gln-Gly-Met-Leu-Pro-Val-Cys-Pro-Leu
122–137[b]	Lys-Thr-Cys-Met-Thr-Thr-Ala-Gln-Gly-Thr-Ser-Met-Tyr-Pro-Ser-Cys
141–146[c]	Lys-Pro-Thr-Asp-Gly-Asn
139–147[d]	Cys-Thr-Lys-Pro-Thr-Asp-Gly-Asn-Cys

[a] Lerner et al. (1981)
[b] Dreesman et al. (1982)
[c] Prince et al. (1982)
[d] Bhatnager et al. (1982)

plasmid containing a vaccinia marker gene. The plasmid was transferred to a whole vaccinia virus by being put into cells infected with normal vaccinia virus. Genetic exchange between the plasmid and the vaccinia produced some recombinant viruses. Cells infected with these recombinant vaccinia viruses synthesized and excreted 22-nm particles similar to those obtained in the medium of hepatoma cell line PLC/PRF/5. Rabbits vaccinated with vaccinia virus recombinants have rapidly produced antibody to HB_sAg. It will be encouraging if a live vaccine for hepatitis can replace an inactvated vaccine.

IV. Chemically Synthesized Polypeptides with HB_sAg Antigenicity

A novel approach to creating a hepatitis B vaccine is to chemically synthesize polypeptides with active immunogenicity against HBV. Several polypeptides, chemicosynthesized according to amino acid sequences of HB_sAg fragments, revealed their antigenicity (Table 5) only on hydrophilic domains (Lerner et al. 1981; Dreesman et al. 1982; Prince et al. 1982; Bhatnager et al. 1982). Chemicopolypeptides showed a weaker immunogenicity than did natural HB_sAg polypeptides. Coagulation of chemicopolypeptides into micelles or conjugation of them onto tetanus toxoid could enhance their immunogenicity markedly (Sanchez et al. 1982). With respect to the possibility of using chemicopolypeptides as hepatitis vaccine, there is still a controversy because it is not known whether chemicopolypeptides with fewer determinants and weaker immunogenicity would be capable of preventing HBV attack.

Studies on hepatitis B vaccine have made great progress in the past 10 years. Besides serum HB_sAg vaccine as a commercial article, HB_sAg polypeptide vaccine, genetic engineering of HB_sAg vaccine, and chemicopolypeptide vaccine, are all being developed very quickly. Prevention of hepatitis and a decline in the incidence of primary hepatocellular carcinoma can be expected with the wide use of hepatitis B vaccine among the human population.

References

Almeida JD, Rubenstein D, Scott EJ (1971) New antigen-antibody system in Australia antigen-positive hepatitis. Lancet 2: 1225–1227

Bhatnagar PK, Papas E, Blum HE, et al. (1982) Immune response to synthetic peptide analogues of hepatitis B surface antigen specific for the a determinant. Proc Natl Acad Sci USA 79: 4400–4404

Blumberg BS (1964) Polymorphism of serum protein and the development of isoprecipitins in transfused patients. Bull NY Acad Med 40: 377–386

Blumberg BS, London WT (1981) Hepatitis B virus and the prevention of primary hepatocellular carcinoma. New Engl J Med 304: 782–784

Burrell CJ, Mackay P, Greenaway PJ, et al. (1979) Expression in *Escherichia coli* of hepatitis B virus DNA sequences cloned in plasmid PBR 322. Nature 279: 43–47

Cabral GA, Marcino-Cabral F, Funk GA, et al. 1978) Cellular and humoral immunity in guinea pigs to two major polypeptides derived from hepatitis B surface antigen. J Gen Virol 38: 339–350

Charnay P, Poucell C, Louise A, et al. (1979a) Cloning in *Escherichia coli* and physical structure of hepatitis B virion DNA. Proc Natl Acad Sci USA 76: 2222–2226

Charnay P, Mandart E, Hampe A, et al. (1979b) Localization on the viral genome and nucleotide sequence of the gene coding for the two major polypeptides of the hepatitis B surface antigen (HB_sAg). Nucleic Acid Res 7: 335–346

Charnay P, Gervais M, Louise A, et al. (1980) Biosynthesis of hepatitis B virus surface antigen in *Escherichia coli*. Nature 291: 503–506

Dane DS, Cameron CH, Briggs M (1970) Virus-like particles in serum of patient with Australia antigen-associated hepatitis. Lancet 2: 695–698

Dreesman GR, Hollinger FB, Melnick JL (1975) Biophysical and biochemical properties of purified preparation of hepatitis B surface antigen. Am J Med Sci 270: 123–129

Dreesman GR, Hollinger FB, Sanchez Y, et al. (1981) Immunization of chimpanzees with hepatitis B virus-derived polypeptides. Infect Immun 32: 62–67

Dreesman GR, Sanchez Y, Ionescu-Matiu I, et al. (1982) Antibody to hepatitis B surface antigen after a single inoculation of uncoupled synthetic HB_sAg peptides. Nature 295: 158–160

Dubois MF, Poucell C, Pousset S, et al. (1980) Excretion of hepatitis B surface antigen particles from mouse cells transformed with cloned viral DNA. Proc Natl Acad Sci USA 77: 4549–4553

Edman JC, Hallewell P, Valenzuela P, et al. (1981) Synthesis of hepatitis B surface and core antigen in *E. coli*. Nature 291: 503–506

Galibert F, Mandart E, Fitoussi F, et al. (1979) Nucleotide sequence of the hepatitis B virus genome (subtype ayw) cloned in *E. coli*. Nature 281: 646–650

Gerin JL, Shih JWK, Kaplan PM, et al. (1975) Biophysical and biochemical characterization of hepatitis B antigen. Am J Med Sci 270: 115–121

Hilleman MR, Buynak EB, Roehm RR, et al. (1975) Purified and inactivated human hepatitis B vaccine: progress report. Am J Med Sci 270: 401–404

Hilleman MR, Bertland AU, Buynak EB, et al. (1978) Clinical and laboratory studies of HB vaccine. In: Vyas GN, Cohen SN, Schmid R (eds) Viral hepatitis. Franklin Institute Press, Philadelphia, pp 525–538

Hollinger FB, Dreesman GR, Sanchez Y, et al. (1978) Experimental hepatitis B polypeptide vaccine in chimpanzees. In: Vyas GN, Cohen SN, Schmid R (eds) Viral hepatitis. Franklin Institute Press, Philadelphia, pp 557–567

Kaplan PM, Greeman RL, Gerin JL, et al. (1973) DNA polymerase associated with human hepatitis B antigen. J Virol 12: 995–1005

Krugman S, Giles JP (1970) Viral hepatitis. New light on an old disease. JAMA 212: 1019–1029

Krugman S, Giles JP, Hammond J (1971) Viral hepatitis. Type B (MS-2 strain): studies on active immunization. JAMA 217: 41–45

Landers TA, Greenberg HB, Robinson WS (1977) Structure of hepatitis B Dane particle DNA and nature of the endogenous DNA polymerase reaction. J Virol 23: 368–376

Lerner RA, Green N, Alexander H, et al. (1981) Chemically synthesized peptides predicted from the nucleotide sequence of the hepatitis B virus genome elicit antibody reaction with the native envelope protein of Dane particles. Proc Natl Acad Sci USA 78: 3403–3407

Mackay P, Pasek M, Magazin M, et al. (1981) Production of immunologically active surface antigens of hepatitis virus by *Escherichia coli*. Proc Natl Acad Sci USA 78: 4510–4514

Maupas P, Melnick JL (1981) Hepatitis B infection and primary liver cancer. Prog Med Virol 27: 1–5
Maupas P, Goudeau A, Coursaget P (1978) Immunization against hepatitis B in man: a pilot study of two years duration. In: Vyas GN, Cohen SN, Schmid R (eds) Viral hepatitis. Franklin Institute Press, Philadelphia, pp 539–556
Maupas P, Chiron JP, Barin F, et al. (1981) Efficacy of hepatitis B vaccine in prevention of early HB_sAg carrier state in children. Lancet 1: 289–292
Miyanohara A, Toh-E A, Nazaki C, et al. (1983) Expression of hepatitis B surface antigen gene in yeast. Proc Natl Acad Sci USA 80: 1–5
Moriarty AM, Houer BH, Shih JWK, et al. (1981) Expression of the hepatitis B virus surface antigen gene in cell culture by using a simian 40 vector. Proc Natl Acad Sci USA 78: 2606–2610
Neurath AR, Prince AM, Lippin A (1974) Hepatitis B antigen: antigenic sites related to human serum proteins revealed by affinity chromatography. Proc Natl Acad Sci USA 71: 2663–2667
Peterson DL, Roberts IM, Vyas GN (1977) Partial amino acid sequence of two major compenent polypeptides of hepatitis B surface antigen. Proc Natl Acad Sci USA 74: 1530–1534
Prince AM (1981) Hepatitis B virus and hepatocellular carcinoma: Molecular biology provides futher evidence for an etiologic association. Hepatology 1: 73–75
Prince AM, Vnek J, Brotman B, et al. (1978) Comparative evaluations of hepatitis B vaccines in chimpanzees and in man. In: Vyas GN, Cohen SN, Schmid R (eds) Viral hepatitis. Franklin Institute Press, Philadelphia, pp 507–523
Prince AM, Ikram H, Hopp TP (1982) Hepatitis B virus vaccine: Identification of HB_sAg/a and HB_sAg/d but not HB_sAg/y subtype antigenic determinants on a synthetic immunogenic peptide. Proc Natl Acad Sci USA 79: 579–582
Purcell RH, Gerin JL (1975) Hepatitis B subunit vaccine: A preliminary report of safety and efficacy test in chimpanzees. Am J Med Sci 270: 395–399
Purcell RH, Gerin JL (1978) Hepatitis B vaccine: A status report. In: Vyas GN, Cohen SN, Schmid R (eds) Viral hepatitis. Franklin Institute Press, Philadelphia, pp 491–505
Robinson WS (1977) The genome of hepatitis B virus. Ann Rev Microbiol 31: 357–377
Robinson WS, Clayton DA, Greenman RL (1974) DNA of human hepatitis B virus candidate. J Virol 14: 384–391
Sanchez Y, Ionescu-Matiu I, Sparrow JT, et al. (1982) Immunogenicity of conjugates and micelles of synthetic hepatitis B surface antigen peptides. Intervirology 18: 209–213
Shih JWK, Gerin JL (1977) Proteins of hepatitis surface antigen: Amino acid compositions of the major polypeptides. J Virol 21: 1219–1222
Skelly J, Howard CR, Zuckerman AJ (1979) Analysis of hepatitis B antigen components solubilized with Triton x-100. J Gen Virol 44: 679–689
Skelly J, Howard CR, Zuckerman AJ (1981) Hepatitis B polypeptide vaccine preparation in micelle form. Nature 290: 51–54
Smith GL, Mackett M, Moss B (1983) Infectious vaccinia virus recombinants that express hepatitis B virus surface antigen. Nature 303: 490–495
Sninsky JJ, Siddiqui A, Robinson WS, et al. (1979) Cloning and endonuclease mapping of the hepatitis B viral genome. Nature 279: 364–368
Stratowa C, Doehmer J, Wang Y, et al. (1982) Recombinant retroviral DNA yielding high expression of hepatitis B surface antigen. EBMO J 1: 1573–1578
Summers J, O'Connell A, Millman I (1975) Genome of hepatitis B virus: Restriction enzyme cleavage and structure of DNA extracted from Dane particles. Proc Natl Acad Sci USA 72: 4597–4601
Szmuness W (1979) Large-scale efficacy trials of hepatitis B vaccine in the USA baseline: data and protocols. J Med Virol 4: 327–340
Szmuness W, Stevens CE, Harley EJ, et al. (1980) Hepatitis B vaccine. Demonstration of efficacy in a controlled clinical trial in a high-risk population in United States. N Engl J Med 303: 833–841
Szmuness W, Stevens CE, Zang EA, et al. (1981) A controlled clinical trial of the efficacy of the hepatitis B vaccine (Heptavax B): a final report. Hepatology 1: 377–385
Tabor E, Howard CR, Skelly J, et al. (1982) Immunogenicity in chimpanzees of experimental hepatitis B vaccines prepared from intact hepatitis B virus, purified polypeptide or polypeptide micelles. J Med Virol 10: 65–74

Tao QM, Wang JQ, Feng BF, et al. (1980) Further research on the HB vaccine. J Beijing Med College 12: 223–226[1]
Valenzuela P, Gray P, Quiroga M, et al. (1979) Nucleotide sequence of the gene coding for the major protein of hepatitis B virus surface antigen. Nature 280: 815–819
Valenzuela P, Medina A, Rutter WT, et al. (1982) Synthesis and assembly of hepatitis B virus surface antigen particles in yeast. Nature 298: 347–350
Wang Y, Stratowa C, Schaefer-Ridder M, et al. (1983) Enhanced production of the hepatitis B surface antigen in NIH 3T3 mouse fibroblasts by using extrachromosomally replicating bovine papillomavirus vector. Mol Cell Biol 3: 1032–1039
Wu XF, Zhou YZ, Feng ZM, et al. (1983) Cloning and restriction mapping of human HBV genome serotype adr. Scientia Sinica 2: 162–167[1]
Young P, Vaudin M, Dixon J, et al. (1982) Preparation of hepatitis B polypeptide micelles from human carrier plasma. J Virol Meth 4: 177–185
Zhou YZ, Gu BC, Xia SY, et al. (1980) Antigenicity of hepatitis B surface antigen polypeptides. Shanghai Med J 3: 7–12[1]
Zuckerman AJ (1975) Hepatitis vaccine: A note of caution. Nature 255: 104–105

1 Chinese

23 Alpha-Fetoprotein During Ontogenesis and Oncogenesis: Gene, Regulation of Gene Expression, and Phenotypic Structure

Zhen Qing-yi

Alpha-fetoprotein (AFP), a major constituent of fetal serum in all mammalian species, decreases drastically with the progress of gestation. At birth, the value of AFP in serum decreases markedly to a very low level, only several hundredths of the highest amount in the fetus. It further decreases to a basal level of the adult within several months after birth.

Re-elevation of AFP in the adult occurs under a selected number of pathological conditions: liver injury, including viral and chemical injury as well as partial hepatectomy, hepatocarcinomas, teratomas, etc. In addition, lymphoproliferative disease, a number of congenital birth defects including congenital nephrosis, severe Rh-hemolytic disease, and several open neutral tube defects are associated with the abnormal appearence of AFP. These striking and reproducible elevations of AFP in carcinomas of liver and germ cells, in regenerative liver disease, and in fetal abnormalities in humans have been widely used for clinical and other scientific purposes, even for early diagnosis and treatment of subclinical hepatocellular carcinoma in China.

Besides the clinical diagnosis, serum AFP measurement has been widely employed in the mass survey of populations for detecting primary liver cancer in China. Since 1970, over 4 million people have been screened by means of several tests, such as double diffusion, CIEP, rocket immunoradioautography, and/or hemoagglutination (Coordinating Group for the Research of Liver Cancer, China 1974, 1979). It was found that more than 400 persons who had no clinical signs or symptoms had abnormal AFP levels and were finally proved to be liver cancer patients; some of them have since been cured (Shanghai Coordinating Group for Research on Liver Cancer, 1979).

It has been proven that almost all mammals are able to produce AFP, with common chemical and immunological properties (except for species specificity), as well as identical dynamics during ontogenesis and oncogenesis. The association of AFP decline with maturation and its elevation with pathogenesis of hepatocytes has generated great interest in the mechanism of regulation of AFP gene expression in vivo and in vitro, and experimental model systems have been established. Cell-free systems have also been developing rapidly in recent years with the aid of the techniques and concepts of molecular genetics. It is conceivable that further understanding of the mechanisms controlling the AFP gene will be of prime importance for elucidation of the hepatocarcinogenesis mechanism.

AFP and albumin show somewhat reciprocal dynamics during ontogenesis and oncogenesis. Parallel studies on AFP and albumin at various levels such as gene expression and regulation, gene evolution and location, and primary and secondary polypeptide structure have been carried out extensively in recent years, and have brought about some valuable results.

Compared with that in mammals, AFP found in birds and sharks shows similar physicochemical properties and common dynamics during ontogenesis. The shark is ovoviviparous and has existed on earth for several hundred million years. The continued existence and relative conservation of the AFP gene in its evolution suggest that AFP may play a role in some biological functions.

An extensive literature has been accumulated since 1963, when Abelev and Tatarinov found AFP in mice and humans respectively. This chapter reviews the studies on the AFP gene, AFP gene expression and regulation, and its fine structure.

The references cited here are mainly limited to those closely associated with the above-mentioned aspects, mainly published in recent years. Several reviews of AFP are available (Abelev 1971, 1974; Hirai et al. 1973; Ruoslahti et al. 1974; Zhen 1975; Lamerz and Fateh-Moghadam 1975; Lau and Linkins 1976; Nørgaard-Pedersen 1976; Tomasi 1977; Zhang and Zhen 1977; Abelev et al. 1979; Hirai 1979; Stillman and Sell 1979; Smith and Kelleher 1980; Tang and Yang 1981; Zhen and Zhang 1981; Zhou and Xu 1982), in which a considerable number of papers are cited.

Table 1. AFP-mRNAs

AFP-mRNA sources	AFP-mRNA sequences / Total poly(A) containing RNAs (%)	Purity (%)	Nucleotide length	Reference
Mouse				
Yolk sac	23	98	2700	Miura et al. (1979)
Rat				
Yolk sac	22	90	2527	Chiu et al. (1979)
Yolk sac	20			Liao et al. (1980a)
Fetal liver	2–4			Liao et al. (1980b)
Morris hepatoma 7777	11	97	2700	Innis and Miller (1977)
Morris hepatoma 7777	11	99	2235	Sala-Trepat et al. (1979a)
BERH-2 hepatoma	4–1.5		(22 S)	Shu et al. (1980); Li et al. (1981)
AH-66 ascites hepatoma			2700	Choi and Higashi (1981a)
Man				
Fetal liver	1	40		Huang et al. (1980)

I. AFP Structure Gene

AFP-mRNAs from several species have been purified and characterized. These mRNAs have been reversely transcribed to their corresponding complementary DNAs (cDNA), and cloning has been achieved in many laboratories. The characteristics of several AFP-cDNA clones have been successfully studied.

A. AFP-mRNAs from Different Sources

The contents and some characteristics of AFP-mRNAs from fetuses and hepatomas are listed in Table 1.

B. Clonings of cDNAs Corresponding to Several AFP-mRNAs and Characterization

AFP-mRNAs from several species and sources have been reversely transcribed, thus the cDNAs may be obtained and cloned in bacteria. The details are listed in Table 2.

Structurally, AFP-cDNA reversely transcribed from AFP-mRNA can more or less represent the AFP gene. Cloned AFP-cDNA in bacteria may proliferate in large amounts, providing enough AFP genes for various scientific purposes.

C. AFP Structural Gene

Studies of the structures of AFP genes have been and are being carried out extensively as an important step toward elucidating the basis of AFP gene regulation during ontogenesis and oncogenesis. Among the studies listed in Table 1 and Table 2, mouse yolk sac AFP gene has been investigated in more detail. Somatic cell hybrids containing various combinations of mouse chromosomes, together with a constant set of hamster chromosomes, have been tested for the presence of both AFP and serum albumin genes, using DNA restriction mapping techniques. Both these genes are now known to be mapped on chromosome 5. A 35-kb genomic DNA containing a 22-kb AFP gene and a 24-kb of DNA which contains an 18-kb albumin gene have been isolated and characterized without any overlapping sequences being encountered. This suggests that the AFP gene is one with single copy (D'Eustachio et al. 1981). Both AFP and albumin genes are organized similarly into 15 coding segments interrupted by 14 intervening sequences (Kioussis et al. 1981). They are closely linked in tandem on the same stranded DNA, the AFP gene being 13.5 kb pairs away from the 3′ side of the albumin gene (Ingram et al. 1981).

In addition, the AFP gene in rat AH-66 ascites hepatoma cell nuclei can be preferentially digested by DNase I, whereas that in rat liver cell nuclei can not. Perhaps the AFP gene exists in a relaxed conformation in hepatomas and in a more condensed structure in rat liver (Choi and Higashi 1981 b).

Table 2. Cloning of AFP structural gene in plasmid vector pBR 322

AFP-cDNA	AFP-mRNA-coding insert	Reference
Mouse		
Yolk sac	15.75 kb segment of DNA, over 85% of AFP coding sequence	Tilghman et al. (1979); Gorin et al. (1981)
Yolk sac	Entire sequence from 3′region of the AFP-mRNA	Law and Dugaiczyk (1981)
Rat		
Yolk sac	Sequence of 3′-terminal untranslated region and a portion of the coding region of the AFP mRNA	Liao et al. (1980b)
McA-RH 7777, a Morris hepatoma 7777 cell line	825 base pair of unique sequence, transcribed from 3′end of the AFP-mRNA	Innis et al. (1979) Innis and Miller (1980)
Morris hepatoma 7777	Most sequence of the AFP-mRNA	Jagodzinski et al. (1981)
Human		
Fetal liver	A partial sequence of the AFP-mRNA	Beattie and Dugaiczyk (1982)
Testicular embryonal carcinoma	900 nucleotide sequence from 3′end of the AFP-mRNA	Morinaga et al. (1982)

Nucleotide sequences of AFP structural genes from cloned cDNAs have been examined. AFP-mRNA sequences and AFP polypeptide sequences have been also deduced on the basis of the nucleotide sequences of AFP structural genes for mice, rats, and man by Law and Dugaiczyk (1981), Gorin et al. (1981), Jagodzinski et al. (1981), Liao et al. (1980b), and Beattie and Dugaiczyk (1982).

II. AFP Gene Expression and Regulation

The control of AFP gene expression in mammalian ontogenesis and oncogenesis will provide a powerful model for probing eucaryotic gene regulation in the context of differentiation and carcinogenesis. The first important question in this field is whether the regulation of the levels of polysomal AFP-mRNA molecules is due to transcriptional control, to modulation at the level of processing and transport, or to gene amplification-deletion mechanisms. Sala-Trepat et al. (1979b) have shown that the processes responsible for the changes in AFP phenotypic expression associated with hepatocarcinogenesis do not involve permanent changes in gene number and arrangement. Furthermore, several laboratories have provided evidence that regulation occurs at the transcriptional and/or pretranscriptional levels, rather than owing to the changes in gene number and arrangement.

A. Expression and Regulation at the Transcriptional Level

AFP has a very high concentration in the body fluid of both mammalian fetuses and adults with liver cancer or germ cell-derived tumors, while the level is negligible in healthy adults. AFP-mRNA levels also provide dynamic changes coincident with those at body fluid AFP levels during ontogenesis and oncogenesis. The dynamics of AFP-mRNA levels in mouse liver during late gestation and early neonatal life is shown in Fig. 1 (Tilghman and Belayew 1982). The changes of AFP-mRNA levels in rat yolk sac and liver during pre- and postnatal development are similar (Liao et al. 1980a), paralleling the dynamics of AFP during pre- and postnatal development of the rat mentioned in previous reports (de Nechaud and Uriel 1971; Cheng et al. 1976a). During rat hepatocarcinogenesis by 3′-MeDAB the increases in AFP-mRNA concentrations coincide with those in AFP biosynthesis (Schwartz et al. 1982b; Cheng et al. 1976b) (see Fig. 2).

B. Methylation of AFP Gene: Possible Pretranscriptional Regulation

5′-Methylcytosine (5′Cm) is the only modified base in eucaryotic DNA, comprising 1%–3% of the total cytosine and predominating within the dinucleotide sequence 5′CC. It has recently been postulated that DNA methylation may play a role in the hierarchy of controls which regulate gene expression and differentiation in eucaryotes (for review, see Razin and Riggs 1980). Perhaps methylation is utilized primarily to stabilize memory of a differentiated state through DNA replication, a process that might otherwise disrupt delicate protein-DNA and protein-protein interactions. This possibility is suggested by the observation that some organisms in which differentiated cells do not continue replication may not utilize 5′Cm-DNA modification.

Andrews et al. (1982a) and Kunnath and Locker (1983) have recently investigated the parallel correlation of AFP-mRNA and 5′-methylation of cytosines in the AFP gene of the mouse and the rat. The mouse AFP-mRNA is present at high levels in yolk sac endoderm, fetal liver, and an AFP-producing hepatoma, whereas it is greatly reduced in yolk sac mesoderm and not detected in adult liver, brain, or a non-AFP-producing hepatoma. In each tissue studied there is a striking correlation between expression and hypomethylation at six CCGG sites of the AFP gene, which indicates that the regulation of AFP-mRNA biosynthesis may be closely associated with the presence of CmCGG in the AFP gene. The rat AFP gene is also heavily methylated at 18 days' gestation, and it develops demethylated regions at the 3′ half of the gene in the adult. It is not yet clear what factor controls the methylation of six CCGG sites in the AFP gene.

C. Stability of AFP-mRNA: Possible Transcriptional and/or Post-transcriptional Regulation

The stability of AFP-mRNA is a part of studies of the regulation of AFP gene expression. Andrew et al. (1982b) have observed the stability of AFP-mRNA during mouse yolk sac development. Their experimental results show that the half-life of

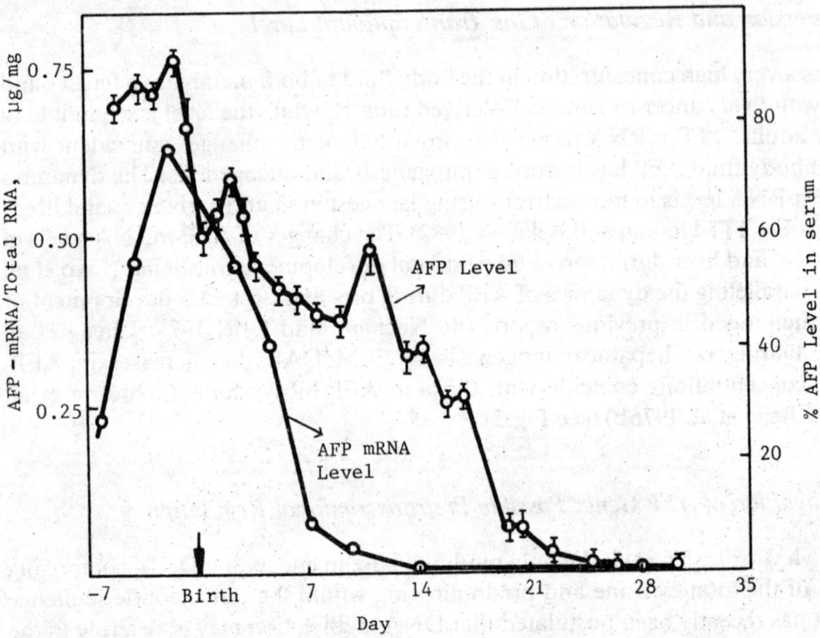

Fig. 1. AFP level in murine serum and AFP-mRNA level in murine liver during pre- and postnatal development. (de Nechaud and Uriel 1971; Tilghman and Belayew 1982)

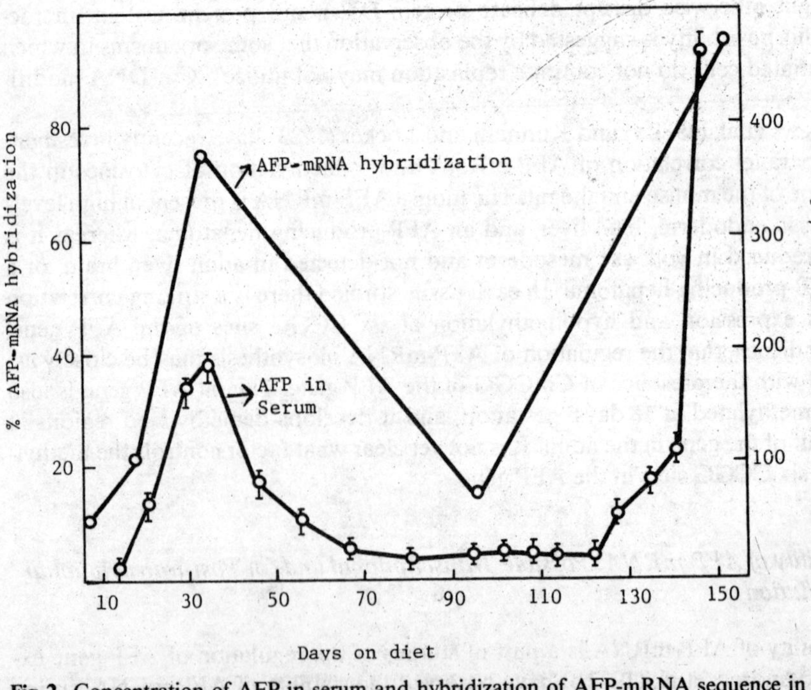

Fig. 2. Concentration of AFP in serum and hybridization of AFP-mRNA sequence in total liver cytoplasmic RNA of rats fed with diet containing 3′MeDAB. (Schwartz et al. 1982b)

AFP-mRNA is at least five times greater than that of the majority of yolk sac mRNAs, and that there are no changes in the stability of AFP-mRNA from day 11.5 to day 17.5 of gestation. These results indicate that a selective stabilization of AFP-mRNA is involved in AFP pretranslational regulation. Further studies are needed on the mechanism of AFP-mRNA selective stabilization and to determine what enables AFP-mRNA to be highly stable.

D. Specific Factor(s) in Regulation of AFP Gene Expression

Only the natural factor(s) that influence AFP biosynthesis will be illustrated here. Both naturally stimulating and suppressing factors have been reported, but none has been purified.

1. AFP-mRNA Synthesis-Stimulating Factor(s)

Selten et al. (1981) reported an interesting phenomenon, that a species-specific serum factor or factors were needed in AFP-mRNA synthesis of the rat hepatoma cell line (SY/1/80). SY/1/80 was derived from a liver cell tumor induced with diethylnitrosoamine. This original tumor was capable of producing AFP; however, in in vitro-propagated hepatoma cells, after passages in growth medium containing newborn calf serum, the AFP and AFP-mRNA were undetectable. Supplementation with rat serum instead of calf, horse, or human sera in growth medium for this cell line led to resynthesis of AFP-mRNA. These findings suggest that a species-specific serum factor or factors play an important role in the regulation of AFP gene expression, although the nature of the factor(s) and the mechanism of action remain to be investigated.

2. AFP Production-Suppressing Factor(s)

Tumyan et al. (1975) reported that the serum and extracts from various organs of adult mice were able to suppress AFP synthesis in newborn mice. They have provided evidence that there was a factor(s) in the serum and in the small and large intestine, liver, lung, brain, thymus, spleen, and kidneys of adult mice which suppressed AFP production in neonatal mice. The nature of the factor(s) is not yet known.

E. Glucocorticoid Suppression of AFP-mRNA Synthesis: A Model of Negative Regulation

Belanger et al. (1981) and Chiu et al. (1981b) have studied the effect of dexamethasone, one of the glucocorticoids, on AFP synthesis in newborn rat liver. They found that the hormone selectively and abruptly interrupted AFP-mRNA synthesis and turnover rate at the transcriptional level, but exerted no effects on albumin and albumin-mRNA synthesis. The glucocorticoid action was reversible. After dexamethasone withdrawal, the AFP-mRNA level rose again, and hepatic production of AFP was reinitiated. Selective inhibition of AFP-mRNA synthesis by dexamethasone has also been found in regenerating rat liver (Chiu et al. 1981a) and in cultured hepatoma 7777 cells (Schwartz et al. 1982a). Therefore, suppression of AFP synthesis by glucocorticoids may provide a suitable model of negative gene regulation exploitable at the molecular level, in case hepatocarcinogenesis and AFP reproduction induced by various carcinogens may be regarded as a model of positive regulation of AFP gene expression – which has not been illustrated in this chapter (for review, see Stillman and Sell 1979; Zhou and Xu 1982).

III. AFP Fine Structure

The microheterogeneity of AFP from several species has been found by means of isoelectrofocusing (Zhen and Ji 1981), chromatography on lectins (for review, see Smith and Kelleher 1980), or affinity radio-immunoelectrophoresis (Xu and Zhou 1982). Although the biochemical bases of the heterogeneity have not been elucidated to date, a great amount of information about AFP structure has been accumulated, such as the amino acid sequences, the carbohydrate units, and the binding of fatty acids.

A. Primary and Secondary Structures of AFP Polypeptide Chain

Earlier studies showed N-terminals of about 25 amino acid sequences of AFPs from mice, rats, and human subjects, using Edman chemical degradation (Aoyagi et al. 1977; Yachnin et al. 1977; Peter et al. 1978). The AFPs from several species are very similar in their N-terminal sequences, despite the fact that the sequences are not homogeneous (Aoyagi et al. 1977).

Thereafter, Liao et al. (1980b) and Innis and Miller (1980) deduced the COOH-terminal sequence of rat AFP from its corresponding cDNA and mRNA sequences. Law and Dugajczyk (1981), Gorin et al. (1981), and Jagodzinski et al. (1981) have deduced the full amino acid sequence of mouse and rat AFP from the nucleotide sequences of their chimeric plasmids containing overlapping segments of cDNA. The results obtained were essentially identical, the similarity between amino acid sequence of rat and mouse AFP being over 80%. In addition, using the regular-spaced position of cysteine bridges generated a two-dimensional structure which revealed the presence of three closely related domains within the AFP molecule. A comparison of the amino acid sequence with that of either human or bovine albumin revealed in each case a 32% conservation of the primary sequence. More recently, Beattie and Dugaiczyk (1982), Morinaga et al. (1983) deduced the sequence of human AFP from the human AFP-cDNA sequence. With regard to the variants of the AFP polypeptide chain, subtle differences cannot be excluded at the present time.

B. Glycan Structures in the AFP Molecule and Its Assemblage

AFP was first proven to be a glycoprotein by Ruoslahti and Seppälä in 1971. Yoshima et al. (1980) further demonstrated that human hepatoma AFP contained asparagine-linked glycans, and that the glycans could be quantitatively released from the polypeptide moiety by hydrazinolysis and recovered as oligosaccharides after N-acetylation. On the other hand, AFP could be separated with concanavalin A (Con-A)affinity chromatography into subfractions: a Con-A-reactive variant and a Con-A-nonreactive variant (Smith and Kelleher 1980; Bayard and Kerckaert 1977; Lai and Lorscheider 1978). The proportion of Con-A-nonreactive AFP was found to be higher in amniotic fluid than in circulating fluid of fetus (Ruoslahti et al. 1978). Con-A-nonreactive variant was presumed to be of yolk sac origin, the reactive variant, of liver origin (Ruoslahti and Adamson 1978). In fact, the AFP variants may be used in some cases to differentiate between liver cancer and nonmalignant liver diseases (Breborowicz et al. 1981; Xu and Zhou 1982; Zhen et al. 1983). These studies have laid a basis and aroused great interest in further investigation of the carbohydrate structures in AFP molecules.

1. Glycans in Human Hepatoma AFP

Asparagine-linked glycans of AFP from human hepatoma contain a nutral (N) and two acidic (A-1, A-2) components. Each molecule of AFP contains only one asparagine-linked glycan (Yoshima et al. 1980). The proposed structures are shown in Fig. 3.

2. Glycans in Rat Amniotic Fluid AFP

The glycans in AFP from rat amniotic fluid (at 14 days of gestation) are fractionated on Con-A-Sepharose into two kinds: Con-A-reactive and -nonreactive. Each AFP variant contains either two reactive or two nonreactive glycans – not at random, but a pair of identical carbohydrate chains at two glycosylation sites (Bayard and Kerckaert 1981). The proposed structures are shown in Fig. 4.

N:

±Fucα1 ↓ 6

Galβ1→4GlcNAcβ1→2Manα1 ↘
⁶₃Manβ1→4GlcNAcβ1→4GlcNAc→Asn
Galβ1→4GlcNAcβ1→2Manα1 ↗

A1:

±Fucα1 ↓ 6

Galβ1→4GlcNAcβ1→2Manα1 ↘
⁶₃Manβ1→4GlcNAcβ1→4GlcNAc→Asn
NeuAcα2→6Galβ1→4GlcNAcβ1→2Manα1 ↗

A2:

±Fucα1 ↓ 6

NeuAcα2→6Galβ1→4GlcNAcβ1→2Manα1 ↘
⁶₃Manβ1→4GlcNAcβ1→4GlcNAc→Asn
NeuAcα2→6Galβ1→4GlcNAcβ1→2Manα1 ↗

Fig. 3. Proposed structures of glycans *N*, *A-1*, and *A-2* in AFP of human hepatoma. *Gal*, galactose; *Man*, mannose; *Fuc*, fucose; *GlcNAc*, N-acetylglucosamine; *NeuAc*, N-acetylneuraminic acid; *Asn*, asparagine

Manα1 ↘
[NeuAcα2→3(6)Galβ1→4GlcNAc]n→ $^{3}_{6}$Manβ1→4GlcNAcβ1→4GlcNAc→Asn
Manα1 ↗

n = 1, Con-A reactive AFP
n = 2, Con-A nonreactive AFP

Fig. 4. Proposed structures of Con-A-reactive and -nonreactive glycans in AFP of rat amniotic fluid

Con-A reactive

NeuAcα2→3/6Galβ1→4GlcNAcβ1→2Manα1 ↘
$^{3}_{6}$Manβ1→4GlcNAcβ1→4GlcNAcβ1→Asn
NeuAcα2→6/3Galβ1→4GlcNAcβ1→2Manα1 ↗

Con-A nonreactive

NeuAcα2→3/6Galβ1→4GlcNAcβ1→2Manα1 ↘
$^{3}_{6}$Manβ1→4GlcNAcβ1→4GlcNAcβ1→Asn
NeuAcα2→3/6Galβ1→4GlcNAcβ1→2Manα1 ↗

NeuAcβ2→6/3Galβ1→4GlcNAcβ1 ↗ 4

Fig. 5. Proposed structures of Con-A-reactive and -nonreactive glycans in AFP of fetal calf serum

3. Glycans in Fetal Calf AFP

The glycans in AFP from fetal calf serum are fractionated on Con-A-Sepharose into reactive glycan and nonreactive glycan; the proposed structures are shown in Fig. 5. Fetal calf AFP exists in three molecular variants, differing in their types of glycans; both glycans are triantennary in 75% of the total AFP molecules; 20% of AFP molecules have one triantennary and one biantennary glycan and 5% contain two biantennary glycans (Krusius and Ruoslahti 1982).

From the data obtained so far, the carbohydrate units of AFPs from different species and sources are similar; the core structure, however, is the same and is also found in other complex-type glycans:

±Fuc
|
Man ╲
Man ╱ Man — GlcNAc — GlcNAc — Asn-peptide

The outer chains may be monoantennary in rat amniotic fluid (see Fig. 4); biantennary in human liver cancer, rat amniotic fluid, and calf fetus (see Figs. 3, 4, and 5); and triantennary in calf fetus (see Fig. 5). Furthermore, each AFP molecule contains one N-glycosidic carbohydrate unit in human liver cancer, two units in both rat amniotic fluid and fetal calf serum. In addition, two glycan units in each variant of rat amniotic fluid AFP are identical with one another, whereas two glycan units in each variant of fetal calf AFP may be two tri-, two bi-, or one tri- and one biantennary glycan.

The fucose-containing glycans and tri- or tetra-antennary glycans are found only in abnormal cells. Malignant cells differ from normal cells in their glycosylation process, perhaps because of their tendency to revert to developmentally earlier glycosylation patterns. It is expected that glycosylation variants of AFP may serve as clinical markers.

4. Position of Assemblage of AFP Carbohydrate Chains in Hepatoma Cells

Mano and Chou (1982) studied the formation of AFP variants in cultured Mc-A-RH-7777 rat hepatoma cells. They found that the intracellular 68000-dalton polypeptide might consist of polypeptides with apparent molecular weights ranging from 68000 to 70000. The 68000-dalton polypeptide in cells was mostly bound to Con-A-Sepharose, whereas the 69000-dalton polypeptide consisted of Con-A-bound and unbound variants. The 68000-dalton polypeptide was the precursor of the mature polypeptides of apparently 69000 and 73000 daltons in cells and medium. Their experiments led to the following conclusions: (a) Glycosylation takes place in cells, (b) molecular variants of AFP are formed before the excretion of the cells, and (c) only processed AFP is secreted into the medium.

C. Fatty Acids on the AFP Molecule

The specific binding of fatty acids to AFP has been widely found in human beings and other mammals (Parmelee et al. 1978; Nagai et al. 1982). The fatty acids binding to AFP are now known to be noncovalent. Because of the close association of fatty acids with AFP biological functions the fatty acids in AFP are here considered as a portion of the AFP molecule.

Parmelee et al. (1978), Nagai et al. (1982), and Lampreave et al. (1982) have adopted a milder procedure for purifying AFP from human fetal tissue, human hepatoma serum, rat fetus, rat maternal serum, Morris 7777 hepatoma serum, and fetal pigs. The major AFP component has an isoelectric point pI 4.7, the minor component pI 5.3. The pI 4.7 contains about 2.4 mol of fatty acids/mol of AFP, whereas the minor is fat-free.

The levels of fatty acids in various human AFP preparations are listed in Table 3. The levels of fatty acids in various rat AFP preparations from different sources are listed in Table 4.

AFPs isolated from human fetuses contain ≥2 mol of fatty acids, of which C20:4 (12%–39%) and C22:6 (16%–42%) constitute more than half of the total. However, the situation in rat maternal and hepatoma AFP and in two of three human hepatoma AFPs seems to be different. Perhaps some fatty acid-bearing AFPs are responsible for certain definite biofunctions.

AFPs from some species are known to be able to combine with steroid hormones; however, the combination has not been discussed here because it is not a common characteristic of all AFPs. For example, human AFP does not combine with steroid hormones.

Table 3. Molecular ratios of fatty acids on human AFP [after Parmelee et al. (1978) and Nagai et al. (1982)]

AFP sources	mol fatty acid/mol AFP						
	C16:0	C18:0	C18:1	C18:2	C20:4	C22:6	Total
Fetal tissue							
Isolate 1	0.21	0.05	0.66	0.17	0.29	1.01	2.39±0.07
Isolate 2	0.20	0.14	0.28	0.17	0.99	0.88	2.66±0.17
Isolate 3	0.33	0.11	0.15	0.46	1.20	0.49	3.09±0.11
Hepatoma serum							
Case 1	0.49	0.14	0.49	0.26	0.56	0.18	2.12
Case 2	0.18	0.04	0.09	0.06	0.08	0.00	0.45
Case 3	0.35	0.02	0.20	0.13	0.00	0.00	0.40

C16:0, Palmitic acid; C18:0, stearic acid; C18:1, oleic acid; C18:2, linoleic acid; C20:4, arachidonic acid; C22:6, 4, 7, 10, 13, 16, 19-docosahexenoic acid

Table 4. Molecular ratios of fatty acids on rat AFP [Nagai et al. (1982)]

AFP sources	mol fatty acid/mol AFP						
	C16:0[a]	C18:0	C18:1	C18:2	C20:4	C22:6	Total
Fetus	0.16	0.03	0.29	0.16	0.16	0.15	0.93
Maternal serum	0.16	0.07	0.28	0.05	0.02	0.00	0.58
Morris 7777 hepatoma serum	0.22	0.09	0.43	0.08	0.04	trace	0.86

[a] For fatty acids, see Table 3.

IV. Monoclonal Antibodies to Human AFP

The hybrid cell lines secreting monoclonal antibodies to human AFP are produced by fusion of a mouse myeloma cell line with spleen cells from mice (mostly BALB/c) immunized with purified or partially purified human AFP (Uotila et al. 1980, 1981; Stenman et al. 1981; Heyningen et al. 1982; Hunter et al. 1982; Nomura et al. 1982; Zhou et al. 1982). Monoclonal antibodies may be of IgG1 or IgA subclasses. The monoclonal antibodies obtained by Nomura et al. (1982) and Uotila et al. (1981) reacted with two different antigenic determinants, those obtained by Heyningen et al. (1982) with three different antigenic determinants. A mixture of the monoclonal antibodies exhibited cooperativeness; however, the sensitivity of the RIA with pooled monoclonals was not as good as that with conventional antiserum. There may be six different antigenic determinants on the surface of the natural AFP molecule (Zhen 1979; Zhen and Ji 1982). Experiments are in process on directing monoclonal antibodies to all different epitopes on human AFP, and their cooperative action will be reevaluated. The therapy of hepatoma and localization of cancer nodules with monoclonal antibodies to human AFP have not yet been attempted, although a few trials with polyclonal antibodies have been done, and these seem to be beneficial (Hirai 1981; Liu et al. 1983). Chemotherapy by intravenous administration of daunomycin conjugates with monoclonal and conventional anti-rat-AFP antibodies has been reported by Tsukada et al. (1982). Daunomycin conjugates with anti-AFP were capable of delaying rat hepatoma development efficiently and produced a long-term survival rate of 60%.

V. Concluding Remarks

The expression of fetal products by tumor cells is consistent with a variety of theories of cancer origin, such as dedifferentiation, blocked ontogeny, embryonal rests, or oncogene activation. Oncodevelopmental gene expression during ontogenesis and oncogenesis represents a model system which can be used to answer basic questions about the nature of carcinogenesis. The most typical oncofetal protein is AFP. In this article we have reviewed the current advances in studies of AFP gene structure and AFP phenotypic structure and of AFP gene expression and regulation. We believe that AFP is a hepatoma marker that is valuable for exploring alterations in gene expression and regulation during experimental hepatocarcinogenesis and clinical process. We hope that studies of AFP can be exploited to answer questions concerning the nature and mechanism of hepatocarcinogenesis and some clinical questions, as well as to advance the early diagnosis and treatment of liver cancer.

References

Abelev GI (1971) α-Fetoprotein in ontogenesis and its association with malignant tumors. Adv Cancer Res 14: 295–358

Abelev GI (1974) α-Fetoprotein as a marker of embryo-specific differentiations in normal and tumor tissue. Transplant Rev 20: 3–37

Abelev GI, Engelhardt NV, Elgort DA (1979) Immunochemical and immunohistochemical micromethods in the study of tumor-associated embryonic antigen (α-fetoprotein). Methods Cancer Res 18: 1–37

Andrews GK, Dziadek M, Tamaoki T (1982 a) Expression and methylation of the mouse α-fetoprotein gene in embryonic, adult, and neoplastic tissues. J Biol Chem 257: 5148–5153

Andrews GK, Janzen RG, Tomaoki T (1982 b) Stability of α-fetoprotein messenger RNA in mouse yolk sac. Dev Biol 89: 111–116

Aoyagi Y, Ikenaka R, Ichida F (1977) Comparative chemical structures of human α-fetoproteins from fetal serum and from ascites fluid of a patient with hepatoma. Cancer Res 37: 3663–3667

Bayard B, Kerckaert JP (1977) Characterization and isolation of nine rat alpha-fetoprotein variants by gel electrophoresis and lectin affinity chromatography. Biochem Biophys Res Commun 77: 489–495

Bayard B, Kerckaert JP (1981) Uniformity of carbohydrate chains within molecular variants of rat α-fetoprotein with distinct affinity for concanavalin A. Eur J Biochem 113: 405–414

Beattie WG, Dugaiczyk A (1982) Structure and evolution of human α-fetoprotein deduced from partial sequence of cloned cDNA. Gene 20: 415–422

Belanger L, Frain M, Baril P, Gigras Mc, Bartkowiak J, Sala-Trepat JM (1981) Glucocorticosteroid suppression of α-fetoprotein synthesis in developing rat liver. Evidence fc selective gene expression at the transcriptional level. Biochemistry 20: 6665–6672

Breborowicz J, Mackiewicz A, Preborowicz D (1981) Microheterogeneity of alpha-fetoprotein in patient serum as demonstrated by lectin affino-electrophoresis. Scand J Immunol 14: 15–20

Cheng PJ, Zhen QY, Sun C, Liu SL, Li TY (1976 a) The normal development and AFP dynamics of embryonic rat liver. Acta Biochim Biophys Sinica 8: 271–280[1]

Cheng PJ, Zhen QY, Sun C, Li TY, Liu SL (1976 b) Localization of AFP in rat liver tissue in correlation to the dynamics of serum AFP during 3′MeDAB carcinogenesis. Acta Biochim Biophys Sinica 8: 49–60[1]

Chiu JF, Decha-Umphai W, Commer P (1979) α-Fetoprotein mRNA of rat yolk sac and hepatoma. Nucleic Acids Res 7: 239–249

Chiu JF, Gabryelak T, Commers P, Massari R (1981 a) The elevation of α-fetoprotein messenger RNA in regenerating rat liver. Biochem Biophys Res Commun 98: 250–254

Chiu JF, Massari RJ, Schwartz CE, Meister NT, Thanassi W (1981 b) Hormonal modulation of α-fetoprotein gene expression in newborn rat livers. Nucleic Acids Res 9: 6917–6933

Choi NH, Higashi T (1981 a) Isolation of α-fetoprotein messenger ribonucleic acid from AH-66 ascites hepatoma cells. Chem Pharm Bull (Tokyo) 29: 3305–3310

Choi NH, Higashi T (1981 b) Studies on the activity of α-fetoprotein gene. Chem Pharm Bull (Tokyo) 29: 3311–3319

Coordinating Group for the Research of Liver Cancer, China (1974) Application of serum alpha-fetoprotein assay in mass survey of primary carcinoma of liver. Advances in Tumour Prevention, Detection and Characterization 2: 655–658

Coordinating Group for Research on Liver Cancer, China (1979) Studies on alpha-fetoprotein IV. Further studies on alpha-fetoprotein in mass surveys and follow-up studies on primary hepatocellular carcinoma. Advances in Medical Oncology, Research and Education 4: 291–295

de Nechaud B, Uriel J (1971) Transitory cell antigens of rat liver. I. The secretion and synthesis of fetospecific serum proteins during hepatic development and regeneration. Int J Cancer 8: 71–80

D'Eustachio P, Ingram RS, Tilghman SM, Ruddle FH (1981) Murine α-fetoprotein and albumin: two evolutionary linked proteins encoded on the same mouse chromosome. Somatic Cell Genet 7: 289–294

Gorin MB, Cooper DL, Eiferman F, Rijn P, Tilghman SM (1981) The evolution of α-fetoprotein and albumin. I. A comparison of the primary amino acid sequences of mammalian α-fetoprotein and albumin. J Biol Chem 256: 1954–1959

Heyningen VV, Barron L, Brock DJH, Crichton D, Lawrie S (1982) Monoclonal antibodies to human α-fetoprotein: analysis of the behaviour of three different antibodies. J Immunol Methods 50: 123–131

Hirai H (1979) Model systems of AFP and CEA expression. Methods Cancer Res 18: 39–97

Hirai H (1981) An approach to the immunotherapy of patients with hepatoma using antibody to alpha-fetoprotein. Foundation for Basic Research of Oncology, Tokyo, Japan

Hirai H, Nishi S, Watabe H, Tsukada Y (1973) In: Hirai H, Miyaja T (eds) Alpha-fetoprotein and hepatoma. Gann Monograph No 14. Tokyo, University of Tokyo Press, pp 19–32

Huang DP, Li BG, Ding CR, Zhu CR (1980) Isolation of AFP polysomes of human embryonic livers by several immunoprecipitation methods. Acta Biochim Biophys Sinica 12: 171–180[1]

Hunter WM, Bennie JG, Brock DJH, Heyningen VV (1982) Monoclonal antibodies for use in an immunoradiometric assay for α-fetoprotein. J Immunol Methods 50: 133–144

Ingram RS, Scott RW, Tilghman SM (1981) α-Fetoprotein and albumin genes are in tandem in the mouse genome. Proc Natl Acad Sci USA 78: 4694–4698

Innis MA, Miller DL (1977) Quantitation of rat α-fetoprotein messenger RNA with a complementary DNA probe. J Biol Chem 252: 8469–8475

Innis MA, Miller DL (1980) α-Fetoprotein gene expression. Partial DNA sequence and COOH-terminal homology to albumin. J Biol Chem 255: 8994–8996

Innis MA, Harpolled MM, Miller DL (1979) Amplification of α-fetoprotein-complementary DNA by insertion into a bacterial plasmid. Arch Biochem Biophys 195: 128–135

Jagodzinski LL, Sargent TD, Yang M, Glackin C, Bonner J (1981) Sequence homology between RNAs encoding rat α-fetoprotein and rat serum albumin. Proc Natl Acad Sci USA 78: 3521–3525

Kioussis D, Eiferman F, Rijin P, Gorin MB, Ingram RS, Tilghman SM (1981) The evolution of α-fetoprotein and albumin. II. The structures of the α-fetoprotein and albumin genes in the mouse. J Biol Chem 256: 1960–1967

Krusius T, Ruoslahti E (1982) Carbohydrate structure of the concanavalin A molecular variants of α-fetoprotein. J Biol Chem 257: 3453–3457

Kunnath L, Locker J (1983) Developmental changes in the methylation of the rat albumin and α-fetoprotein genes. EMBO J 2: 317–324

Lai PCW, Lorscheider FL (1978) Separation and characterization of two bovine alpha-fetoprotein molecular variants by concanavalin A-Sepharose chromatography. Biochem Biophys Res Commun 82: 492–497

Lamerz R, Fateh-Moghadam A (1975) Carcinofetale Antigene. I. Alpha-fetoprotein (Übersichten). Klin Wochenschr 53: 147–169
Lampreave F, Calvo M, Nval J, Pineiro A (1982) Long-chain fatty acids bound to α-fetoprotein and to serum albumin from fetal and adult pig. Comp Biochem Physiol 73B: 823–827
Lau HL, Linkins SE (1976) Alpha-fetoprotein. Am J Obstet Gynecol 124: 533–554
Law SW, Dugaiczyk A (1981) Homology between the primary structure of α-fetoprotein, deduced from a complete cDNA sequence, and serum albumin. Nature 291: 201–205
Li M, Shu LX, Li WY (1981) Isolation and purification of alpha-fetoprotein messenger RNA from rat transplantable hepatoma BERH-2. Acta Biol Exp Sinica 14: 145–152[1]
Liao WSL, Conn AR, Taylor JM (1980a) Changes in rat α-fetoprotein and albumin mRNA levels during fetal and neonatal development. J Biol Chem 255: 10036–10039
Liao WSL, Hamilton RW, Taylor JM (1980b) Amino acid sequence homology between rat α-fetoprotein and albumin at the COOH-terminal regions. J Biol Chem 255: 8046–8049
Liu YK, Yang KZ, Wu YD, Gang YQ, Zhu DN (1983) Treatment of advanced primary hepatocellular carcinoma by 131-I-anti-AFP. Lancet 1: 531–532
Miura K, Law SWT, Nishi S, Tamaoki T (1979) Isolation of α-fetoprotein messenger RNA from mouse yolk sac. J Biol Chem 254: 5515–5521
Mano T, Chou JY (1982) Biosynthesis of α-fetoprotein in cultured hepatoma cells. J Biol Chem 257: 5827–5830
Morinaga T, Sakai M, Wegmann TG, Tamaoki T (1982) α-fetoprotein messenger RNA in human embryonal carcinoma grown in nude mice, and cloning of its complementary DNA. Oncodev Biol Med 3: 301–313
Morinaga T, Sakai M, Wegmann TG, Tamaoki T (1983) Primary structures of human α-fetoprotein and its mRNA. Proc Natl Acad Sci USA 80: 4604–4608
Nagai N, Becker JL, Deutsch HF (1982) The fatty acid levels of rat alpha-fetoprotein derived from fetuses, pregnancy and hepatoma sera. Oncodev Biol Med 3: 343–350
Nomura M, Imai M, Nakamura T, Miyakawa Y, Mayumi M (1982) Demonstration of two distinct antigenic determinants on human α-fetoprotein by monoclonal antibodies. Mol Immunol 19: 1691–1697
Nørgaard-Pedersen B (1976) Human alpha-fetoprotein. A review of recent methodological and clinical studies. Scand J Immunol [Suppl] 4
Parmelee DC, Evenson MA, Deutsch HF (1978) The presence of fatty acids in human α-fetoprotein. J Biol Chem 253: 2114–2119
Peter EH, Nishi S, Tamaoki T (1978) Murine alpha-fetoprotein: N-terminal amino acid sequence and C-terminal residue. Biochem Biophys Res Commun 83: 75–82
Razin A, Riggs AD (1980) DNA methylation and gene function. Science 210: 604–610
Ruoslahti E, Adamson E (1978) Alpha-fetoproteins produced by the yolk sac and the liver are glycosylated differently. Biochem Biophys Res Commun 85: 1622–1630
Ruoslahti E, Seppälä M (1971) Studies of carcino-fetal proteins: physical and chemical properties of human α-fetoprotein. Int J Cancer 7: 218–225
Ruoslahti E, Pihko H, Vaheri A, Seppälä M, Virolainen M, Konnttinen A (1974) In: Beer RF, Tilghman RC, Bassett EG (eds) The role of immunological factors in viral and oncogenic process. Johns Hopkins University Press, Baltimore, Maryland, pp 249–255
Ruoslahti E, Engvall E, Pekkala A, Seppälä H (1978) Developmental changes in carbohydrate moiety of human alpha-fetoprotein. Int J Cancer 22: 515–520
Sala-Trepat JM, Dever J, Sargent K, Thomas K, Sell S (1979a) Changes in expression of albumin and α-fetoprotein genes during rat liver development and neoplasia. Biochemistry 18: 2167–2178
Sala-Trepat JM, Sargent TD, Sell S, Bonner J (1979b) α-Fetoprotein and albumin genes of rats: no evidence for amplification, deletion, or rearrangement in rat liver carcinogenesis. Proc Natl Acad Sci USA 76: 695–699
Schwartz CE, Burkhardt AL, Huang DP, Chiu JF (1982a) The effects of dexamethasone on α-fetoprotein and albumin synthesis in cultured hepatoma 7777 cells. Biosci Rep 2: 777–784
Schwartz CE, Gabryelak T, Smith CJ, Taylar JM, Chiu JF (1982b) The expression of α-fetoprotein and albumin genes in rat liver during chemical carcinogenesis. Biochem Biophys Res Commun 107: 239–245
Selten GCM, Selten-Versteegen AME, Yap SH (1981) Expression of alpha-fetoprotein and albu-

min in a rat hepatoma cell line SY/1/80: evidence for the need of species-specific serum factors. Biochem Biophys Res Commun 103: 278–284
Shanghai Coordinating Group for Research on Liver Cancer, China (1979) Diagnosis and treatment of primary hapatocellular carcinoma in early stage. Advances in Medical Oncology, Research and Education 4: 285–289
Shu YC, Liu HH, Hsu L, Li WY (1980) Quantitation of mRNA levels of alpha-fetoprotein and albumin in transplantable rat hepatoma BERH-2. Acta Biol Exp Sinica 13: 353–360[1]
Smith CJP, Kelleher PC (1980) Alpha-fetoprotein moelcular heterogeneity. Physiological correlations with normal growth, carcinogenesis and tumor growth. Biochim Biophys Acta 605: 1–32
Stenman UH, Sutinen ML, Selander RK, Tontti K, Schröder J (1981) Characterization of a monoclonal antibody to human alpha-fetoprotein and its use in affinity chromatography. J Immunol Methods 46: 337–345
Stillman D, Sell S (1979) Models of chemical hepatocarcinogenesis and oncodevelopmental gene expression. Methods Cancer Res 18: 135–168
Tang ZY, Yang BH (1981) Clinical studies on α-fetoprotein. In: Tang ZY (ed) Primary liver cancer. Shanghai Science and Technical Press, Shanghai, pp 176–192[1]
Tilghman SM, Kioussis D, Gorin MB, Ruiz JPG, Ingram RS (1979) The presence of intervening sequences in the α-fetoprotein gene of the mouse. J Biol Chem 254: 7393–7399
Tilghman SM, Belayew A (1982) Transcriptional control of the murine albumin/α-fetoprotein locus during development. Proc Natl Acad Sci USA 79: 5254–5257
Tomasi TB (1977) Structure and function of alpha-fetoprotein. Ann Rev Med 28: 453–465
Tsukada T, Hurwitz E, Kashi R, Sela M, Hibi N, Hara A, Hirai H (1982) Chemotherapy by intravenous administration of conjugates of daunomycin with monoclonal and conventional anti-rat-alpha-fetoprotein antibodies. Proc Natl Acad Sci USA 79: 7896–7900
Tumyan BG, Svet-Moldavsky GG, Karmanova NV (1975) Factors suppressing α-fetoprotein production in newborn mice. Nature 255: 244–245
Uotila M, Engvall E, Ruoslahti E (1980) Monoclonal antibodies to human alpha-fetoprotein. Mol Immunol 17: 791–794
Uotila M, Ruoslahti E, Engvall E (1981) Two-site sandwich enzyme immunoassay with monoclonal antibodies to human alpha-fetoprotein. J Immunol Methods 42: 11–15
Xu KL, Zhou J (1982) Studies of human AFP variants by Concanavalin A affinity radioimmunoelectrophoresis. Biochem Biophys 6: 30–32[1]
Yachnin S, Hsu R, Heinrikson RL, Miller JB (1977) Studies on human α-fetoprotein, isolation and characterization of monomeric and polymeric forms and amino-terminal sequence analysis. Biochim Biophys Acta 493: 418–428
Yoshima H, Mizuochi T, Ishii M, Kobata A (1980) Structure of the asparagine-linked sugar chains of α-fetoprotein purified from human ascites fluid. Cancer Res 40: 4276–4281
Zhang XY, Zhen QY (1977) Progress in alpha-fetoprotein research. Acta Biochim Biophys Sinica 9: 321–338[1]
Zhen QY (1975) Studies on human α-fetoprotein in China. Biochem Biophys 3: 7–12[1]
Zhen QY, Ji RH (1981) Microheterogeneity of alpha-fetoprotein in human fetal serum. Kexue Tonbao 26: 463–466
Zhen QY, Ji RH (1982) Application of the equation T/B – (Ag) for radioimmunoassay in estimating the number of antigenic determinants. Acta Biochim Biophys Sinica 14: 105–112[1]
Zhen QY (1979) A linear standard curve for radioimmunoassay. The T/B versus (Ag) plot. Acta Biochim Biophys Sinica 11: 181–186[1]
Zhen QY, Zhang XY (1981) Basic research on α-fetoprotein. In: Tang ZY (ed) Primary liver cancer. Shanghai Science and Technical Press, Shanghai, pp 163–175[1]
Zhen QY, Ji RH, Engst K (1983) Microheterogeneity of alpha-fetoprotein in human fetuses and patients with liver cancer as well as partial characterization. Cancer Res Prev Treat 10: 209–212[1]
Zhou JX, Xu B (1982) Influence of bio-active substances on AFP gene expression in liver carcinogenesis. Biochem Biophys 6: 1–6[1]
Zhou GY, Wu GD, Hu SZ, Zeng YF (1982) Hybridoma cell lines producing monoclonal antibodies specific for human α-fetoprotein (HAFP). Acta Biochim Biophys Sinica 14: 417–420[1]

1 Chinese

24 Pathology of Subclinical Hepatocellular Carcinoma

Ying Yue-ying, Zhai Wei-rong

In contrast to conventional HCC, subclinical hepatocellular carcinoma (SCHCC) denotes a particular type of case in which the obvious symptoms or signs relating to HCC are lacking; therefore, SCHCC in its proper sense is a clinical rather than a pathological concept. These symptomless or "occult" cases of HCC can be discovered only by serum-AFP survey or serial AFP monitoring of subjects with chronic liver diseases (CLD) (Tang et al. 1980; Purves 1976; Okuda et al. 1975; Zhu 1981; Johnson and Williams 1980; Kata et al. 1978). Diagnosis of HCC before the occurrence of symptoms is indeed a remarkable advance in improving the ultimate outcome of this disease, which for centuries had a grave prognosis owing to the deep location of the tumor in the liver and the lack of specific diagnostic tools for early detection. Since AFP was discovered and proven to be a useful marker for HCC, early detection of HCC has been rendered possible by serum AFP survey or monitoring, especially in cases of CLD, which usually constitute the background for the development of HCC. Consequently, the identification of SCHCC increases ten fold following AFP survey.

It is worth noting that SCHCC is relative early liver cancer, complete resection of which is possible. A low operative mortality (2.1%) and an encouraging ultimate outcome, with a 5-year survival rate of up to 64.4% had been reported by Tang et al (1983). In spite of the fact that most SCHCC are small HCC, not all of these cases are in their early stage. This chapter reports the pathological characteristics and background of SCHCC and its biological behavior.

I. Material and Methods

A total of 69 cases of SCHCC had been encountered at Zhong Shan Hospital of the Shanghai First Medical College from 1973 to 1980. The majority of cases in this series were detected by serum AFP survey. The final diagnosis of HCC was based on pathological examination of either aspiration biopsies or surgical resection specimens (67 cases) or of autopsy materials (two cases).

All specimens were fixed in 10% formalin, tissue blocks were embedded in paraffin, and sections were routinely stained with H and E., orcein (for HB_sAg) (Shikata et al. 1974; Deodhar et al. 1975; Ying et al. 1980), and immunoperoxidase (for Hb_sAg and HB_cAg) (Zhai and Ying 1981; Ye et al. 1982; Yamada and Nakane 1977), while von Gieson (for collagen fiber) and Gordon-Sweet (for reticulin fiber) stains were done when indicated.

II. Clinical Findings

A. Age and Sex

The 69 patients included 63 men and six women, the ratio being 9.5:1. The age at the time of diagnosis of HCC ranged from 21 to 65 years, the average being 43.9. The distribution of cases in various age groups is shown in Fig. 1.

B. Clinical Manifestations

Of the 69 patients, 34 had a history of viral hepatitis from 3 years up to 20 years, and five patients had been alcoholics for 10–20 years. The clinical signs that led to the detection of HCC were obtained mainly by means of serum AFP survey.

Serological tests for Hb_sAg in 42 cases gave 26 positive results, the positive rate being 61.9%.

III. Gross Pathology

HCC was found more commonly in the right than in the smaller left lobe. Of the 69 cases in this series, the tumor was found in the right lobe in 35, in the left lobe in 28, in the caudate lobe in one, and diffusely distributed in the remaining four; one was unknown. In 54 cases the tumor could be visualized and measured directly, and it was distinctively small in 40, varying from 0.8 to 5 cm in diameter. In these 40 cases there were 38 single nodules and only two double nodules with a spherical volume less than 65.5 cm^3. One could see the majority of cases had small HCC (Ying and Zhai 1979; Okuda et al. 1977b). In another 12 cases, the diameter of the tumor was larger, varying from 6 to 8 cm. In the remaining two autopsied cases, the

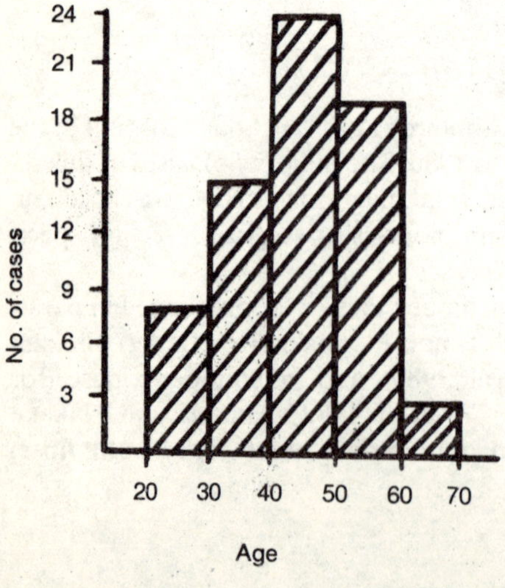

Fig. 1. Age distribution of SCHCC

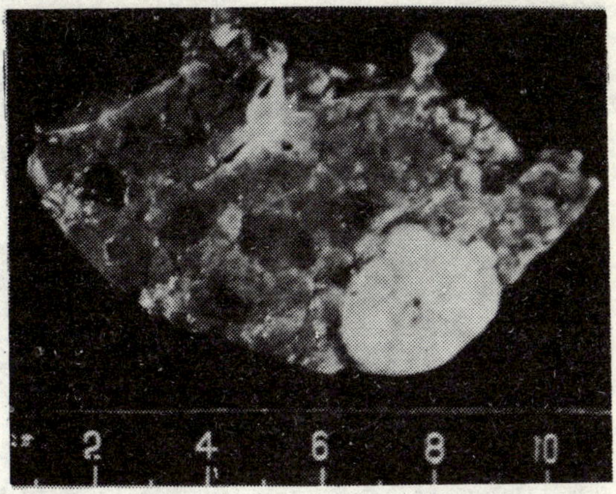

Fig. 2. Small HCC with fibrous capsule

main tumor was massive, with a diameter of 10 cm or more and multiple nodules scattered in the neighboring parenchyma.

One of the characteristic features of small HCC in this series was the presence of fibrous capsules, which were usually thin; some were complete and distinct (Fig. 2), while others were incomplete, with local disruption by the protruding tumor growths. However, these protruding nodules were usually found later to be encapsulated. The tumor tissue was usually brownish in color, with connective stroma having a lobular appearance. The larger tumors in this series were different from the small HCC in that necrosis and hemorrhage were present in the tumor proper. Satellite nodules surrounding the main tumor mass were frequently encountered; some of these even showed multiple tumor nodules scattered diffusely (Edmondson 1958; Ying et al. 1981; Cameron 1976).

IV. Microscopic Pathology

The HCC in this series were mostly well differentiated; according to the classification of Edmondson (1958), 37 of the 69 cases were grade II, 32 grade III. No grade I or grade IV was found. A comparison between small HCC and large HCC tumors of the same series showed no difference in the degree of differentiation.

The polygonal tumor cells were arranged in cords or plates producing trabecular patterns (Fig. 3) or having a pseudoglandular appearance (Fig. 4). In areas of macrotrabecular growth the cancer cells often grew solidly, without any particular patterns. Cytologically, besides varying degrees of pleomorphism of the tumor cells, clear cells (Fig. 5) and giant cells were found in some cases (Fig. 6). The characteristic stroma of HCC composed of sinusoids lined by the attenuated endothelial cells was found in the majority of tumors, but the stroma of some encapsulated small HCC was composed of dense connective tissue (Fig. 7), and sclerosing HCC were not seen in this series (Peters 1976; Ying et al. 1963).

Fibrous capsule surrounding the tumor was either complete or incomplete; in the latter situation the invasion of tumor cells into the capsule was commonly seen, usually followed by disruption of the capsule and invasion of the tumor cells into

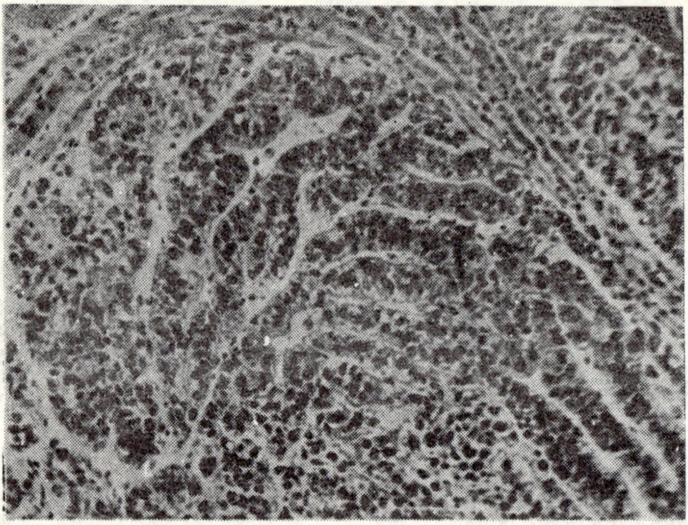

Fig. 3. Well-differentiated HCC showing trabecular pattern. H. and E., × 125

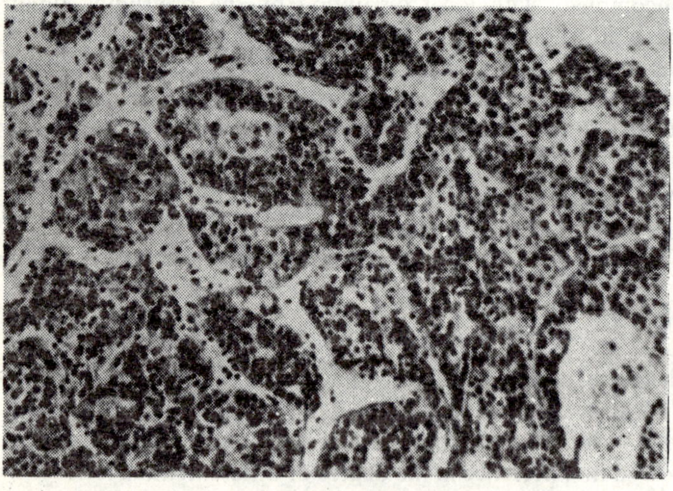

Fig. 4. Pseudoglandular pattern of HCC. H. and E., × 125

the surrounding parenchyma (Fig. 8). Lymphocytic infiltrations were often seen at the margin of the invading cancer cells in direct contact with the surrounding liver tissues, and the number of infiltrated lymphocytes varied from case to case (Fig. 9).

Microscopic tumor thrombi (Fig. 10) were found in even the smallest HCC in this series, measuring 0.8 cm in diameter.

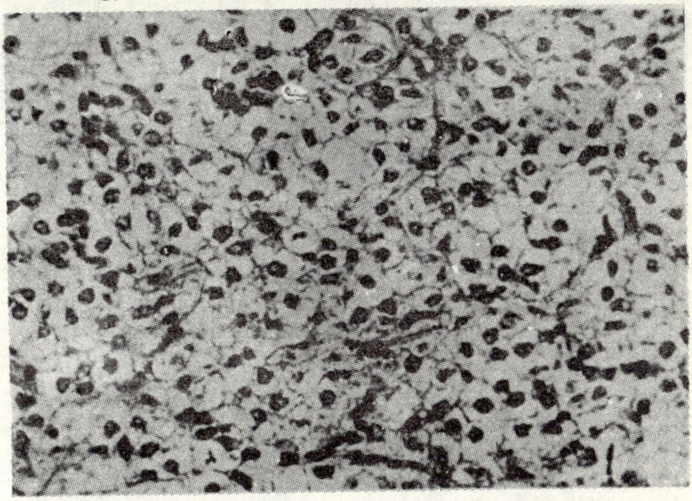

Fig. 5. HCC composed of 'clear cells.' H. and E., × 160

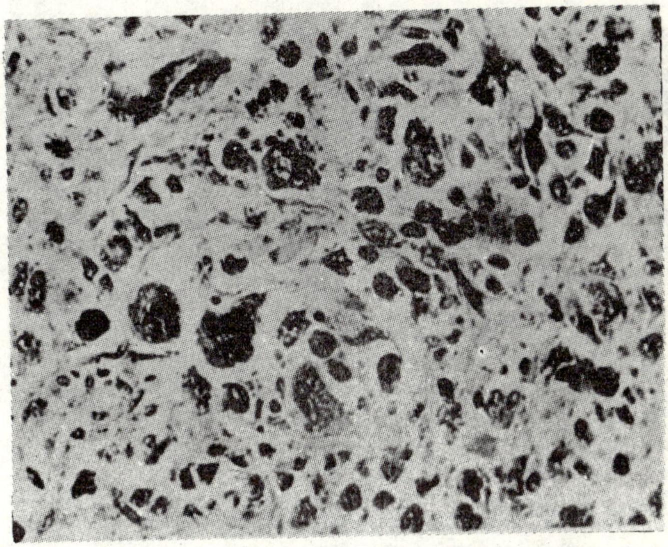

Fig. 6. HCC showing anaplastic giant tumor cells. H. and E., × 400

V. Pathology of Non-cancerous Portion of Liver

The noncancerous portion of the liver in HCC usually showed CLD changes, which might set the stage for the development of liver cell cancer. Of all the CLD, chronic viral hepatitis and cirrhosis are most frequently encountered (Anthony 1976b; Shikata 1976; Zhai et al. 1982).

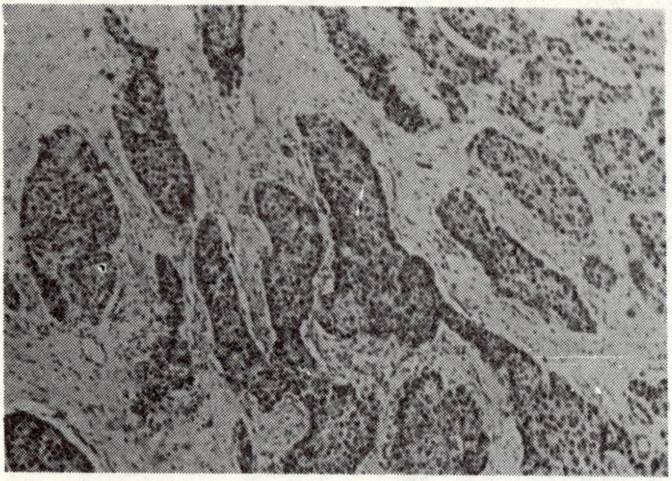

Fig. 7. HCC with dense-connective-tissue stroma. H. and E., ×63

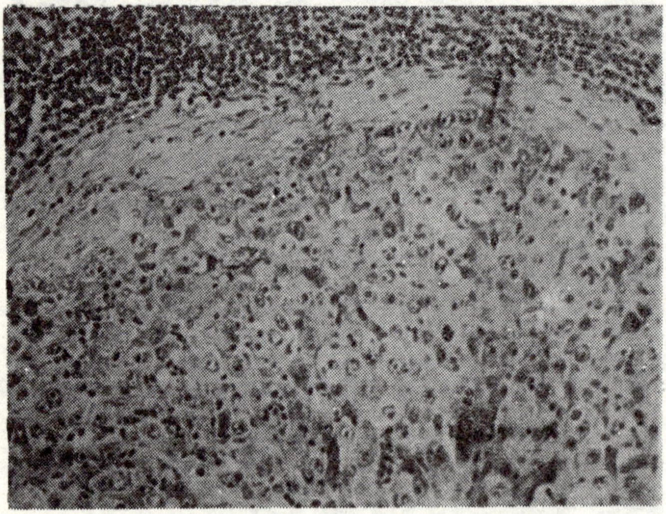

Fig. 8. HCC showing fibrous encapsulation. H. and E., ×160

A. Chronic Hepatitis

According to the morphology described by Ishak (1976) and Hadziyannis (1974), of the 51 surgically resected specimens in our series, 35 showed hepatitis changes, of which 21 were chronic active hepatitis (CAH), six chronic persistant hepatitis (CPH), and eight non-specific reactive hepatitis; 25 of the 27 cases of CAH and CPH showed positive intracellular HB_sAg. In some cases the CAH changes were fairly prominent with a large amount of lymphocytic infiltration of the portal

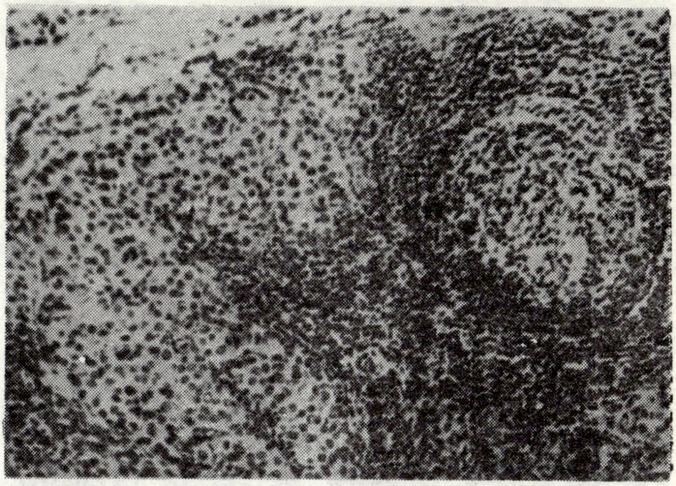

Fig. 9. Marked lymphocytic infiltration with lymphoid follicle formation at the margin of the invading cancer cells. H. and E., ×125

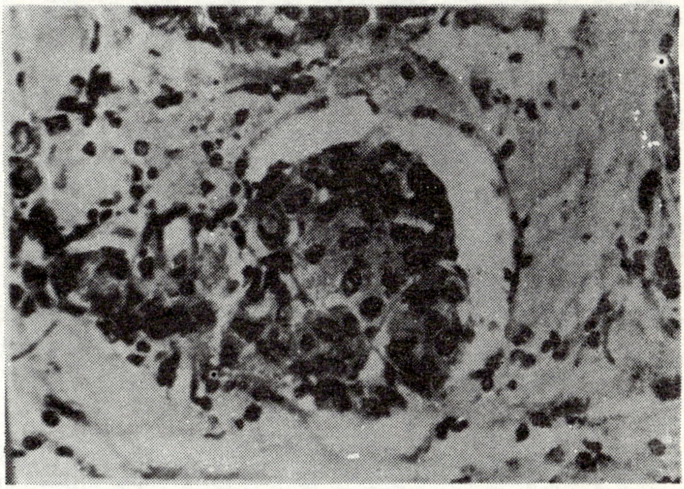

Fig. 10. Tumor thrombus. H. and E., ×320

spaces, disruption of the hepatic plates, piecemeal necrosis of the adjacent hepatic cells, and inflammatory infiltration involving the hepatic lobules accompanied by filbrous septal formation (Fig. 11).

Nonspecific reactive hepatitis (Patric and McGee 1980) is characterized by the presence of large numbers of lymphocytes in the portal spaces, but the adjacent liver parenchyma is usually well preserved. These changes are found in the liver tissue close to the tumor nodules.

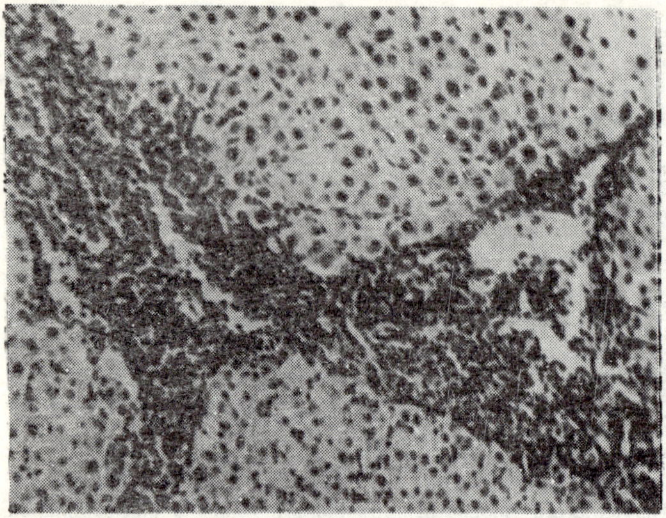

Fig. 11. CAH in noncancerous portion of the liver in HCC. H. and E., × 160

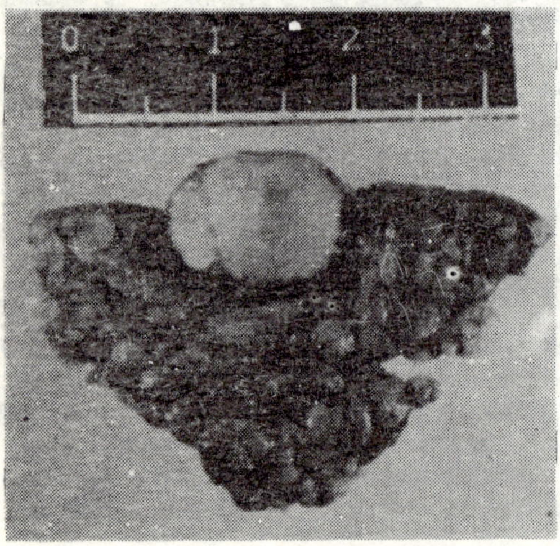

Fig. 12. HCC associated with macronodular cirrhosis with thin septae

B. Liver Cirrhosis

HCC is usually associated with cirrhosis (Anthony et al. 1977; Popper 1972); this was also the case in 45 of 51 cases (88.2%) in the present series. The majority of cases of cirrhosis are of the macronodular type, with thin septae (Fig. 12). Microscopically, nodules are composed of multiple hepatic lobules surrounded by thin fibrous septae, some of which show incomplete septal formation and are known as the "incomplete septal type". No evidence of alcoholic cirrhosis was found in those with a long history of alcohol addiction (10–20 years) in this series.

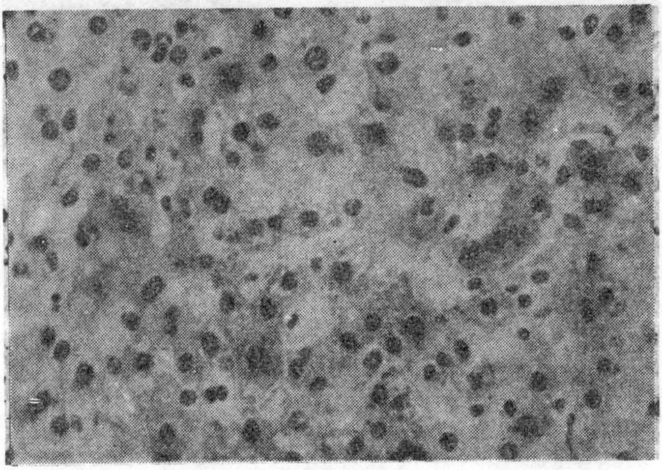

Fig. 13. Liver cell dysplasia. H. and E., ×320

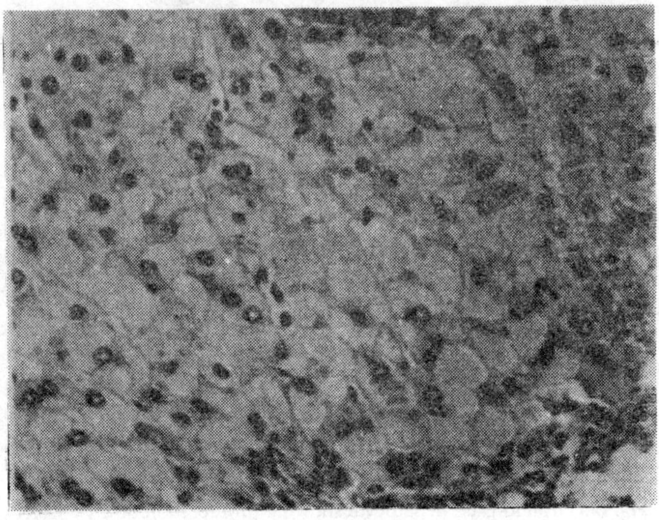

Fig. 14. Ground-glass hepatocytes. H. and E., ×320

C. Liver Cell Dysplasia

Liver cell dysplasia is characterized by large cells with abundant and often polychromaphilic cytoplasm and bizzarre hyperchromatic or multiple nuclei, the N/C (the ratio of neucleus to cytoplasm) being within the normal limit (Fig. 13) (Anthony et al. 1973; Anthony 1976a). They may be scattered sparsely or occur in groups. In this series the majority of dysplastic liver cells were found in areas of actively progressing cirrhosis accompanied by CAH, and orcein staining was occasionally positive.

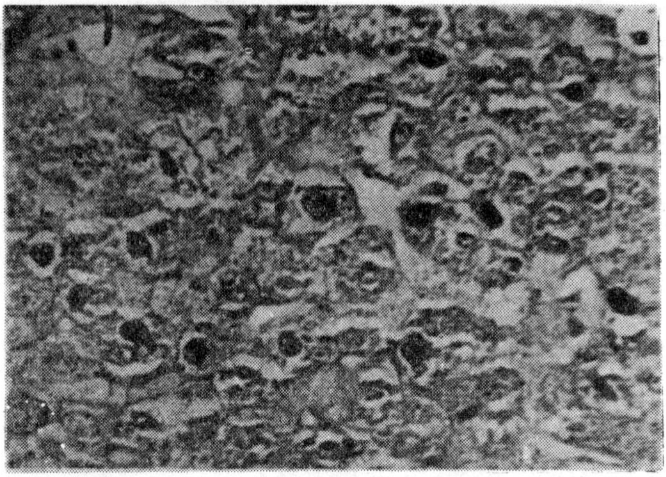

Fig. 15. Ground-glass hepatocytes showing positive orcein stain. ×400

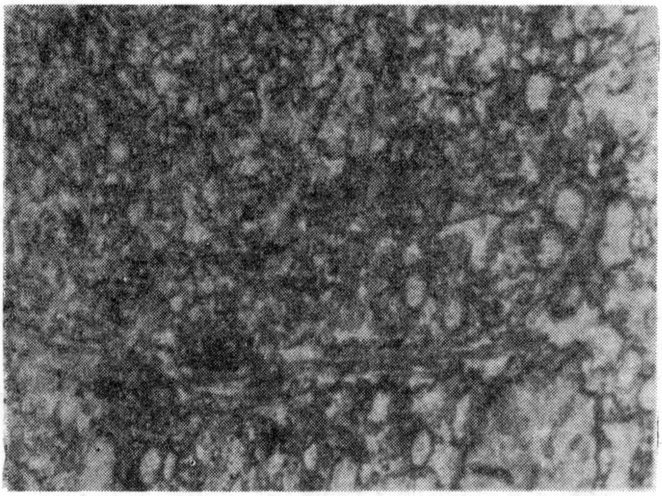

Fig. 16. Ground-glass hepatocyte showing proliferation of SER which contain filamentous HB_sAg uranyl acetate and lead citrate ×75000

D. Ground-glass Hepatocytes

Ground-glass hepatocytes are characterized by bulky, pale, eosinophilic granular cytoplasm (Fig. 14) and stain quite distinctly with orcein (Fig. 15); marked proliferation of smooth endoplasmic reticulum (SER) containing abundant HB_sAg can be shown under electron microscopy (Fig. 16). These cells are arranged either scattered and single or in groups or clusters, seen particularly in cases of CAH or actively progressing cirrhosis with positive serum or intracellular HB_sAg (Hadziyannis 1981; Popper 1975).

VI. Problems

The pathology of SCHCC is a relatively new and interesting area in medical science. For decades pathologists seldom had the chance to see liver cancer in its early stages, especially in the stage before the occurrence of clinical symptoms. The majority (74.0% of SCHCC in the present series were small HCC, each tumor having a diameter less than 5 cm, but the remaining 25.9% were moderate or late stage cancers. Therefore, SCHCC is not synonymous with early liver cancer.

A. The Biological Characteristics of SCHCC

All SCHCC belonged to grades II–III, both highly or poorly differentiated tumors being absent in this series. Though the biological characteristics of SCHCC in this series were not universal, the following points are worth discussing.

Small HCC (74.5% in the present series) are usually encircled by thin fibrous capsules. This encapsulation usually impedes the growth of the tumor mass, especially its degree of expansion (Nakashima 1976). While invasion of the cancer cells which disrupt the thin fibrous capsule is a common occurrence, reencapsulation of the invading cancer cells may not infrequently be observed. Therefore, the alternating processes of encapsulation, invasion, and reencapsulation of the cancer accompany the growth of the tumor. The thick fibrous stroma in the interior of the tumor nodules, giving them the lobular appearance, is the result of the growth of paracapsular tumor satellites which are reencapsulated at the boundary of the liver parenchyma.

Large or massive HCC, constituting 24.5% of the present series, is the group which deserves special consideration because of the peculiar absence of clinical symptoms. It should be noted that in nearly half of our cases (6/14) in this group the main tumor masses were rather well demarcated and encapsulated, but the capsules are usually found to be invaded by the tumor and become disrupted and incomplete. Such encapsulated HCC is rare in the Western (Edmondson and Steiner 1954) and African reports (Berman 1954), but it is comparatively more common in Japan; of 156 autopsied cases of HCC (Okuda et al. 1977a), 16 (10.3%) were found to be encapsulated. In the department of pathology of the Shanghai First Medical College, none of the 220 HCC autopsied cases showed encapsulation of the tumors (Ying et al. 1981). According to Edmondson and Steiner (1954) and Peters (1976) the expanding growth pattern of HCC is the one that produces a distinct boundary forming a fibrous capsule. Although it has not been established whether expanding growth is less malignant than inductive growth (Nakashima et al. 1974), it seems that the appearance of fibrous capsule tends to indicate the slow growth of the tumor. In fact, most cases of encapsulated HCC are relatively well differentiated, and none in the present series appeared to be anaplastic. According to Okuda's observation, the encapsulated HCC are slowly growing tumors; the incidence of tumor growth in the portal vein branches is lower with encapsulated than with nonencapsulated HCC, being 71.4% and 90% respectively. The clinical course of the early stage is protracted, and if the tumor is detected early, the patient may be a good candidate for surgery.

B. Pathological Background of SCHCC

The predominant pathological background for the development of HCC is liver cirrhosis. In the present series 88.2% of HCC cases were associated with cirrhosis, and incidence slightly higher than in the 220 autopsied HCC cases (85.5%) reported by the authors in 1980. Most of the cirrhosis associated with SCHCC in this series was the macronodular type with thin septae; all cirrhotic changes were mild and the fibrous septae were fairly thin and sometimes incomplete. Many cases with cirrhosis proved to be the result of HB-CAH with positive serum and intracellular HB_sAg markers (Ying et al. 1981; Coordination Group on Pathology of Liver Cancer 1982).

The presence of ground-glass hepatocytes in the cirrhotic liver parenchyma of HCC could be implicated in the development of HCC associated with chronic HBV infection. These hepatocytes show partial resistance to the growth of HBV, permitting the replication of HB_sAg only; therefore, a large amount of HB_sAg is found in the proliferated SER (Hadziyannis 1980, 1982; Popper 1975). Recently Okita et al. in Japan (1977) and Thung et al. in the U.S.A. (1979) reported that these cells could produce AFP and that they retained α_1-antitrypsin. However, the production of the antigens was detected mainly in ground-glass hepatocytes located at the cirrhotic areas of the superimposed HCC. The changes suggested that these hepatocytes have some of the characteristics of embryonic liver cells. As shown by the study of experimental liver carcinogenesis, the putative premalignant cells might have the morphological and functional characteristics of embryonic cells. Therefore, ground-glass hepatocytes could be considered 'transferred' or premalignant cells, although, morphologically, they are not indentical to the dysplastic cells described by Anthony et al. (1973). Histochemical studies revealed that the dysplastic cells show decreased activity of G-6-P on the one hand and increased GT activity on the other hand (Kalengaji and Desmet 1978; Parke and Gay 1978). However, a preliminary study has shown that there is increased rather than decreased G-6-P activity in the ground-glass cells (Hardonk et al. 1979). Further studies to explore the properties of the ground-glass cells have been carried out in recent years, investigating plasma membrane alteration (Popper 1977).

The pathological background of SCHCC is different from that of clinical HCC only in the degree of cirrhosis involved. Of our patients with SCHCC, 62.2% (28/45) also have mild cirrhosis and 37.8% (17/45) moderate or severe cirrhosis, while cirrhosis is mild in 30% (12/40) of those with clinical HCC, and moderate or severe in 70% (Ying and Zhai 1979; Ying 1981). Statistically, there is a marked difference between these two groups ($P < 0.01$). These data show that the cirrhosis in SCHCC is relatively mild, and the liver is therefore better compensated functionally; this might be the pathological basis for the low number or absence of clinical symptoms in this group of cases.

C. Host Reaction to Growing HCC

The host reaction to growing HCC is rather strong in SCHCC cases of the present series, as shown by active lymphocytic infiltration along the margin of the invading tumor. The reaction is so marked in some cases that the portal spaces are greatly enlarged by the collection of large numbers of lymphocytes, even the formation of lymph follicles. The phenomenon of lymphocytic infiltration and the close contact with the cancer cells may be a sign of the reaction of lymphocytes to the target cancer cells. Cell culture studies have proven that the direct contact of lymphocytes with the target cells is a prerequiste for the occurrence of cell lysis caused by lymphocyte-mediated cytotoxicity (Perlman and Helm 1969). Such processes can be seen by means of electron microscopy; lymphocytes, with their protruding cytoplasmic processes, are found to be in close contact with tumor cells, and lysis of the cell membrane can be found at the point of contact (Sasaki et al. 1981). Such a host reaction is especially marked in SCHCC cases. It should be noted that the growing tumor in the liver parenchyma remains so 'silent' that there is no sign of cellular reaction. The strong host reaction in SCHCC might be responsible for the slow progression of tumor growth, and hence for the retarded development of clinical symptoms. This symptomless 'lag' varies according to the interaction of tumor growth with host reaction. Therefore, either suppression of tumor growth or enhancement of the host immune reaction toward the growing tumor may prolong the 'lag' of SCHCC. Since this 'lag' represents a relative balance between the cancer growth and the host reaction, it may be considered the critical period when successful therapy can be expected.

References

Anthony PP (1976a) Precursor lesions for liver cancer in humans. Cancer Res 36: 2579–2683

Anthony PP (1976b) The background to liver cell cancer. In: Cameron HM, Linsell DA, Warwick GP (eds) Liver cell cancer. Elsevier, Amsterdam, pp 93–117

Anthony PP, Vogel CL, Barker LF (1973) Liver cell dysplasia. A premalignant condition. J Clin Pathol 26: 217–223

Anthony PP, Ishak KG, Nayak NC, Poulsen HE, Scheuer PJ, Sobin LH (1977) The morphology of cirrhosis: Definition, nomenclature and classification. Bull WHO 55: 521–540

Berman C (1954) Primary carcinoma of the liver. Lewis, London, pp 21–26

Cameron HM (1976) The pathology of liver cell cancer. In: Cameron HM, Linsell DA, Warwick GP (eds) Liver cell cancer. Elsevier, Amsterdam, pp 17–41

Coordination Group on Pathology of Liver Cancer, China (1982) (Ying YY et al. 1982) The relationship between hepatocellular carcinoma, liver cirrhosis and hepatitis. Natl Med J China 62: 257-261[1]

Deodhar KP, Tapp E, Scheuer PJ (1975) Orcein staining of hepatitis B surface antigen in paraffin sections of liver biopsies. J Clin Pathol 28: 66–70

Edmondson HA (1958) Tumor of the liver and intrahepatic bile ducts. Atlas of tumor pathology. Sect. 7, Fascicle 25, AFIP, Washington DC

Edmonson HA, Steiner PE (1954) Primary carcinoma of the liver. A study of 100 cases among 48900 necropsies. Cancer 7: 462–503

Hadziyannis SJ (1980) HCC and type B hepatitis. Clin Gastroenterol 9: 117–130

Hadziyannis SJ (1981) The ground-glass hepatocytes: an aid to diagnosis, a challenge to pathophysiology, In: Berk PD, Chalmers TC (eds) Frontiers in liver diseases. Thieme-Stratton, New York, pp 106–121

Hardonk MJ, Houthoff HJ, Koudstaal J, et al. (1979) Histochemistry of enzyme activities in hepatitis B antigen-containing liver cells. In: Proc. of the 14th meeting of the EASL, Düsseldorf, p 19

Ishak KG (1976) Light-microscopic morphology of viral hepatitis. Am J Clin Pathol 65: 787–827

Johnson PT, William R (1980) Serum alpha-fetoprotein estimation and doubling time in hepatocellular carcinoma: Influence on therapy and possible value in early detection. J Natl Cancer Inst 64: 1329–1332

Kata Y, Okuda K, Musha H, Nakashima T (1978) Detection of hepatocellular carcinoma during a clinical follow-up of chronic liver diseases. Gastroenterology 74: 578–582

Kalengaji MMR, Desmet UJ (1978) Liver cell populations and histochemical patterns of adult- and fetal-type proteins during aflatoxin B_1 hepatocarcinogenesis. In: Remmer H, Belt HM, Bannasch P, Popper H (eds) Primary liver tumors. MTP Press, Lancaster, pp 467–483

Nakashima T, Kojiro M, Sakamoto K, Okuda K, Shimokawa Y, Kubo Y (1974) Studies of primary liver carcinoma. Proposal of new gross anatomical classification of primary liver carcinoma. Acta Hepatol Jpn 15: 279–291 (in Japanese)

Nakashima T (1976) Vascular changes and hemodynamics in hepatocellular carcinoma. In: Okuda K, Peters PL (eds) Hepatocellular carcinoma. Wiley, New York, pp 169–203

Okita K, Kodama T, Harada T, Noda K, Fukumoto Y, Takenami T, Shigeta K, Mizuta M, Takemoto T (1977) Early lesion and development of primary HCC in man – association with HBV infection. Gastroenterol Jpn 12: 51–57

Okuda K, Kotoda K, Obata H, Hayashi N, Hisamitsu T, Tamiya M, Kubo Y, Yakushiyi F, Nagata E, Jinnouchi S, Shimokawa Y (1975) Clinical observation during a relative early stage of hepatocellular carcinoma, with special reference to serum AFP levels. Gastroenterology 69: 226–234

Okuda K, Musha H, Nakajima Y, Kubo Y, Shimokawa Y, Nagasaki Y, Sawa Y, Jinnouchi S, Kaneko T, Obata H, Hisamitsu T, Motoike Y, Okazaki N, Kojiro M, Sakamoto K, Nakashima T (1977a) Clinicopathologic features of encapsulated hepatocellular carcinoma (a study of 26 cases). Cancer 40: 1240–1245

Okuda K, Nakashima T. Obata H, Kubo Y (1977b) Clinocopathological studies of minute hepatocellular carcinoma – analysis of 20 cases, including four with hepatic resection. Gastroenterology 73: 109–115

Parke DV, Gay TJB (1978) A comparative study of the enzyme and morphological changes of liver of rat fed butylated hydroxytoluene, safrole, pon-ceau MX or 2-acetamidefluorene. In: Remmer H, Belt HM, Bannasch P, Popper H (eds) Primary liver tumors. MTP Press, Lancaster, pp 321–346

Patric RS, McGee JOD (1980) Biopsy pathology of the liver. Chapman and Hall, London, pp 116–117

Perlman P, Holm G (1969) Cytotoxic effects of lymphoid cells in vitro. Adv Immunol 11: 117–193

Peters PL (1976) Pathology of HCC. In: Okuda K, Peters PL (eds) Hepatocellular carcinoma. Wiley, New York, pp 57–71

Popper H (1972) Pathologic aspect of cirrhosis: a review. Am J Pathol 87: 228–258

Popper H (1975) The ground-glass hepatocytes as a diagnostic hint. Human Pathol 6: 517–520

Popper H (1977) Summary. In: Popper H, Bianchi L (eds) Membrane alterations as basis of liver injury. MTP Press, Lancaster, pp 372–377

Purves LR (1976) Alpha-fetoprotein and the diagnosis of liver cell cancer. In: Cameron HM, Linsell DA, Warwick GP (eds) Liver cell cancer. Elsevier, Amsterdam, pp 61–79

Sasaki H, Ichida F, Kamimura T, Kojima T (1981) Ultrastructural interaction of lymphocytes and hepatocytes bearing HB antigens. In: Berk PD, Chalmers TC (eds) Frontiers in liver diseases. Thieme-Stratton, New York, pp 196–207

Shikata T (1976) Primary liver carcinoma and liver cirrhosis. In: Okuda K, Peters RL (eds) Hepatocellular carcinoma. Wiley, New York, pp 53–71

Shikata T, Uzawa T, Yashiwara N, Akatsuka T, Yamazaki S (1974) Staining method of Australia antigen in paraffin section. Detection of cytoplasmic inclusion bodies. Jpn J Exp Med 44: 25–36

Tang ZY, Yang BH, Tang CL, Yu YQ, Lin ZY, Weng HZ (1980) Evaluation of population screening for hepatocellular carcinoma. Chin Med J 93: 795–799

Tang ZY, Yu YQ, Zhou XD, Zhou NQ (1983) Surgical treatment of subclinical hepatocellular carcinoma (HCC) and its ultimate outcome – a comparative study of 74 cases of subclinical HCC and 229 cases of clinical HCC undergone surgery. J Exp Clin Cancer Res 3: 261–268

Thung SM, Gerber MA, Sarno E, Popper H (1979) Distribution of 5 antigens in liver tissue: light- and electron-microscopic location by peroxidase-labeled antibody method. Lab Invest 41: 101–106

Yamada G, Nakane PK (1977) Hepatitis B core and surface antigens in liver tissue: light- and electron-microscopic location by peroxidase-labeled antibody method. Lab Invest 36: 649–659

Ye ZR, Zhang XR, Zhai WR (1982) A comparative study of PAP and double bridge PAP method for detection of Hb Ag in liver tissue. Acta Acad Med Primae Shanghai 9: 49–54

Ying YY (1981) Pathology of hepatocellular carcinoma. In: Tang ZY (ed) Primary liver cancer. Shanghai Science and Technical Publishers, Shanghai, pp 115–150[1]

Ying YY, Zhai WR (1979) Pathology of small hepatocellular carcinoma. Natl Med J China 59: 410–414[1]

Ying YY, Ma CC, Xu YT, Lei HH, Linag SF, Liu CH, Ku CY (1963) Primary carcinoma of liver (with special reference to histogenesis and its relationship to liver cirrhosis). Chin Med J 82: 279–294

Ying YY, Zhang YE, Zhai WR, Ma JY, Hu XQ (1980) Hepatocellular carcinoma and hepatitis B antigen. Acta Acad Med Primae Shanghai 7: 241–246[1]

Ying YY, Zhai WR, Song QL, Hu XQ, Ma JY, Xu YD (1981) Hepatocellular carcinoma, liver cirrhosis and hepatitis B. Tumor 1: 1–5[1]

Zhai WR, Ying YY (1981) Distribution of HB_sAg in hepatic tissue with comparison of different methods for manifestation. Acta Acad Med Primae Shanghai 8: 181–187[1]

Zhai WR, Ying YY, Song QL, Hu XQ, Ma JY, Xu YD, Ye ZR (1982) Primary hepatocellular carcinoma and chronic liver disease. Chin J Pathol 11: 283–287[1]

Zhu YR (1981) AFP serosurvey and early diagnosis of liver cell cancer in the Qi-dong area. Chin J Oncol 3: 35–37[1]

1 Chinese

25 Experimental Hepatoma in China

Wang Heng-wen, Xu He

Work on experimental hepatoma in China has centered mostly on the problems of etiology, pathogenesis, diagnosis, treatment, and prevention of human hepatocellular carcinoma. Less work has been done with this material for the investigation of carcinogenesis or tumor biochemistry in general (see Chaps. 26 and 27).

I. Transplantable Hepatomas

A. Establishment of an AFP-positive Transplantable Rat Hepatoma

Discovery of the value of serum AFP monitoring for the diagnosis of primary hepatocellular carcinoma in man encouraged scientists to search for a similar animal model. In 1978 a dynamic change in serum AFP levels in Wistar rats during diethylnitrosamine hepatocarcinogenesis was followed by means of RIA (Ke et al. 1978). Before long, it was reported that a transplantable AFP-positive rat hepatoma, BERH-2, had been established from primary hepatocellular carcinoma induced in a Wistar rat with diethylnitrosamine treatment (Chiang et al. 1978). Sera of Wistar rats bearing the primary hepatoma and the transplanted tumors were shown to contain AFP. Furthermore, a positive correlation was found between the growth rate of this hepatoma and the amount of AFP in the host serum. In the karyotype analysis and G-banding study of marker chromosomes, it was found that BERH-2 hepatoma cells were aneuploid, with a model number of 72 chromosomes. An abnormal metacentric chromosome of large size occurred with high frequency. It was composed of the long arms of no. 4 and no. 7, and was considered to be a marker chromosome of BERH-2, its chromosome formula being t (4:7) (7qter→7cen: : 4cen: : 4q22→4qter) (Chiang 1981). An in vitro cell line (CBRH 7919) was established from BERH-2 (Chu et al. 1980). AFP was present in the cytoplasm of cells of early passages, as shown by immunoperoxidase labeling, but it failed to appear on further cell passages. However, organ culture of BERH-2 seemed to maintain the ability to synthesize AFP for a longer period of time, as demonstrated by immunoelectrophoretic assay (Lu et al. 1978).

B. The Influence of Normal Liver RNA on Growth and Malignant Characteristics of Hepatoma Cells

Since BERH-2 has the ability to synthesize AFP, it has proven to be especially useful in studies on the influence of normal liver mRNA on the growth and malignant characteristics of hepatoma cells. It was reported in Shanghai in 1978 that active normal mouse liver mRNA could inhibit nucleic acid and protein synthesis of mouse ascitic hepatoma cells in culture. Similarly, human liver mRNA was found to be able to slightly inhibit the growth of human hepatoma cells in culture (BEL 7402). At the same time, albumin synthesis in both mouse and human hepatoma cells was found to be stimulated (Li et al. 1978). These findings were considered to support the view that errors in gene expression might be the primary change in carcinogenesis, and that normal mRNA might be a logical means of reversing cancer cells to normal differentiation, at least to a certain extent and for a short period of time (Fishman and Sell 1976). With the establishment of BERH-2 in Wistar rats, more exacting experiments were made to test the influence of mRNA on cellular activity and differentiation. AFP-mRNA was isolated and purified from BERH-2 (Li et al. 1981), and in the same way albumin mRNA was isolated and purified from the same tumor; both mRNAs were quantitated by means of translation of the mRNA in the cell-free protein synthesizing systems of wheat-germ, followed by specific antibody precipitation of the ^{3}H-labeled, newly synthesized AFP and albumin, and polyacrylamide gel analysis of the dissociated immune complex. AFP and albumin mRNA levels of BERH-2 were thus compared with those of normal rat liver. It was found that both mRNA levels were elevated in hepatoma as compared with normal liver. The results obviously differed from reports in previous publications that AFP and its mRNA usually increased with simultaneous decrease in albumin and its mRNA in hepatoma (Hsu et al. 1980). At about the same time, another Shanghai laboratory also reported that stimulation of albumin synthesis of hepatoma cells by normal liver RNA did not persist on cell passages without further RNA treatment (Guo et al. 1981). This was also a readjustment of a viewpoint based on previous observations made in the same laboratory (Ku et al. 1966).

C. Establishment of a Transplantable Hepatoma in Inbred Mice

In 1980 it was reported that a transplantable hepatoma had been established in inbred 615 mice (the mouse strain had been established in Tianjing) from a hepatoma arising spontaneously (Fan et al. 1980). It was demonstrated histochemically that γ-GTP was present in varying amounts in the cytoplasm of hepatoma cells, according to their degree of dedifferentiation. The enzyme was also present in the cortex of the mouse kidney and in liver cells of neonatal animals (Fan et al. 1982). In spite of the undoubted superiority of transplantable hepatoma in inbred animal strains for metabolic and other cancer studies, reports of this category continued to appear with the use of transplantable hepatomas long passaged in random-bred animals (Zhang et al. 1982). This was probably a result of the limited availability of specific inbred animal strains.

II. Chemically Induced Hepatomas

A. AFP in Liver and Hepatoma Cells and Other Early Changes During Chemical Hepatocarcinogenesis

Studies with chemically induced hepatomas were also directed mostly at the appearance and location of AFP in cancer and liver cells during hepatocarcinogenesis. With the application of immunoperoxidase labeling of AFP, its presence in the rat liver during 3'MeDAB hepatocarcinogenesis was investigated (Cancer Research Group 1976). It was found that not all hepatoma cells contained AFP in the cytoplasm. AFP was not detected in the well-differentiated hepatoma cells, but was present in cancer cells with moderate and high dedifferentiation; its amount varied with the growth rate of the cells.

In an experiment reported more recently, pathohistological, histochemical, immunofluorescent, and electron-microscopic observations were made during various stages of hepatocarcinogenesis in the rat by 3'MeDAB feeding (Xu et al. 1982). Oval cell proliferation was prominent during the early stage, and these cells were probably undifferentiated stem cells of the liver that were capable of further differentiation. Some of them were found capable of transforming into transitional cells, with the potential to develop into small AFP-containing hepatocytes. With the latter, further differentiation into both mature hepatocytes and cholangiolar cells could be observed. Transitions from oval cells to small hepatocytes and to precancerous lesions (hyperplastic areas, hyperplastic nodules, etc.) were observed. Precancerous lesions consisted of immature hepatocytes showing depletion of functional enzymes of mature hepatocytes, such as G-6-Pase and ATPase, but the presence of enzymes of embryonic hepatocytes such as γ-GTP. These findings showed that cells of precancerous lesions were immature hepatocytes.

Histological and histochemical observations of the appearance and distribution of γ-GTP were made during rat hepatocarcinogenesis by aflatoxin administration (Xu et al. 1981). γ-GTP was found to be nonhomogeneous and more intensely stained in liver cancers, precancerous lesions, and γ-GTP positive extrahepatic foci than in any embryonic or neonatal rat liver. However, hepatoma cells with very little differentiation were sometimes free of γ-GTP. Observation of oval cell proliferation and the associated lesions showed a distribution pattern of γ-GTP activity similar to that of the cholangiolar system, thus suggesting their cholangiolar origin. Other observations suggested the transition of oval cells to small hepatocytes and then to proliferative nodules. However, no systematic observations were reported of early liver changes during hepatocarcinogenesis by threshold doses of carcinogens other, than the feeding of 0.06% 3'MeDAB with the rat diet, or rather large oral doses of aflatoxin.

B. Experimental Synergistic Carcinogenesis of the Liver

In an experiment studying the synergistic action of the chronic administration of *N*-phenyl-2-naphthylamine (PBNA) with small weekly oral doses of CCl_4 in rats, the relationship between cirrhosis and cancer of the liver was incidentally demonstrated (Wang and Wang 1981). PBNA was found to be carcinogenic to the rat, inducing carcinomas in various internal organs except the liver after long-term gastric intubation of large doses (Wang et al. 1981). However, when PBNA was given to male albino rats by repeated gastric intubation before and after weekly intubation of 0.09–0.15 ml/kg CCl_4, portal cirrhosis of the liver occurred early in 60% of the experimental animals, and 67.5% of the cirrhotic rats (45.5% of the experimental rats)later developed complications of cholangiolar and/or hepatocellular carcinomas. Female rats had a lower frequency of cirrhosis by the same treatment, with only one case of cholangioma in 15, while five of the others developed carcinomas of the lungs and ovaries. Since CCl_4 controls of both sexes developed cirrhosis of the liver much less frequently than the experimental animals receiving the combined treatment, and rats fed only PBNA showed no histological changes in the liver, with normal ALT levels, the synergistic action of PBNA and CCl_4 was demonstrated both by increased cancer incidence and by preferential organotropism for the liver in the experimental male rats (Wang and Wang 1981). In this group, oval cell proliferation was also observed during an early stage of the combined treatment. It was presumed after this experiment that PBNA must be an inhibitor of liver cell proliferation, thus facilitating the cirrhogenic process caused by CCl_4.

In a later experiment, PBNA was given to male Wistar rats prior to subtotal hepatectomy. Liver cell proliferation was found to be inhibited in comparison with hepatectomy controls not given PBNA previously (Wang et al. 1982). These experiments may have some implication as regards the importance of multiple etiological factors in the genesis of human liver cancer.

For the chemoprevention of aflatoxin hepatocarcinogenesis, chronic experiments on rats were done to study the effects of the food additive BHA (butylated hydroxyanisole) and riboflavin on this induced liver cancer (Chen et al. 1981; Su et al. 1981) BHA was found to exert a definite effect, in the postponement of the appearance of proliferative lesions as well as in the reduction of their incidence and extent. The final rate of liver cancer was also significantly reduced and the appearance of extrahepatic cancers noticeably delayed by BHA administration. Riboflavin treatment was found to accelerate the appearance of precancerous hepatic lesions, although it inhibited their further development. In the end, it did not exert any inhibitory effect on hepatic and extrahepatic cancers induced by aflatoxin.

III. Search for Better Experimental Models of Etiology and Pathogenesis of Human Primary Hepatocellular Carcinoma

For years the rat has been the animal of choice in experimental studies on liver cancer and on carcinogenesis in general. Recently , epidemiological and pathomorphological evidence has suggested the important role that hepatitis B virus may play in the genesis of human liver cancer, in addition to aflatoxins and other environmental pollutants (Gao et al. 1981; Mai et al. 1982; Sun et al. 1979; Yen et al. 1981; Ying et al. 1981). These findings prompted a search for animals in which the interaction between hepatitis virus and chemical carcinogens may be better investigated. It was reported that, in a county with a high prevalence of human liver cancers home-raised ducks, also had high frequency of liver cancer; preliminary studies showed that the prevalence of duck liver cancer varied from one commune to another in parallel with the incidence of human liver cancer in the various communes (Zhang et al. 1981). In a later investigation on ducks in the same hyperendemic area, virus-like particles were found by means of electron microscopy in the serum of 17 of 35 2-year-old ducks. All 17 showed liver lesions varying from hepatitis to hepato- and cholangiocellular proliferation to liver cancer (Wang et al. 1980). A recent paper reported that such virus-like particles were found to be about 50 nm in diameter, and contained endogenous DNA polymerase, as do DNA viruses in general. All ducks with such particles in the serum showed various pathological changes of the liver. Some virus-containing serum samples exerted an inhibitory effect upon the interaction of HB_sAg with its antibody. The virus-like particles were also agglutinated by anti-HB_sAg antibody. The authors suggested the existence of a group of viruses in nature that are related to hepatitis and liver cancers of various animal species, including human beings. The reported duck virus was considered to be a possible member of this virus group, since it possessed determinants similar to those of HB_sAg (Zhou et al. 1980). Though studies of duck liver diseases and duck viruses are still in the early stage, the use of inbred ducks, free of vertical and transverse virus infections, to study the interaction of virus infection with various chemical factors in the etiology and pathogenesis of primary liver cancer is being seriously contemplated. Such scientific research would need a great deal of basic work and the close collaboration of workers in animal breeding, pathology, biochemistry, virology, and other disciplines.

References

Cancer Research Group. Shanghai Inst of Biochemistry, Academia Sinica (1976) Localization of AFP in rat liver in correlation with the dynamics of serum AFP during 3'MeDAB carcinogenesis. Acta Biochem Biophys Sinica 3: 49–60[1]

Chen ZY, Yan RC, et al. (1981) Experimental studies on inhibition of BHA and riboflavin on induction of rat liver cancers by aflatoxin. I. Observations on precancerous lesions. In: National Symposium on Fungal Toxins and Cancers[1]

Chiang CM (1981) Studies on a transplantable rat hepatoma BERH-2. II, Karyotype analysis and G-banding of marker chromosomes. Acta Biol Exp Sinica 14: 65–70[1]

Chiang CM, Ji WX, Sun LY, et al. (1978) Studies on transplantable rat hepatoma BERH-2. I. The establishment of the tumor line and its morphology, ultrastructure, and alpha-fetoprotein production. Acta Biol Exp Sinica 11: 87–96[1]

Chu TH, Yeh HJ, Chen JM (1980) Establishment and some biological characteristics of a rat hepatoma cell line (CBRH-7919). Acta Biol Exp Sinica 13: 113–115[1]

Fan WK, et al. (1980) Establishment of a transplantable hepatoma (H615) in inbred 615 mice from hepatoma arising spontaneously. Proceedings of the 3rd National Symposium of Pathophysiologists, p 47[1]

Fan WK, et al. (1982) Histochemical demonstration of γ-glutamyl-transpeptidase (γ-GT) in a transplantable hepatoma (H615) of inbred 615 mice. Tumor 2: 12–14[1]

Fishman WH, Sell S (1976) Conference report of regulation of gene expression in development and neoplasia. Cancer Res 36: 4205

Gao RN, Tu JT, Gao YT (1981) A preliminary report of etiological and epidemiological studies on primary liver cancer in Chongming country of Shanghai. Tumor 1: 4–7[1]

Guo C, Tang JC, Hong WN, et al. (1981): Study on the genetic stability of hepatoma cells reversed by normal mouse liver RNA. Tumor 1: 11–13[1]

Hsu YC, Liu HH, Hsu L, et al. (1980) Quantitation of mRNA levels of alpha-fetoprotein and albumin in transplantable rat hepatoma BERH-2. Acta Biol Exp Sinica 13: 353–360[1]

Ke SJ, Hsu HS, Shi WK, et al. (1978) Alpha-fetoprotein in rat during diethylnitrosamine carcinogenesis. Acta Biol Exp Sinica 11: 106–108[1]

Ku JR, et al. (1966) Biological effects of normal cell RNA on cancer cells. Natl Med J China 52: 209–223[1]

Li M, Shu LX, Li WY (1981) Isolation and purification of alpha-fetoprotein messenger RNA from rat transplantable hepatoma BERH-2. Acta Biol Exp Sinica 14: 145–152[1]

Li WY, et al. (1978) Translation of normal liver mRNA and its transforming effects on hepatoma cells in vitro. Acta Biol Exp Sinica 11: 109–124[1]

Lu JH, Yeh HJ, Chen JM (1978) Preliminary observation of the rat hepatoma (BERH-2) in organ culture. Acta Biol Exp Sinica 11: 137–146[1]

Mai K, et al. (1982) A study on the immune state of human populations to HBV. I. The prevalence of anti-HB_s and its significance. Acta Virol Sinica 1: 49–53[1]

Su CC, Yan RC, et al. (1981) Experimental studies on inhibition of BHA and riboflavin on induction of rat liver cancers by aflatoxin. II. Observations on formation of liver cancer and other cancers. In: National Symposium on Fungal Toxins and Cancers.[1]

Sun ZT, et al. (1979) Pathological and serological investigation on early primary hepatocellular carcinoma and its liver disease background. Chin J Oncol 1: 13–19[1]

Wang HW, Wang D (1981) The synergistic action of antioxidant D and carbon tetrachloride on rat liver. Acta Biol Exp Sinica 14: 372–377[1]

Wang NJ, Sun ZT, Pang QF, et al. (1980) Liver cancer, liver disease background and virus-like particles in serum among ducks from high-incidence area of human hepatocellular carcinoma. Chin J Oncol 2: 174–176[1]

Wang HW, Wang D, Tang PX, et al. (1981) The carcinogenic activity of antioxidant D on albino rats. Acta Biol Exp Sinica 14: 77–85[1]

Wang D, et al. (1982) Comparison of carcinogenic activities of antioxidant D in TA1 and ICR mouse strains. Shanghai Communication on Animal Husbandry and Veterinary Medicine 2: 9–11[1]

Xu W, Yen RC, et al. (1981) Observations on liver histology and γ-GT histochemistry during rat hepatocarcinogenesis by AFT administration. In: National Symposium on Fungal Toxins and Cancers[1]

Xu YD, Ying YY, Wu AJ (1982) Experimental pathological study of liver carcinogenesis. Tumor 2: 1–3[1]

Yen RC, et al. (1981) Relationship between liver cell cancer, liver cirrhosis and B hepatitis antigen: a histochemical analysis of 462 livers. Chin J Oncol 3: 143[1]

Ying YY, et al. (1981) The relationship between hepatitis B virus, liver cirrhosis and primary hepatocellular carcinoma. Tumor 1: 1–5[1]

Zhang RY, Chen CC, Ze WY, et al. (1981) A preliminary analysis of the epidemiology, pathology, morphology, and etiology of duck liver cancer in Qidong country of Kiangsu. Tumor 1: 8–11[1]

Zhang YL, et al. (1982) Comparative study on activity of cyclic nucleotide phosphodiesterases in mouse liver and hepatoma ascites cells. Tumor 2: 10–12[1]

Zhou YZ, et al. (1980) A virus possibly related to duck hepatitis and duck liver cancer. Shanghai Med 3: 1–3[1]

1 Chinese

26 Experimental Liver Carcinogenesis

Zhang Yu-yan, Yao Zhen

Rodent liver is an excellent target organ for the studies of the processes and mechanisms of carcinogenesis. Our understanding of the pathogenetic, biological, and biochemical characteristics of liver cancer induced by chemical carcinogens is continuously expanding, although some problems such as the genetic mechanism of hepatocarcinogenesis still await solution. In this chapter we will briefly cover some aspects of pathogenesis, the change of phenotypic expression, and some genetic mechanisms of hepatocarcinogenesis.

I. Pathogenesis

Under the influence of chemical carcinogens or hepatitis virus infection, the liver of rodents of certain strains can develop hepatocellular carcinomas progressively through a series of changes, including toxicity, hyperplasia, preneoplastic lesions, and finally cancer formation. Laird and Barton (1961) were the first to note that hepatocarcinogenesis can be divided into two stages: initiation and promotion (Farber 1980; Williams 1980; Pitot and Sirica 1980; Emmelot and Scherer 1980).

A. Initiation

Toxic changes are the early reactions of liver to the damaging actions of carcinogenic substances, the cytotoxic action being more pronounced in the central portion of the hepatic lobule. These changes are increasingly severe with increasing doses of carcinogen, and vary with the type of carcinogen used. The changes include the general inhibition of DNA and RNA synthesis, as indicated by the decrease of thymidine and cytidine incorporation (Rajewsky 1967, 1968), in spite of the fact that the synthesis in some parenchymal cells is increased.

Cells resistant to the cytotoxic action of hepatotoxins and carcinogens proliferate and develop to form distinct focal and nodular hyperplastic lesions. Farber (1973) was the first to emphasize the importance of the hyperplastic nodule in preneoplastic lesions. In the liver of rats fed with diethylnitrosamine (DENA) Friedrich-Freksa et al. (1969) first observed altered foci that were devoid of histochemically demonstrable G-6-Pase activity; this was later confirmed by others (Schauer and Kunze 1968; Rabes et al. 1972). These foci are often located near periportal regions of the liver, and they consistently show a drecrease in the activities of other enzymes, including ATPase, nucleoside polyphosphatase, β-glucuronidase, and serine dehydratase (Kitagawa and Pitot 1974). On the other hand, glycogen storage, disturbance in iron uptake or metabolism, the thymidine-labeling index, and ^{3}H-cytidine incorporation of cells from such foci are often greater than those of the surrounding normal parenchyma cells (Schauer and Kunze 1968; Simard and Daoust 1966; Rabes and Szymkowiak 1979). One of the most interesting biochemical markers for preneoplastic and neoplastic liver lesions in the rat is the increased activity of fetal hepatocyte enzyme γGTP (Fiala and Fiala 1973). Staining for γ-GTP is the most useful method of counting the number of foci or nodules or proliferating hepatocytes, since between 90% and 95% of the foci and nodules are positive at all stages in the preneoplastic phase (Farber 1980).

Preneoplastic foci induced during the first 2 weeks of carcinogen treatment cannot, by themselves, transform into a malignant tumor (Barbason and Betz 1981). This is to some extent a reversible process, and subsequent action of the carcinogen is necessary to break the normal homeostatic regulatory mechanism of liver cell proliferation, changing the foci into irreversible malignancy.

B. Promotion and Liver Cancer Induction

Hyperplastic nodules derived from altered foci grow progressively into persistent hyperplastic nodules from which cancers later arise. Craddock (1976) and Cayama et al. (1978) suggested that cell replication and cell proliferation plays an essential role in the induction of cancer. Substances that normally do not induce liver cancer in intact animals, especially in a single dose, become carcinogenic after partial hepatectomy. The stimulus of partial hepatectomy therefore appears to act as a promoting agent for liver carcinogenesis, and the single dose of carcinogen is regarded as an initiating agent (Pound and McGuire 1978). On the other hand, under certain conditions a single-dose treatment does induce liver cell cancer in situations where the rate of cell replication is high, as in newborn animals, or in adult animals in which restorative hyperplasia of the liver has been induced by treatment with certain hepatotoxins.

Pitot et al. (1978) used phenobarbital to promote liver cancer induction. Solt et al. (1983) concluded that 2 weeks' exposure to dietary 2-acetylaminofluorene (AAF) plus partial hepatectomy or the administration of CCl_4 had a strong promoting effect on liver carcinogenesis. Wang et al. (1981) and Wang and Wang (1981) reported that repeated gastric intubations of a sesame-oil solution of crude antioxidant D, before and after small weekly oral doses of carbon tetrachloride given to male albino rats, induced early occurrence of portal cirrhosis of the liver in 60% of the animals they studied; 67.5% of them had complications of cholangioma and/or hepatocellular carcinoma. However, no cholangiomas or hepatocellular carcinomas were induced when rats were treated with antioxidant D but without CCl_4. The administration of phenobarbital and carbon tetrachloride provided a condition to promote selective proliferation of hyperplasia nodules. To produce liver cell cancer in the absence of an independent stimulus for mitosis, chronic administration of the carcinogen was usually necessary.

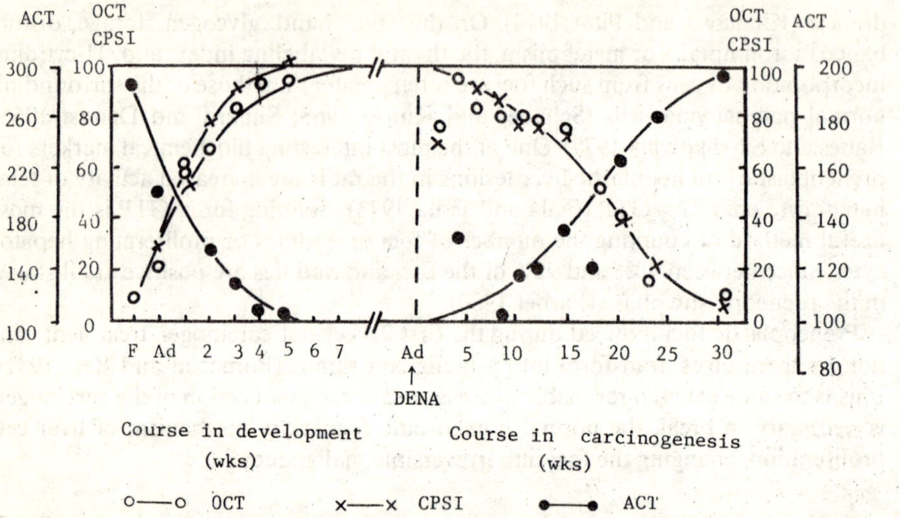

Fig. 1. The relative changes in aspartate carbamyl transferase *(ACT)*, ornithine carbamyl transferase *(OCT)*, and carbamyl phosphate synthetase *(CPSI)* during hepatocarcinogenesis induced by DENA. *F*, fetal; *Ad*, adult

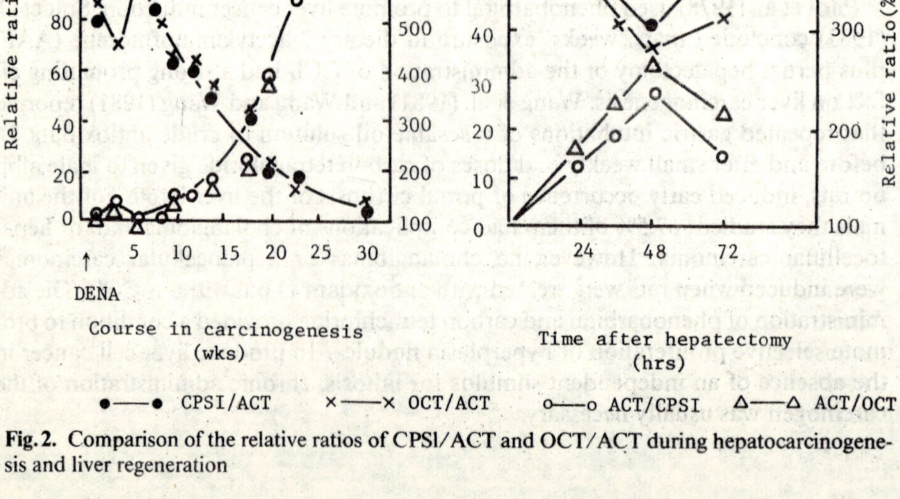

Fig. 2. Comparison of the relative ratios of CPSI/ACT and OCT/ACT during hepatocarcinogenesis and liver regeneration

II. Characterization of Gene Expression During Hepatocarcinogenesis

A. At Early Stage

1. Changes in Proliferating and Tissue-specific Enzyme Activities

Li et al. (1977) studied the interrelationship between the changes in proliferating enzyme activities of rat liver, such as aspartate carbamyl transferase (ACT) – a key enzyme in pyrimidine biosynthesis – and in tissue-specific enzymes, such as ornithine carbamyl transferase (OCT) and carbamyl phosphate synthetase (CPS 1) – key enzymes in the urea cycle – during ontogenesis and during carcinogenesis by DENA. They observed that the activities of CPS 1 and OCT decreased while that of ACT increased in the course of DENA-induced carcinogenesis. The pattern of the relative changes in these enzyme activities was just the reverse of what was observed during ontogenesis (Fig. 1). Results obtained with RIA suggested that the change of CPS 1 activity in rat liver during DENA-induced carcinogenesis might be attributed to the alteration of the rates of enzyme synthesis (Huang et al. 1983). Comparisons made between the relative ratio of CPS 1 to ACT and that of OCT to ACT during hepatocarcinogenesis and liver regeneration indicated a drop in both CPS 1/ACT and OCT/ACT after rats had been fed DENA for 2–4 weeks and then returned to normal in the 6th week. After that, the ratio dropped again and never recovered. The changes of ratios before the 6th week of feeding with DENA were similar to those found in regenerating liver (Fig. 2).

The three pathways in ornithine metabolism, i.e. the urea cycle, polyamine synthesis, and ornithine transamination (OTA), were also studied after the injection of a single dose of DENA (200 mg/kg body wt.) or feeding a small dose of the carcinogen (15 mg/kg/day) to rats. The results indicated that the activity of hepatic ornithine decarboxylase (ODC) was increased while that of OCT and OTA was decreased. Furthermore, the changes could also be reversed to the normal levels at the early stage of DENA treatment. The reversibility of changes in OTA activities was noted when the administration of DENA (5 mg/kg/day) was stopped after 6 weeks' feeding (Li et al. 1982).

Based on their studies of the pathology and enzymatic changes of liver, Li et al. divided the process of carcinogenesis into three stages: the first 6 weeks of DENA feeding could be considered the stage of simple hyperplasia, at whicn the changes in the relative ratio of enzyme activity were reversible, similar to those observed in regenerating liver; from the 6th to the 16th week of carcinogen feeding began the stage of malignant transformation with the irreversibility of changes in the relative ratio of enzyme activity. The final stage was the formation of hepatocellular carcinoma. Quantitative immunological titration indicated that the decrease in CPS 1 activity in hepatoma, DENA-fed liver, and neonatal liver was due to a decrease in the level of enzyme protein, without significant alteration in the immunological properties of CPS 1 from these different tissues (Huang et al. 1982).

2. Reexpression of Fetal Proteins

In normal growth and development, some proteins were present in fetal liver but absent, or present only in minimal amounts, in adult liver. However, they usually reappeared or were present in large quantities in hepatocellular carcinoma – for instance, AFP and γ-GTP, appeared, and there were changes in the pattern of aldolase isozyme. These characteristics are now utilized as very important markers for the detection of the process of hepatocarcinogenesis and the formation of hepatoma.

a. The association of AFP with malignant hepatocellular carcinoma was first observed by Abelev (1971). Its dynamic reappearance in rats during hepatocarcinogenesis induced by various agents such as 3'-MeDAB (Cancer Research Group et al. 1976), DENA (Ke et al. 1978), ethionine (Hancock et al. 1976), and aflatoxin B_1 (Kroes et al. 1972) has also been studied. In general, as time went on the amount of AFP increased gradually after carcinogen feeding; it was also found to be elevated in toxic liver (Smuckler et al. 1976; Ikehera 1973; Sell et al. 1974b) and in regenerating liver (Sell et al. 1974a), but in much smaller amounts than in carcinogen-induced liver. Early increase of serum AFP was also observed in spontaneous hepatocarcinogenesis in C3H/A/BOM and C3HeB/FeJ mice (Jalanko et al. 1978). Boss et al. (1977) detected AFP in the urine of rats exposed to 3'-methyl-4-dimethyl-aminoazobenzene.

Immunofluorescent localization of AFP-containing cells in the liver was achieved with Fischer rats fed 0.05% AAF; approximately 1% of the oval cells contained AFP (Sell 1978). AFP-positive reactions were also detected in small liver cells (Stratil et al. 1978) and in poorly differentiated liver cell carcinomas after 3'-MeDAB feeding (Cancer Research Group et al. 1976).

b. Membrane-associated fetal antigen in rat hepatoma were observed by Xu et al. (1984) in our laboratory. Absorbed antiserum against the surface antigens isolated from 10–15 day rat fetal cells with 3M KCl-PBS was used to compare the immune reaction of cells of fetal rat liver, primary rat hepatoma induced by DENA, transplantable rat hepatoma BERH-2, and normal rat liver by the unlabeled immunoperoxidase method. The results showed that a membrane-associated fetal antigen in rat hepatoma was also present on the cell surface and in the cytoplasm of fetal liver cells. The immunoenzymatic reaction was stronger in 13–14 day fetal liver (Fig. 3c) than in 19-day fetal liver. In the liver of newborn rats the antigen was still present on the cell surface. It was decreased or had disappeared in normal adult rat liver (Fig. 3e) and reappeared in hepatomas (Fig. 3a and b). Similar findings were reported for cultured human hepatoma cells (Shi et al. 1977) and surgical hepatoma specimens (Tsung et al. 1980).

c. Gamma-GTP is an enzyme present in large amounts in fetal and neonatal liver, but only in minimal amounts in normal adult rat liver. During aflatoxin B_1-induced carcinogenesis, the appearance of hyperplastic liver cell foci was followed by strong γ-GTP activity localized on the cell membranes and in the cytoplasm. The focal reappearance of γ-GTP occurred before the development of true carcinomas and

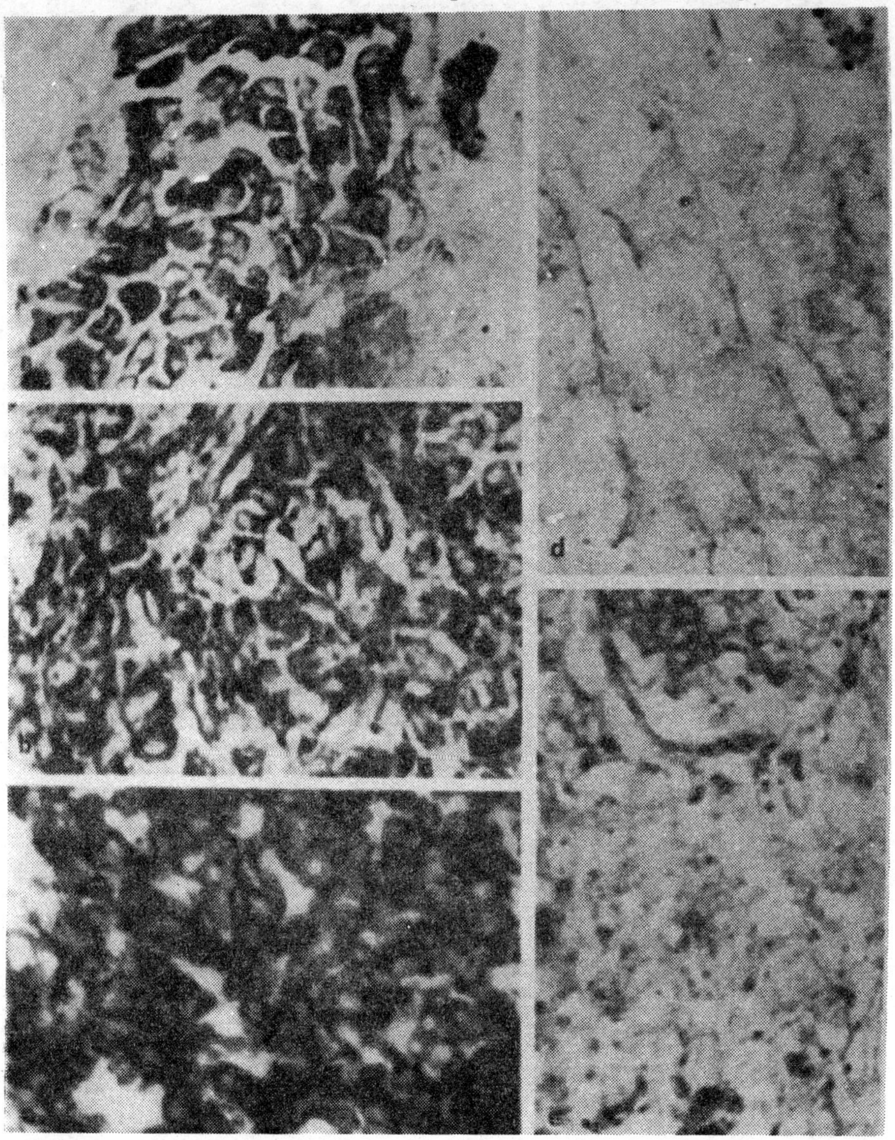

Fig. 3a–e. Membrane-associated fetal antigen in rat hepatoma. **a** Section of a primary hepatoma showing positive cell surface enzmye reaction in a neoplastic focus and weak reaction in cytoplasm. Normal liver cells around the neoplastic focus give only a weak or negative reaction. **b** Transplantable hepatoma showing positive reaction on cell surface and weak reaction in some cytoplasm. **c** Liver section of a 13-day-old fetus. **d** Control section of rat transplantable hepatoma treated with normal rabbit serum instead of with specific antiserum; negative reaction. **e** Normal liver section from an adult rat showing negative reaction

then persisted in the tumor tissue (Kalengayi et al. 1975). The reappearance of γ-GTP during hepatocarcinogenesis was not as early as that of AFP. Using rabbit anti-γ-GTP antibody, γ-GTP-positive hepatocytes could be isolated from male F344 rats fed AAF during the early stage of hepatocarcinogenesis (Hanigan and Pitot 1982).

d. Aldolase is an enzyme highly active on fructose-1,6-phosphate (FDP), and it therefore plays a crucial role in the metabolism of fructose in liver. There are three forms of aldolase in mammalian tissues: types A, B, and C. The genes of aldolase subunits show some heteromeric properties (Penhoet et al. 1966; Penhoet and Rutter 1971). Endo et al. (1970) observed that muscle-type aldolase activity was increased in rat liver in the early stage of 3'-MeDAB-induced hepatocarcinogenesis. In our laboratory, Xu et al. (1978) made an observation of the changes in aldolase activity and its isozyme pattern in rat liver during DENA-induced hepatocarcinogenesis. The results indicated that the aldolase activity for F1P decreased rapidly in liver within the first 8 weeks of DENA administration and then remained at a relatively low level. The aldolase activity for fructose-1, 6-diphosphate (FDP) in liver appeared unchanged within the first 16 weeks of DENA treatment, but rose quickly thereafter (Fig. 4). The ratio of FDP/F1P is shown in Table 1.

The isozyme pattern of aldolase was analyzed using electrophoresis on acetate cellulose membrane. The results showed that the decrease in activity of aldolase B was accompanied by the appearance of aldolase A in rats that were fed DENA for 4 and 8 weeks. Then the activity of aldolase C appeared in the liver of rats fed DENA for 12 weeks. Among the six rats with primary hepatoma so far analyzed, A_3, A_1C_4,

Table 1. Comparison of aldolase activities during DENA induced hepatocarcinogenesis

Tissue	Aldolase activities[a]		FDP/F1P
	FDP substrate	F1P substrate	
Normal adult rats			
Muscle	12.10	0.35	34.60
Liver	1.05	1.02	1.03
Liver of rats fed DENA for			
4 weeks	1.18	0.70	1.69
8 weeks	0.93	0.41	2.27
12 weeks	1.02	0.47	2.17
16 weeks	1.06	0.40	2.65
20 weeks[b]	1.63	0.36	4.53
Transplantable hepatoma BERH-2[c]	0.88	0.12	7.33
Fetal liver of rats			
14–15 days	0.49	0.17	2.88
18–19 days	1.03	0.61	1.69

[a] Unit of enzyme activity: μM/1 g tissue/min
[b] All rats listed at 20 weeks had primary hepatoma
[c] Transplantable hepatoma BERH-2 was derived originally from a primary hepatoma of rat fed DENA (Chiang et al. 1978).

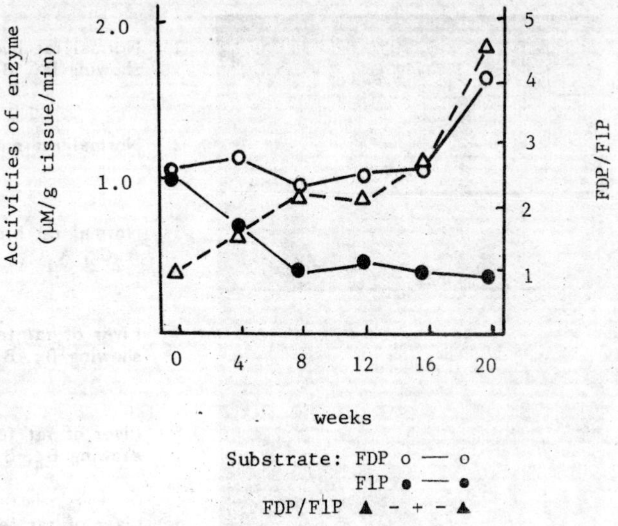

Fig. 4. Change in aldolase activities of liver in DENA-fed rats

and C_4 bands are present in four of them, and only A_3 and A_1C_4 bands in the other two (Fig. 5).

e. Pyruvate kinase (PK) plays an important role in the regulation of glycolysis and gluconeogenesis and possesses three isozymes (L, K, and M types). The three types display some differences in electrophoretic mobility, isoelectric point, kinetics, and immunological properties, and are the products of three different genes. The L-type isozyme in rat liver during hepatocarcinogenesis was progessively decreased and the K-type isozyme increased. Changes in isozyme pattern and specific activity of PK were detectable before histological alterations appeared (Silber et al. 1978).

B. At Late Stage and in Hepatoma

Many of the characteristics which appeared in the early stage of hepatocarcinogenesis were also observed in the late stage and in hepatoma.

There was a positive correlation between the growth rate of AFP-positive transplantable BERH-2 hepatoma and the amount of AFP found in the serum of tumor-bearing rats (Chiang et al. 1978). The BERH-2 hepatoma cells were aneuploid, with a model number of 72 chromosomes (Chiang 1981). Sell and Morris (1974) demonstrated that the amount of AFP in Morris hepatomas with different growth rates was correlated with their growth rate and chromosome composition. On the other hand, the albumin synthesis in Morris hepatoma was decreased as compared with that of normal adult rats (Schreiber et al. 1976).

The abnormal expression of the aldolase isozyme pattern in rat hepatoma cells was correlated with their degree of differentiation. The expression of type-A isozyme aldolase was highest in the poorly differentiated hepatoma, while its expression in highly differentiated hepatoma was the same as that in adult normal liver

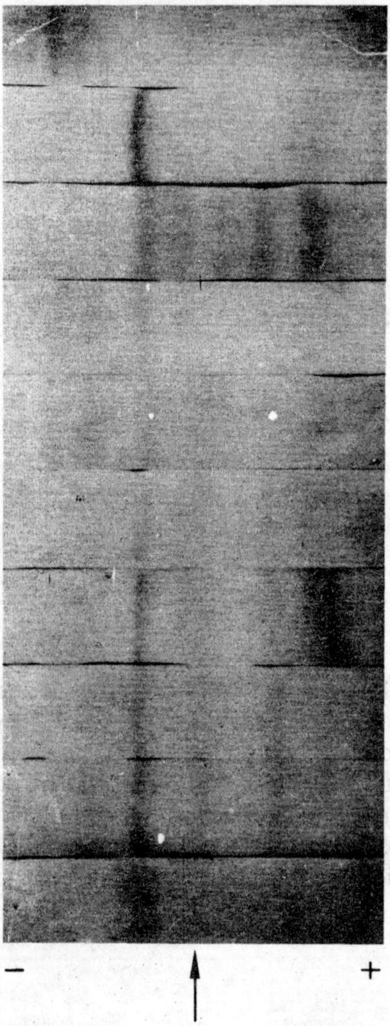

1 Normal rat liver, showing B_4, B_3A_1 bands

2 Normal rat muscle, showing A_4 band

3 Normal rat brain, showing A_4, A_3C_1, A_2C_2, A_1C_3, C_4 bands

4 Liver of rat fed DENA for 4 weeks, showing B_4, B_2A_2, A_4 bands

5 Liver of rat fed DENA for 8 weeks, showing B_4, B_2A_2, A_4 bands

6 Liver of rat fed DENA for 12 weeks, showing B_2A_2, A_4, A_1C_3 bands

7 Rat primary hepatoma, showing A_4, A_1C_3, C_4 bands

8 Rat primary hepatoma, showing A_4, A_1C_3 bands

9 Rat transplantable hepatoma BERH-2, showing A_4, A_1C_3 bands

10 14-day rat fetal liver, showing A_4 bands

Fig. 5. Changes in aldolase isozyme gene expression during hepatocarcinogenesis

(Weinhouse 1973). The starch electrophoretic patterns of glucose-ATP phosphotransferases of fetal and neonatal liver and hepatoma and the isoelectric pattern of PK isozymes of rat liver and hepatoma manifested the same relationship as that between the degree of differentiation of hepatoma and isozyme patterns (Weinhouse et al. 1972). The results suggested that a "switching on" of genes coded for fetal proteins in hepatoma cells was followed by the "switching off" of genes for the products of the differentiated cells, but this was not a general rule. Carbamylphosphate synthetase and threonine dehydrase, which are also liver-specific enzymes related to differentiated functions of the liver, showed remarkably higher activities in hepatomas than in normal liver (Ono et al. 1972).

III. Abnormality of Gene Expression Control and Genome of Rat Liver During Hepatocarcinogenesis

Genome structure and the control of gene expression are the keys to the mechanism of hepatocarcinogenesis.

A. Observations on Hepatoma Genome

1. Genome Analysis Using Restriction Endonucleases

Parker et al. (1979, 1981) compared the nuclear and nucleolar DNA of Novikoff hepatoma cells and normal rat liver cells using *Eco*RI restriction endonuclease and agarose gel electrophoresis. Three *Eco*RI fragments were found in the Novikoff hepatoma DNA: fragment A, 3.6 megadaltons; fragment B, 1.3 megadaltons; and fragment C, 0.91 megadaltons. Fragments B and C appeared in equal amounts in both nuclear and nucleolar DNA of rat liver and hepatoma cells. The reiteration frequencies of fragment A in Novikoff hepatoma and rat liver were 6600 and 30 respectively, which means a 220-fold enrichment of fragment A in the Novikoff hepatoma genome. Fragment A was localized to the nucleolus. Sequencing of a subfragment (~300 bp) of fragment A digested by endonuclease *Pst*I indicated the presence of a repetitive "island". The homology of DNA fragment in rat strains and tumor cell lines with the amplified 5.8-kb *Eco*RI fragment of the Novikoff hepatoma cell was not complete. A 7.2-kb band in ACT rat DNA, a 7.2-kb band and a 9.4-kb band in both hepatoma 7777 and hepatoma 252 DNA were able to hybridize with the 5.8-kb *Eco*RI fragment. Rothblum et al. (1981) suggested that the 5.8-kb, 7.2-kb, and 9.4-kb fragments might be the results of genetic drift over relatively short periods of time.

2. DNA Damage

The degree of DNA damage of hepatoma cells in situ was analyzed by means of the alkaline elution technique. Three hours after the treatment of male mice with 1,2-dibromoethane (25–75 mg/kg), dose-dependent DNA single-strand breaks could be observed (White et al. 1981). Elution of DNA from rats treated with four cycles of AAF was 71% more than that from normal rats (Stout and Becker 1980). Later, Stout and Becker (1982) demonstrated that the occurrence of progressive DNA damage was coincident with the appearance of foci of altered hepatocytes including those that were γ-GTP positive.

Using a new viscosimetric technique, Brambilla et al. (1983) reported that a single i.p. dose of carcinogen could induce a statistically significant reduction of the time [t_{95}: the time required for $^{\eta}$red to reach 95% of ($^{\eta}$red) max] required for $^{\eta}$red (specific viscosity/DNA concentration) to reach its maximal value. The dose used was so small that it did not produce significant alteration in the pharmacokinetic behavior of these compounds.

3. DNA Alkylation

Margison (1980) suggested that the carcinogenicity of alkalating agents was correlated with their capacity to bind DNA at the O^6 position of guanine. The distribution of 7-methylguanine (Galbraith et al. 1978) and of O^6-methylguanine (Galbraith et al. 1980) was found to occur at random between the repetitive and unique sequences of liver DNA of rats given carcinogen. The half-life of ethylated DNA of intact and regenerating rat liver treated with 10 mg ^{14}C-DENA/kg body wt. was as follows: O^6-ethylguanine, 3–4 h; 7-ethylguanine, 120 h; ethyladenine, 10 h; O^2-ethylthymidine, ~1000 h; phosphotriesters, ~1000 h. The half-life of radioactive purine present in foci (50–100 h) seemed to correspond to that of 7-ethylguanine. Therefore, 7-ethylguanine might be relevant to foci induction (Emmelot and Scherer 1980).

DNA modified by the carcinogen N-acetoxy- 2-acetylaminofluorene was used as an antigen to induce antibodies which reacted only with the modified DNA (Leng et al. 1978). This suggests that the modified DNA had changed its template properties and antigenicity. Pegg (1978) and Stumpf et al. (1979) reported that an enzyme which could remove O^6-methylguanine from liver DNA was inhibited by a carcinogen. Enzymatic release of 7-methylguanine from methylated DNA by rodent liver extracts has been reported by Margison and Pegg (1981).

Eucaryotic DNA can be methylated by DNA methyltransferase to form 5-methylcytosine. This process occurs subsequent to DNA replication and DNA repair. Therefore, undermethylation of DNA can persist for a period of time ranging from several minutes to a few hours after strand synthesis. The 5-methylcytosine content of nuclear DNA can be directly estimated during chemical hepatocarcinogenesis and in the resulting carcinomas. The following degrees of hypomethylation during liver cancer induction were found by Lapeyre and Becker (1979): premalignant nodules, 20%; primary hepatocellular carcinoma induced by AAF, 45%; and primary hepatocellular carcinoma induced by DENA, 32.5%. The DNAs from spontaneous tumors of a certain strain of C_3H mice and those from AAF-, chlordane-, or 3'-Me--DAB-induced tumors in $C_{57}BL$ and B6 C3 mice were all undermethylated as compared with normal liver DNA samples. However, DNA methylase activity from tumor nuclei was found by Lapeyre et al. (1981) to be higher than normal, so that undermethylation of DNA found in the tumors could not be explained by the inactivation of the enzyme, or by a significant deficiency of it. Lapeyre et al (1981) suggested that the resulting undermethylation might be due to an altered chromatin configuration or to a change in the specificity of DNA methyltransferase during carcinogenesis.

B. Alteration of Gene Expression Control

Chromatin structure plays an important role in the control of replication and transcription. Therefore, many observations concerning components, nonhistone protein (NHP) analysis, and transcriptional activity of the chromatin of hepatoma cells have been made. Rodriguez et al. (1979) found that ten nonhistone chromosomal proteins (NHCP), ranging from 55000 to 220000 daltons, were present in the tumors but absent from normal liver. When the chromosomal proteins of chromatin from normal liver, liver of tumor-bearing animals, and spontaneous primary hepatocellular carcinomas of C_3H/HeN mice were analyzed, these authors found no quantitative or qualitative differences in histone contents, but observed more NHCP in the chromatin of tumor and liver of tumor-bearing animals than in that of normal liver (Rodriguez and Becker 1979). Comparison of chromatin nonhistone proteins (NHP) of rat hepatoma BERH-2 and normal rat liver by two-dimensional gel electrophoresis – combining isoelectric focusing with SDS-PAGE and the silver stain method – showed that the two-dimensional pattern of normal liver NHP had a higher relative percentage of spots in the regions of higher molecular weight and higher isoelectric point, while that of hepatoma had a higher relative percentage of spots in the regions of lower molecular weight and lower isoelectric point. Furthermore, there were some protein spots found only in hepatoma or in normal liver (He et al. 1982). The increase in NHP was detected before the appearance of pathomorphological changes (He et al. 1980). Yeoman et al. (1976) reported that a fetal glycoprotein had been detected in the chromatin of Novikoff hepatoma cells. Tsanev and Hadjiolov (1978) observed an increase in the amount of two proteins, of 43 000 and 63 000 daltons, and a decrease in the histone subfraction H1° in the chromosomal protein of primary hepatoma. The above-cited observations indicated that there was a change in the NHP fractions in hepatoma which might, in some way, be related to the change in nuclear enzymes or regulatory proteins. Chromatin isolated from the liver of DENA-fed rats was found to have a higher transcriptional activity in a cell-free system with either *Escherichia coli* RNA polymerase or RNA polymerase II from rat liver than normal liver chromatin. The increase in transcriptional activity was parallel to the development of liver cancer during DENA-induced hepatocarcinogenesis (Hao et al. 1983).

The regulation of the AFP gene in hepatoma cells was used as a marker to study gene control in tumor cells. The levels of AFP-mRNA in normal liver and in Morris hepatoma 7777 were compared by the RNA-cDNA hybridization technique. It was found that at the Rot valve, where 50% of the AFP- cDNA probe hybridized to hepatoma mRNA, less than 1% of the probe hybridizid to poly $(A)^+$-containing RNA from adult rat liver polysomes. It was thus demonstrated that the amount of functional AFP-mRNA was very low in adult liver (Innis and Miller 1977). In one cell line from Morris hepatoma 7777 (AFP-positive), the production of AFP decreased progressively after 8 months in vitro, but the cell retained many malignant characteristics. This suggested that the control mechanism of AFP production in hepatoma is an epiphenomenon (Yoo et al. 1979). On the other hand, in vitro translation or hybridization to an albumin-specific cDNA sequence strongly indicated that the albumin gene was not transcribed in Novikoff hepatoma cells (Capetanaki et al. 1982). However, it was found that the mRNA level of AFP was 2.5–7 times higher in transplantable rat hepatoma BERH-2 than in liver, but that the mRNA level of albumin in hepatoma BERH-2 was only twice that in liver, as studied in an in vitro system. (Hsu et al. 1980). No amplification of the AFP gene was observed (Sala-Trepat et al. 1979), but the polymorphism of the albumin and AFP genes was observed in various inbred strains of rats (Ga'l et al. 1982).A study of AFP gene structure deduced from a complete cDNA sequence revealed an extensive sequence homology to the serum albumin gene (Law and Pugaizyk 1981). These results might suggest that the reappearance of AFP during hepatocarcinogenesis was a *result* of abnormality in gene expression, and not a change in the gene itself.

Gene amplification was observed in ribosomal RNA genes of a rat hepatoma cell line, H4-II E-C3; a ten fold excess of 18S and 28S rRNA genes was found in amplified chromosome regions. Antibodies to 5-methylcytidine could be bound to the DNA of these regions. Most of the amplified rRNA genes were transcriptionally inactive. The 5′-C-C-G-G-3′ sequence in most of the amplified rRNA genes was methylated (Tantravahi et al. 1981).

C. Sequence Complexity of Nucleic Acids During Hepatocarcinogenesis

Some work has been done in our laboratory concerning the changes of sequence complexity during hepatocarcinogenesis induced by DENA. Nucleic acid competitive inhibition experiments indicated that the nucleotide sequence of normal liver nuclear RNA, complementary to the repeated sequence DNA, was partly absent from the nuclear RNA of liver of rats given DENA for 2 weeks, but returned to the normal level after 4 weeks of DENA treatment. The nucleotide sequence seemed to be partly missing again from the nuclear RNA of liver after 8 weeks of DENA treatment, as did that of the transplantable rat hepatoma BERH-2. The changes found in the nucleotide sequence from the 2nd to the 4th week of DENA administration were similar to those found in regenerating liver (Fig. 6) (Zhang et al. 1978). After presaturation competitive inhibition with unlabeled nuclear RNA isolated from the liver of rats fed DENA for 2, 4, 6, 8, and 10 weeks, from primary hepatomas, and from transplantable rat hepatoma BERH-2, the percentages of relative hybridization of labeled liver nuclear RNA were 6.5, 6.7, 5.7, 14.6, 10.8, 46.1, and 41.0 respectively. This indicated that the capacity of nuclear RNA from rat liver for competitive inhibition during DENA-induced hepatocarcinogenesis decreased progressively to about 46% of normal nuclear RNA in the case of primary hepatoma (Fig. 7) (Zhang et al. 1982; Xu and Zhang 1980).

The middle repeated-sequence DNA (Cot 10^{-1}-250) and single-copy-sequence DNA (Cot > 250) were isolated from DNA of rat liver and labeled to be used as a probe to hybridize with excess nuclear RNA. As compared with normal rat liver nuclear RNA, the saturation values of single-copy-sequence DNA complementary to nuclear RNA from the liver of rats fed with DENA for 2, 4, 6, 8, and 10 weeks, and from primary hepatoma, were raised by 41.7%, 86.1%, 86.1%, 2.8%, 13.9%, and 38.9% respectively. The saturation value of single-copy-sequence DNA with nuclear RNA from transplantable rat hepatoma BERH-2 was 61.1% higher than that with nuclear RNA from normal rat liver ($p < 0.005$). These results are shown in Fig. 8 and Table 2 (Xu et al. 1979; Zhang et al. 1982). The saturation values of middle repeated-sequence DNA complementary to nuclear RNA from the liver of rats fed DENA for 4 and 8 weeks, and from primary hepatoma, were found to drop by 20%, 80%, and 90% respectively. The saturation value of middle repeated-sequence DNA with nuclear RNA from transplantable rat hepatoma BERH-2 was 60.0% lower than that with nuclear RNA from normal rat liver ($p < 0.005$). These results are shown in Fig. 9 and Table 3 (Zhang et al. 1982). On the other hand, comparisons of the rRNA present in nuclear RNA with rRNA complementary to repeated-se-

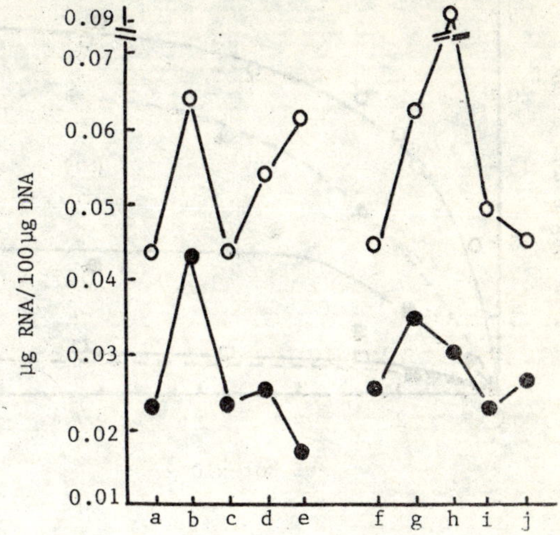

Fig. 6. Hybridization values of labeled nuclear RNA from rat liver cells (○) and hepatoma cells (●) with DNA immobilized on filters after competitive inhibition. *a* Rat liver; *b* liver of rats fed DENA for 2 weeks; *c* liver of rats fed DENA for 4 weeks; *d* liver of rats fed DENA for 8 weeks; *e* primary hepatoma; *f* rat liver (shammed); *g* regenerated liver at 1 day; *h* regenerated liver at 2 days; *i* regenerated liver at 4 days; *j* regenerated liver at 7 days

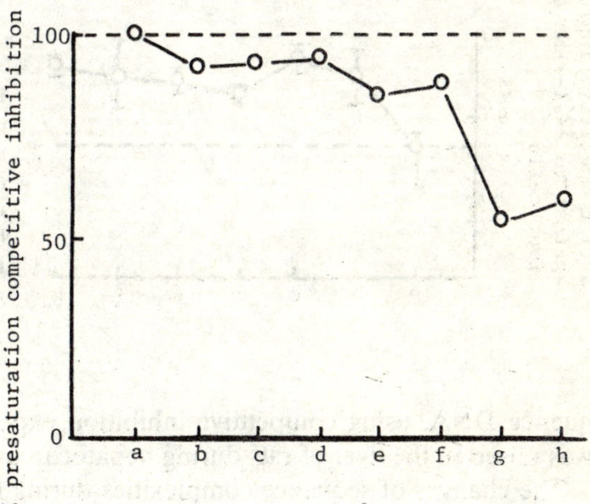

Fig. 7. Comparison of nuclear RNA by presaturation competitive inhibition experiments. *a* Rat liver; *b* liver of rats fed DENA 2 weeks; *c* liver of rats fed DENA 4 weeks; *d* liver of rats fed DENA 6 weeks; *e* liver of rats fed DENA 8 weeks; *f* liver of rats fed DENA 10 weeks; *g* primary hepatoma; *h* transplantable hepatoma BERH-2

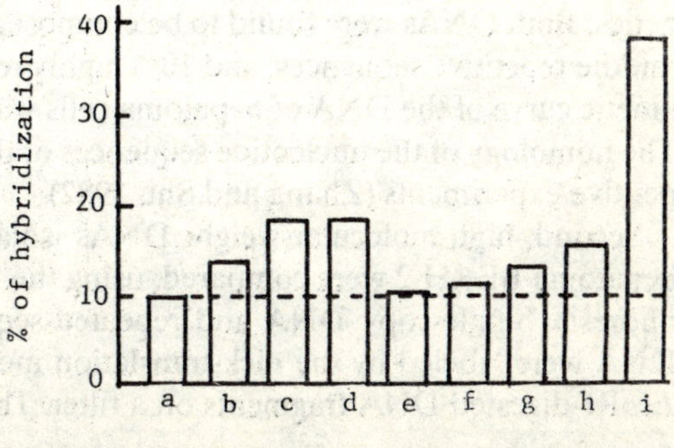

Fig. 8. Value of saturation hybridization of single-copy DNA with nuclear RNA. *a* Rat liver; *b* liver of rats fed DENA for 2 weeks; *c* liver of rats fed DENA for 4 weeks; *d* liver of rats fed DENA for 6 weeks; *e* liver of rats fed DENA for 8 weeks; *f* liver of rats fed DENA for 10 weeks; *g* primary hepatoma; *h* transplantable hepatoma BERH-2; *i* fetal rat liver

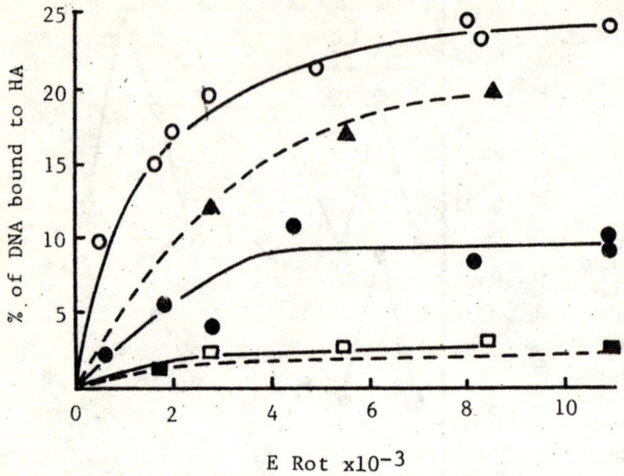

Fig. 9. Saturation hybridization of middle repeated-sequence DNA with nuclear RNA from normal rat liver (○), transplantable hepatome (●), liver of rats fed DENA for 4 weeks (▲) and 8 weeks (□), and primary hepatoma (■)

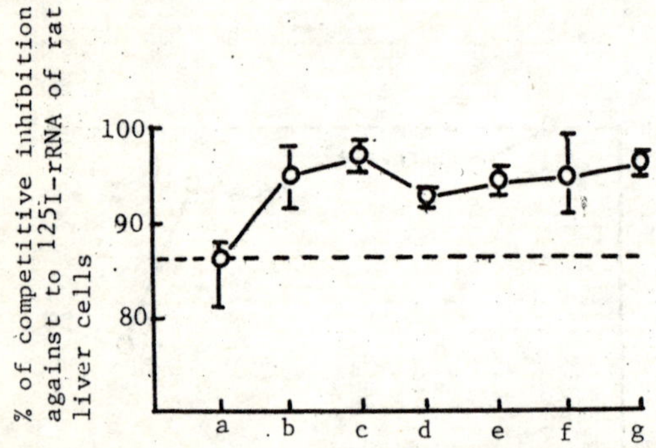

Fig. 10. Comparison of rRNA contained in nuclear RNA by competitive inhibition experiments. *a* Rat liver; *b* liver of rats fed DENA 2 weeks; *c* liver of rats fed DENA 4 weeks; *d* liver of rats fed DENA 8 weeks; *e* liver of rats fed DENA 10 weeks; *f* primary hepatoma; *g* transplantable hepatoma BERH-2

quence DNA, using competitive inhibition experiments, indicated that the latter was raised in the liver of rats during hepatocarcinogenesis (Fig. 10; Xu et al. 1980).

The changes of sequence complexities during hepatocarcinogenesis induced by DENA might be explained by genomic DNA alteration or by abnormal DNA transcription. To discriminate between these alternatives, the DNAs from rat liver and hepatoma were compared in different experiments. First, sequence composition analysis was done, using the hydroxyapatite column method and renaturation kinetics. Both DNAs were found to be composed of 65% single-copy sequences, 25% middle repetitive sequences, and 10% highly repetitive sequences. The renaturation kinetic curve of the DNA of hepatoma cells was similar to that of normal liver cells. The homology of the nucleotide sequences of the two DNAs was evident from competitive experiments (Zhang and Shu 1982).

Second, high-molecular-weight DNAs isolated from normal rat liver and from hepatoma BERH-2 were compared, using the Southern blot technique and electrophoresis. Single-copy DNA and repeated-sequence DNA isolated from rat liver DNA were labeled by the nick-translation method and used to hybridize with the *Eco*RI-digested DNA fragments on a filter. The reactions of the probes with DNA

Table 2. Complexity of nonrepeated-sequence DNA complementary to nuclear RNA

Nuclear RNA	Normal liver	Liver of rats fed DENA: weeks of feeding 2	4	6	8	10	Primary hepatoma	BERH-2 hepatoma
Saturation hybridization value	9.6 ±1.6	13.6 ±1.5	18.3 ±4.4	18.3	9.7 ±1.4	10.8 ±2.5	13.2 ±1.1	15.5 ±1.4
Percentage of total DNA complexity	12.5	17.7	23.8	23.8	12.6	14.0	17.2	20.2
Complexity as kilobases ($\times 10^5$)	3.6	5.1	6.7	6.7	3.7	4.1	5.0	5.8
Increase (%)	0	41.7	86.1	86.1	2.8	13.9	38.9	61.1

Table 3. Complexity of repeated-sequence DNA complementary to nuclear RNA

Nuclear RNA	Normal liver	Liver of rats fed with DENA: weeks of feeding 2	4	6	8	10	Primary hepatoma	BERH-2 hepatoma
Saturation hybridization value	23.7 ±2.1		19.6		2.8		2.4	9.6 ±1.6
Percentage of total DNA complexity	11.9		9.8		1.4		1.2	4.8
Complexity as kilobases ($\times 10^4$)	35		28		4.1		3.5	14
Decrease (%)			20.0		88.2		90.0	60.0
Decrease of[a] inhibition (%)	0	6.5	6.7	5.7	14.6	10.8	46.1	41.0

[a] Competitive inhibition experiments

Table 4. Increase in transport of RNA from nucleus to cytoplasm (in %)

	Normal rat liver	BERH-2 hepatoma	Liver of rats fed with DENA: weeks of feeding 2	4	6	10	Primary hepatoma
Total cytoplasmic[a] RNA	100	123.9	106.5	114.7	120.3	–	–
Total rRNA[a]	100	146.3	125.4	114.6	–	118.2	171.9
Total polysomal RNA[b]	100	185.0					

[a] Competitive inhibition experiments

[b] Saturation hybridization experiments

fragments from rat liver and hepatoma DNA were quite similar. The bands of the probes of Cot 0.01–4 DNA fragments isolated from normal liver DNA and hepatoma BERH-2 DNA hybridizable with *Eco*RI-digested DNA fragments of rat liver and hepatoma DNA were also quite similar. However, when ^{125}I-labeled mercuric nuclear RNAs from rat liver and hepatoma BERH-2 were used as probes to hybridize with *Eco*RI-digested DNA fragments of normal rat liver and hepatoma BERH-2, there seemed to be some difference in the results of hybridization with both probes; the work is still in progress.

D. Transport of RNA from Nucleus to Cytoplasm

Increased transport of RNA from the nucleus to the cytoplasm in hepatoma cells was reported by Drews et al. (1968), Mendecki et al. (1969), and Garrett et al. (1973, 1977). Garrett suggested that the altered transport of RNA might be an important factor in the malignancy process. With DENA-induced hepatocarcinogenesis, the transport of total RNA and rRNA from nucleus to cytoplasm increased gradually during hepatoma development (Zhang et al. 1978; Xu et al. 1980). The amount of total polysomal RNA hybridizable with single-copy-sequence DNA was higher in hepatoma BERH-2 than in normal rat liver (Xu et al. 1979). These results are summarized in Table 4.

A repetitive nuclear RNA (3.5S) was found to exhibit 17% release from the nucleus to the cytoplasm in rats after they had been fed with 3′-MeDAB for 1, 3, and 10 weeks, and a 35% release after 16 weeks (Patel et al. 1979). The percentage of the release of labeled RNA from isolated nuclei of normal liver, regenerating liver, and hepatoma 5123D after incubation with homologous or heterologous cytosol indicated that the cytosol might contain nondialyzable components which could act post-transcription to regulate the nuclear RNA processing and/or transport of mRNA; these factors might differ in normal, regenerating, and neoplastic liver (Schumm et al. 1973). It was suggested that these components might be inactivated by the carcinogen, or that they could transfer the carcinogen into the cell nucleus with the resulting distortion of RNA processing there (Patel et al. 1981).

IV. Conclusion

What is the key point for the transformation of normal cells into cancer cells? Different authors have formulated different hypotheses to explain the process. Early in 1928, Bauer suggested that cancer was caused by somatic mutation. Later, observations concerning the interaction of chemical carcinogens with cellular DNA and the integration of a retrovirus genome into a host genome supported this hypothesis. Loeb et al. (1974) and Sirover and Loeb (1977) suggested that diverse carcinogenic agents could affect DNA so as to cause errors in base pairing during DNA replication. Some of these errors would cause alterations in structural genes for enzymes which function in base selection, and would lead to an expanding number of errors in genetic information. It was proposed that inconsistent DNA replication might be responsible for oncogenesis and tumor progression.

Pitot et al. (Pitot 1968; Pitot et al. 1974, 1976) proposed a membron model which consisted of ribosome, messenger RNA, and the membrane. The experimental evidence indicated that the interaction between the membrane and the polysome gave a structural integrity to the stable mRNA template, which in turn was related to the phenotypic variability. It was suggested that the alteration in template life span and template stability might result from changes in the membron structure, and this hypothesis actually presents a post-transcription mechanism for carcinogenesis.

Comings' (1973) gene-control theory suggested that regulation of the repression and derepression of regulatory genes and structure genes was correlated with cell differentiation and cell growth. Abnormal expression of the regulatory and structural genes might lead to cell transformation.

The concept of Busch (1976) emphasized that the carcinogen might act with a fetal receptor to interact directly with the genome, or might cause a new stimulus within the cell to interact with a receptor that would interact with the genome.

Progress was made when mRNAs for the protein products involved in growth, invasiveness, and metastasis were produced. From observations made on both normal and neoplastic cells by means of electronmicroscopy, Frenster et al. (1976) pointed out a progressive decrease in the number and size of DNA helix openings per cell during cell maturation in vivo which can be correlated with the decreasing rate of proliferation. Therefore, they derived a theory of control of DNA helix opening for carcinogenesis.

Oncogene theory has progressed rapidly over the years. Oncogenes are genes that cause cancer. They were first found in viruses, but their evolutionary history implies that normal vertebrate cells have genes whose abnormal expression can lead to cancerous growth. The studies of the human bladder oncogene by Weinberg (Tabin et al. 1982) and Barbacid (Reddy et al. 1982) in 1982 carry the theory to a new stage. They suggested that a single nucleotide change could convert a normal cellular gene into one capable of causing cancerous transformation. All these theories can be roughly grouped into two categories of cancer cell origin: genetic and epigenetic.

Our own findings on the changes of the total transcriptional products of middle repeated-sequence DNA and single-copy-sequence DNA during DENA induction of liver cancer seemed to suggest that the expression of middle repeated-sequence DNA was partly inhibited while that of single-copy-sequence DNA was enhanced in DENA-induced hepatoma. No deletion of sequence composition from DNA of hepatoma BERH-2 has so far been observed in renaturation kinetics, sequence composition analysis, or analysis of the distribution of single-copy- and repeated-sequence rat DNA on *Eco*RI-DNA fragments of DNAs from rat liver and hepatoma BERH-2. However, hybridizable nuclear RNAs of normal rat liver and rat hepatoma BERH-2 exhibited some difference with *Eco*RI fragments of both DNA. It is supposed that the abnormal expression of genes can play an important role in cancer development, but it is still uncertain whether the alteration of DNA was induced during DENA carcinogenesis. Based on our own published and other unpublished studies, we are of the opinion that some change in DNA – for instance DNA translocation or DNA alkylation – might have occurred during rat hepatocarcinogenesis, which finally led to the abnormal control of gene expression.

References

Abelev GI (1971) Alpha-fetoprotein in ontogenesis and its association with malignant tumours. Adv Cancer Res 14: 295–358

Barbason H, Betz EH (1981) Liver cell control after discontinuation of DENA feeding in hepatocarcinogenesis. Eur J Cancer 17: 149–154

Bauer KH (1928) Mutationstheorie der Geschwulstentstehung. Springer, Berlin

Boss JH, Zajicek G, Okon E, et al. (1977) Excretion of alpha-foetoprotein in the urine of rats during exposure to 3′-methyl-4-dimethylaminoazobenzene. Br J Cancer 35: 100–109

Brambilla G, Carlo P, Finollo R, et al. (1983) Viscometric detection of liver DNA fragmentation in rats treated with minimal doses of chemical carcinogenesis. Cancer Res 43: 202–209

Busch H (1976) A general concept for molecular biology of cancer. Cancer Res 36: 4291–4294

Cancer Research Group. Shanghai Institute of Biochemistry, Academia Sinica (1976) Localization of AFP in rat liver tissue in correlation to the dynamics of serum AFP during 3′-Me-DAB carcinogenesis. Acta Biochim Biophys Sinica 8: 49–59[1]

Capetanaki YG, Flytzanis CN, Alonso A (1982) Repression of the albumin gene in Novikoff hepatoma cells. Mol Cell Biol 2: 258–266

Cayama E, Tsuda T, Sarma DSR, Farber E (1978) Initiation of chemical carcinogenesis requires cell proliferation. Nature 275: 60–62

Chiang CM (1981) Studies on a transplantable rat hepatoma BERH-2 II. Karyotype analysis and G-banding of marker chromosomes. Acta Biol Exp Sinica 14: 65–70[1]

Chiang CM, Ji WX, Sun LY et al. (1978) Studies on transplantable rat hepatoma BERH-2. I. The establishment of the tumor line and its morphology, ultrastructure, and α-fetoprotein production. Acta Biol Exp Sinica 11: 87–96[1]

Comings DE (1973) A general theory of carcinogenesis. Proc Natl Acad Sci USA 70 (part 1): 3324–3328

Craddock VM (1976) Cell proliferation and experimental liver cancer. In: Cameron HM, et al. (eds) Liver cell cancer. Elsevier, Amsterdam, pp 153–201

Drews J, Brawerman G, Morris HP (1968) Nucleotide sequence homologies in nuclear and cytoplasmic ribonucleic acid from rat liver and hepatomas. Eur J Biochem 3: 284–292

Emmelot P, Scherer E (1980) The first relevant cell stage in rat liver carcinogeneses: A quantitative approach. Biochim Biophys Acta 605: 247–304

Endo H, Eguchi M, Yanagi S (1970) Irreversible fixation of increased level of muscle-type aldolase activity appearing in rat liver in the early stage of hepatocarcinogenesis. Cancer Res 30: 743–752

Farber E (1973) Hyperplastic liver nodules. In: Busch H (ed) Methods in cancer research, vol 7. Academic, New York, pp 345–375

Farber E (1980) The sequential analysis of liver cancer induction. Biochem Biophys Acta 605: 149–166

Fiala S, Fiala ES (1973) Activition by chemical carcinogen of γ-Glutamyl transpeptidase in rat and mouse liver. J Natl Cancer Inst 51: 151–158

Frenster JH, Landrum SR, Masek MA et al. (1976) Control of DNA helix opening during in vivo normal and neoplastic cell maturation. In: Fishman WH et al. (eds) Onco-developmental gene expression. Academic, New York, pp 107–114

Friedrich-Freksa H, Gössner W, Börner P (1969) Histochemische Untersuchungen der Cancerogenese in der Rattenleber nach Dauergaben von Diäthynitrosamin. Z Krebsforsch 72: 226–239

Ga'l A, Lucotte G, Nahon JL et al. (1982) Polymorphism of the restriction fragments of the albumin and α-fetoprotein genes in different inbred strains of rats. Acta Biochim Biophys Acad Sci Hungaricae 17: 24

Galbraith AI, Chapleo MR, Itzhaki RF (1978) Distribution of 7′-methylguanine and of replication sites in the different kinetics classes of DNA from rats treated with dimethylnitrosamine. Nucleic Acids Res 5: 3357–3364

Galbraith AI, Itzhaki RF, Craig AW et al. (1980) Removal of O^6-methylguanine from different kinetic classes of rat liver DNA after administration of dimethylnitrosamine. In: Letnansky K (ed) Biology of the cancer cell. Kugler, Amsterdam, pp 17–20

Garrett CT, Gonzalez F, Caine M et al. (1977) Transport of a greater variety of non-reiterated RNA sequences from nucleus to cytoplasm in hepatoma. Proc Am Association Cancer Res (abstracts) 18: 61

Garrett CT, Katz C, Moore RE et al (1973) Competitive RNA-DNA hybridization of nuclear and microsomal RNA during diethylnitrosamine hepatocarcinogenesis. Cancer Res 33: 1662–1669

Hancock RL, Forrester PI, Lorscheider FL et al (1976) Ethionine-induced activation of embryonic genes. In: Fishman WH et al. (eds) Onco-developmental gene expression. Academic, New York, pp 247–251

Hanigan HM, Pitot HC (1982) Isolation of γ-glutamyl transpeptidase-positive hepatocytes during the early stages of hepatocarcinogenesis in the rat. Carcinogenesis 3: 1349–1354

Hao QL, Wang Z, Li SO (1983) Studies on the in vitro transcription of chromatin isolated from liver of rats fed with diethylnitrosamine. Acta Biol Exp Sinica 16: 71–79[1]

He KL, Li MS, Xu YD, et al. (1980) The quantitative changes of chromatin components in the experimental rat hepatoma. Acta Biol Exp Sinica 13: 79–85[1]

He QP, Lin SJ, Song QB, et al. (1982) Comparison of chromatin nonhistone proteins of rat hepatoma and normal liver by two-dimensional gel electrophoresis. Acta Biol Exp Sinica 15: 341–346[1]

Hsu YC, Liu HH, Hsu L, et al. (1980) Quantitation of mRNA levels of alpha-fetoprotein and albumin in transplantable rat hepatoma BERH-2. Acta Biol Exp Sinica 13: 353–360[1]

Huang SH, Li SE, Zan BF, et al. (1982) Studies on the mechanism of carcinogenesis. VI. The immunochemistry of carbamyl phosphate synthetase in rat liver and hepatoma induced by diethylnitrosamine. Acta Biochim Biophys Sinica 14: 407–415[1]

Huang SH, Li SE, Yu Y (1983) Studies on the mechanism of carcinogenesis. VII. Biosynthesis of carbamyl phosphate synthetase I in vivo and in vitro in hepatocellular carcinoma and liver of rats fed with diethylnitrosamine. Acta Acad Med Sinica 5: 21–24[1]

Ikehera H (1973) Changes of serum AFP levels in CCl_4-induced hepatitis. Tumor Res 8: 114

Innis MA, Miller DI (1977) Quantitation of rat α-fetoprotein messenger RNA with a complementary DNA probe. J Biol Chem 252: 8469–8475

Jalanko H, Virtanen I, Engvall E, et al. (1978) Early increase of serum alpha-fetoprotein in spontaneous hepatocarcinogenesis in mice. Int J Cancer 21: 453–459

Kalengayi MMR, Ronchi G, Desmet VJ (1975) Histochemistry of gamma glutamyl transpeptidase in rat liver during aflatoxin B-induced carcinogenesis. J Natl Cancer Inst 55: 579–588

Ke SJ, Hsu HS, Shi WK et al. (1978) α-Fetoprotein in the rat during diethylnitrosamine carcinogenesis. Acta Biol Exp Sinica 11: 105–108[1]

Kitagawa T, Pitot HC (1974) Immunohistochemical study of serine dehydratase (SDH) and its dietary induction in hyperplastic areas and nodules of rat liver during diethylnitrosamine carcinogenesis. In: Proc of XIth International Cancer Congress (abstract), no 3, p 350

Kroes RM, Sontag JM, Weisburger JH et al. (1972) α-Fetoprotein in rats with hepatoma induced by aflatoxin B1. Nature 240: 240–241

Laird AK, Barton AD (1961) Cell proliferation in precancerous liver: relation to presence and dose of carcinogen. J Natl Cancer Inst 27: 827–839

Lapeyre JN, Becker FF (1979) 5-Methylcytosine content of nuclear DNA during chemical hepatocarcinogenesis and in carcinomas which result. Biochem Biophys Res Commun 87: 698–705

Lapeyre JN, Walker MS, Becker FF (1981) DNA methylation and methylase levels in normal and malignant mouse hepatic tissues. Carcinogenesis 2: 873–878

Law SW, Dugaizyk A (1981) Homology between the primary structure of α-fetoprotein, deduced from a complete cDNA sequence, and serum albumin. Nature 291: 201–208

Leng M, Sage E, Fushs RPP et al. (1978) Antibodies to DNA modified by the carcinogen *N*-acetoxy-*N*-2-acetylaminofluorene. FEBS Lett 92: 207–210

Li SO, Fan MC, Ma HS et al. (1977) Studies on the mechanism of carcinogenesis. I. Interrelationship between the changes in proliferating and tissue-specific enzyme activities of rat liver during development and carcinogenesis by diethylnitrosamine. Acta Biochim Biophys Sinica 9: 113–130[1]

Li SO, Fan MC, Li SS et al. (1982) Studies on the mechanism of carcinogenesis. V. Differential changes in activities of enzymes involved in ornithine metabolism in early phase of hepatocarcinogenesis induced by diethylnitrosamine. Acta Acad Med Sinica 4: 141–145[1]

Loeb LA, Springgate CF, Battula N (1974) Errors in DNA replication as a basis of malignant changes. Cancer Res 34: 2311–2321

Margison GP (1980) Carcinogenicity of alkylating agents. In: Letnansky K (ed) Biology of the cancer cell. Kugler, Amsterdam, pp 3–9

Margison GP, Pegg AE (1981) Enzymatic release of 7-methylguanine from methylated DNA by rodent liver extracts. Proc Natl Acad Sci USA 78: 861–865

Mendecki J, Minc B, Choiazy M (1969) Differences in RNA from rat liver and hepatoma revealed by DNA·RNA hybridization. Biochem Biophys Res Commun 36: 494–501

Ono T, Wakabayashi K, Uenoyama K et al. (1972) Regulation of enzyme synthesis relating to differentiation of malignant cells. In: Weinhous S et al. (eds) Gann Monograph on Cancer Research 13, University of Tokyo Press, Tokyo, pp 19–29

Parker DL, Rothblum LI, Busch H (1979) A 3.6-megadalton, highly repetitive *Eco*RI fragment in the genome of Novikoff hepatoma. Cancer Res 39: 1287–1292

Parker DL, Busch H, Rothblum LI (1981) Cloning and characterization of a highly reiterated 5.8-kilobase pair nucleolar *Eco*RI DNA fragment found in Novikoff hepatoma ascites cells. Biochemistry 20: 762–765

Patel NT, Folse DS, Holoubek V (1979) Release of repetitive nuclear RNA into cytoplasm in liver of rats fed 3′-methyl-4-dimethylaminoazobenzene. Cancer Res 39: 4460–4465

Patel NT, Yoshida M, Holoubek V (1981) In vivo incorporation of 3′-methyl-4-dimethylaminoazobenzene into liver nuclei and release of RNA from the nuclei. Cancer Res 41: 743–751

Pegg AE (1978) Dimethylnitrosamine inhibits enzymatic removal of O^6-methylguanine from DNA. Nature 274: 182–184

Penhoet E, Rajkumor T, Rutter WJ (1966) Multiple forms of fructose diphosphate aldolase in mammalian tissues. Proc Nat Acad Sci USA 56: 1275–1282

Penhoet EE, Rutter WJ (1971) Catalytic and immunochemical properties of homomeric and heteromeric combination of aldolase subunits. J Biol Chem 246: 318–323

Pitot HC (1968) Template stability: Its mechanism in liver and its aberration in hepatomas. In: Yamamura Y et al. (eds) Japanese Cancer Association, Gann Monogr 4. Nucleic acids, proteins, and cancer. Maruzen Co., LTD, Tokyo, pp 175–181

Pitot HC, Sirica AE (1980) The stages of initiation and promotion in hepatocarcinogenesis. Biochim Biophys Acta 605: 191–215

Pitot HC, Shires TK, Moyer G et al. (1974) Phenotypic variability as a manifestation of translational control. In: Busch H (ed) The molecular biology of cancer. Academic, New York, pp 523–534

Pitot HC, Barsness L, Goldsworthy T, et al. (1978) Biochemical characterization of stages of hepatocarcinogenesis after a single dose of diethylnitrosamine. Nature 271: 456–458

Pitot HC, Cardelli J, Long B et al. (1976) Intracellular membranes and post-transcriptional regulation in liver and hepatoma. Criss WE et al. (eds) Control mechanisms in cancer. Raven, New York, pp 329–342

Pound AW, McGuire LJ (1978) Repeated partial hepatectomy as a promoting stimulus for carcinogenic response of liver to nitrosamines in rats. Br J Cancer 37: 585–594

Rabes HM, Szymkowiak R (1979) Cell kinetics of hepatocytes during the preneoplastic period of diethylnitrosamine-induced liver carcinogenesis. Cancer Res 39: 1298–1304

Rabes HM, Scholze P, Jantsch B (1972) Growth kinetics of diethylnitrosamine-induced enzyme deficient "preneoplastic" liver cell population in vivo and in vitro. Cancer Res 32: 2577–2586

Rajewsky MF (1967) Changes in DNA snythesis and cell proliferation during hepatocarcinogenesis by diethylnitrorsamine. Eur J Cancer 3: 335–342

Rajewsky MF (1968) Zur RNA-Synthese im Verlauf der Lebercarcinogenesis durch Diäthylnitrosamin. Z Krebsforsch 70: 314–319

Reddy EP, Reynolds RK, Santos E et al. (1982) A point mutation is responsible for the acquisition of transforming properties by the T24 human bladder carcinoma oncogene. Nature 300: 149–152

Rodriguez LV, Becker FF (1979) Alterations in chromosomal proteins in C_3H/HeN mice with spontaneous primary hepatocellular carcinomas. Int J Cancer 24: 806–812

Rodriguez LV, Klein KK, Amoruso M, et al. (1979) Analysis of chromosomal proteins of fractionated chromatin from rat liver and transplantable hepatocellular carcinomas. Int J Cancer 24: 490–497

Rothblum LI, Parker DL, Cassidy B, et al. (1981) Diversity in rat strains and tumor lines of DNA fragments homologous to an amplified 5.8-kilobase *Eco*RI fragment of Novikoff hepatoma cells. Biochem Biophys Res Commun 101: 639–644

Sala-Trepat JM, Sargent TD, Sell S, et al. (1979) α-Fetoprotein and albumin genes of rats: No evidence for amplification, deletion or rearrangement in rat liver carcinogenesis. Proc Natl Acad Sci USA 76: 695–699

Schauer A, Kunze E (1968) Enzymhistochemische und autoradiographische Untersuchungen während der Cancerisierung der Rattenleber mit Diäthylnitrosamin. Z Krebsforsch 70: 252–266

Schreiber G, Urban J, Edwards K, et al. (1976) Mechanism and regulation of albumin synthesis in liver and hepatomas. In: Weber G (ed) Advances in enzyme regulation, vol 14. Pergamon, Oxford, pp 163–184

Schumm DE, Morris HP, Webb TE (1973) Cytosol-modulated transport of messenger RNA from isolated nuclei. Cancer Res 33: 1821–1828

Sell S (1978) Distribution of α-fetoprotein- and albumin-containing cells in the liver of Fischer rats fed four cycles of *N*-2-fluorenylacetamide. Cancer Res 38: 3107–3113

Sell S, Morris HP (1974) Relationship of rat α-fetoprotein to growth rate and chromosome composition of Morris hepatomas. Cancer Res 34: 1413–1417

Sell S, Nichols M, Becker FF et al. (1974a) Hepatocyte proliferation and α-fetoprotein in pregnant, neonatal and partially hepatectomized rats. Cancer Res 34: 865–871

Sell S, Reynolds RD, Reutter W (1974b) Rat αFP: Appearance after galactosamine-induced liver injury. J Natl Cancer Inst 53: 289–291

Shi WK, Lu YL, Ye M, et al. (1977) Membrane-associated embryonic antigen in human hepatocellular carcinoma cells. Acta Zool Sinica 23: 337–344[1]

Silber D, Checisnka E, Rabczynski J et al. (1978) Isozyme pattern of pyruvate kinase during hepatocarcinogenesis induced by 2-acetylaminofluorene in rat liver. Eur J Cancer 14: 729–739

Simard A, Daoust R (1966) DNA synthesis and neoplastic transformation in rat liver parenchyma. Cancer Res 26: 1665–1672

Sirover MA, Loeb LA (1977) A molecular analysis of mutagenesis by oncogenic agents. In: Gallo RC (ed) Recent advances in cancer research: cell biology, molecular biology and tumor virology, vol 1. CRC, Cleveland, pp 49–65

Smuckler EA, Koplitz M, Sell S (1976) α_1-Fetoprotein in toxic liver injury. Cancer Res 36: 4558–4561

Solt DB, Cayama E, Tsuda H et al. (1983) Promotion of liver cancer development by brief exposure to dietary 2-acetylaminofluorene plus partial hepatectomy or carbon tetrachloride. Cancer Res 43: 188–191

Stout DL, Becker FF (1980) Progressive DNA damage in hepatic nodules during 2-acetylaminofluorene carcinogenesis. Cancer Res 40: 1269–1273

Stout DL, Becker FF (1982) Occurrence of progressive DNA damage coincident with the appearance of foci of altered hepatocytes. Carcinogenesis 3: 599–602

Stratil P, Dolezalova V, Nemecek R (1978) Localization of α-fetoprotein by immunofluorescent method during induction of rat liver tumors by 3′-methyl-4-dimethylaminoazobenzene. Neoplasma 25: 171–180

Stumpf R, Margison GP, Montesano R et al. (1979) Formation and loss of alkylated purines from DNA of hamster liver after administration of dimethylnitrosamine. Cancer Res 39: 50–54

Tabin CJ, Bradley SM, Bargmann CI et al. (1982) Mechanism of activation of a human oncogene. Nature 300: 143–149

Tantravahi U, Guntaka RV, Erlanger BF et al. (1981) Amplified ribosomal RNA genes in a rat hepatoma cell line are enriched in 5-methylcytosine. Proc Natl Acad Sci USA 78: 489–493

Tsanev R, Hadjiolov D (1978) Chromosomal proteins in hepatocarcinogenesis. Z Krebsforsch 91: 237–247

Tsung HC, Shi WK, Yao Z (1980) Observations on in situ localization of tumor-associated fetal antigen in human primary hepatoma cells. Acta Biol Exp Sinica 13: 317–324[1]

Wang HW, Wang D (1981) The synergistic action of antioxidant D and carbon tetrachloride on rat liver. Acta Biol Exp Sinica 14: 371–377[1]

Wang HW, Wang D, Tang PX et al. (1981) The carcinogenic activity of antioxidant D on albino rats. Acta Biol Exp Sinica 14: 77–81[1]

Weinhouse S (1973) Metabolism and isozyme alterations in experimental hepatomas. Fed Proc 32: 2162–2167

Weinhouse S, Shatton JB, Criss WE et al. (1972) Isozymes in relation to differentiation in transplantable rat hepatomas. In: Weinhouse S et al. (eds) Gann Mongr Cancer Research 13. Isozymes and enzyme regulation in cancer. University of Tokyo Press, Tokyo, pp 1–17

White RD, Sipes IG, Gandalfi AJ et al. (1981) Characterization of the hepatic DNA damage caused by 1,2-dibromoethane using the alkaline elution technique. Carcinogenesis 2: 839–844

Williams GM (1980) The pathogenesis of rat liver cancer caused by chemical carcinogens. Biochim Biophys Acta 605: 167–189

Xu YH, Peng SF, Xu YN et al. (1978) The changes of aldolase isozyme gene expression in rat liver during hepatocarcinogenesis induced by diethylnitrosamine. Acta Biol Exp Sinica 11: 239–246[1]

Xu YH, Peng SF, Zhang YY (1979) Changes in nuclear RNA and polysomal RNA complementary to the nonrepeated DNA sequence in rat hepatoma. Acta Biol Exp Sinica 12: 238–246[1]

Xu YH, Tsung HC, Peng SF et al. (1984) Membrane-associated fetal antigen in rat hepatoma. Acta Biol Exp Sinica 17: 55–65[1]

Xu YN, Zhang YY (1980) Comparison of nuclear RNAs from rat liver and hepatoma cells by presaturation hybridization experiments. Chin J Cell Biol 2: 12–15[1]

Xu YN, Zhang YS, Zhang YY (1980) Studies on the control mechanism of genetic transcription during rat liver carcinogenesis. II. Comparison of ribosomal RNA. Acta Biol Exp Sinica 13: 371–376[1]

Yeoman LC, Jordan JJ, Busch RK et al. (1976) A fetal protein in chromatin of Novikoff hepatoma and Walker 256 carcinosarcoma tumors that is absent from normal and regenerating rat liver. Proc Natl Acad Sci USA 73: 3258–3262

Yoo T-J, Kuo CY, Patil SR et al. (1979) Loss of alpha-fetoprotein in rat hepatoma culture cells. Int J Cancer 24: 184–192

Zhang YY, Shu XZ (1982) Comparison of nuclear DNAs from normal liver cells and transplantable hepatoma cells of rats by nucleic acid molecular hybridization technique. Acta Biol Exp Sinica 15: 7–13[1]

Zhang YY, Xu YH, Xu YN et al. (1978) Studies on the control mechanism of genetic transcription during rat liver carcinogenesis. I. Comparative study of RNA complementary to the repeated DNA sequence. Acta Biol Exp Sinica 11: 97–104[1]

Zhang YY, Xu YH, Xu YN et al. (1982) Increase of complexity of single-copy-sequence DNA and decrease of complexity of middle repeated-sequence DNA complementary to nuclear RNA during rat liver carcinogenesis. Acta Biol Exp Sinica 15: 137–143[1]

---

1 Chinese

27 Some Biochemical Changes in Experimental Hepatoma

Gu Tian-jue, Chen Hui-li, He Kai-ling, Li Mao-shen*

Many studies have demonstrated that a common feature of carcinogenesis may be abnormal gene expression (Stein et al. 1974; Bonner 1975). In general, a cancer cell has almost the same genes as a normal cell. The abnormalities seen in cancer are due to the malfunctioning of the very complex and undefined mechanisms that dictate the gene expression of a given cell at a particular time in its life cycle. The malfunctioning of these mechanisms would allow the expression or repression of a gene in a manner that is prohibited in the normal differentiated cell (Stein et al. 1978).

Considering the close relationship between carcinogenesis and gene expression, the mechanism of carcinogenesis may be explored by studying gene regulation in the eucaryotic cells.

In our laboratory, investigations have been aimed at elucidating abnormal gene expression and its regulation in hepatoma cells. We have observed and measured some biochemical changes displayed by experimental hepatoma. They are: (a) changes in gene regulation in the nuclei of hepatoma cells, (b) changes in the cell surface membrane of hepatoma, and (c) changes of some isozymes in hepatoma cells.

I. Gene Regulation in the Nucleus

Chromatin, the main material of the nucleus, contains a large number of chromosomal proteins in addition to DNA. Histone constitutes the major chromosomal protein, it is involved in the maintenance of normal chromatin structure and represses gene activity, but it has little action on the specific regulation of gene expression. Nonhistone chromosomal proteins (NHCP), though fewer in number, are made up of hundreds of kinds of individual proteins and possess species and tissue specificity. It seems that nonhistone proteins (NHP) can regulate abnormal gene expression in cancer cells.

---

* We are grateful to our colleagues Drs. Ding Ru-Chuan, Zhu Zheng-mei, and Shao Ming-Chuan for providing us with manuscript material and for their help in the preparation of this review

A. Nonhistone Chromosomal Proteins in Hepatoma and in Normal Liver Cells

In our laboratory, the chromatin components of rat hepatoma induced by *N, N'*-dimethyl-*p*-(*m*-tolylazo)-aniline (3'-MeDAB) were determined in parallel with morphological observation, and the chromosomal proteins of the mouse hepatoma ascites cells (Hep. A cells) were also analyzed.

It was observed in both 3'-MeDAB-induced hepatoma and Hep. A cells that the content of histone was quite constant at a histone-to-DNA ratio of about 1:1 (Table 1), while the ratio of NHP to DNA – not only in cancerous or paracancerous tissue but also at either the early stage (cancer induced for 6 weeks) or the late stage (cancer induced for 15 weeks) – increased markedly with the duration of cancer induction (He et al. 1980; Ding and He 1983a). It should be mentioned that in rat hepatoma induced by 3'-MeDAB for 6 weeks the amount of NHP was higher than that in normal liver, but at that time morphologically distinguishable carcinogenesis of hepatic cells could not be observed. It may be concluded that the increase in NHP content is related to abnormal gene expression and carcinogenesis.

B. Phosphorylation of Nonhistone Chromosomal Proteins

The relationship between chemical modification and the function of chromosomal proteins has been widely investigated recently. The phosphorylation of NHP in particular was thought to play a key role in the regulation of gene expression

Table 1. Changes of chromatin components in rat hepatoma (in mg/mg DNA)

Chromatin	DNA	RNA	Total protein	Histone	Nonhistone protein
Normal rat liver	1	0.03	1.19	1.07	0.79
Precancerous stage					
Early (6 weeks)	1	0.03	2.79	1.11	1.45 $P<0.05$
Late (15 weeks)	1	0.03	2.77	0.92	1.66 $P<0.01$
Cancerous stage (24 weeks)					
Tumor	1	0.04	4.12	1.23	2.75 $P<0.01$
Paracancerous region	1	0.04	2.46	1.33	1.27

Table 2. Chromatin components of normal mouse liver cells and Hep. A cells (in mg/mg DNA)

Chromatin	Total protein	Nonhistone protein	Histone	Phosphorylated nonhistone protein	Phosphorylated NHCP / Total NHCP
Normal mouse liver	1.85±0.10	0.70±0.02	1.15±0.10	0.31±0.01	0.44±0.04
Hep. A cells	2.61±0.06	1.52±0.05	1.08±0.04	1.30±0.03	0.88±0.03
P value	<0.01	<0.01	>0.05	<0.01	<0.01

NHCP, nonhistone chromosomal protein

(Kleinsmith 1978). We found that the content of phosphorylated protein and the ratio of phosphorylated NHP to total NHP in Hep. A cells were higher than those in normal cells by 4.4 and 2.0 times respectively (Table 2). This showed that the total phosphorylation of NHP in Hep. A cells was elevated, while the phosphate groups per weight unit of total nonhistone and phosphorylated nonhistone were decreased by 65% and 32% respectively (Ding and He 1983 b).

It is known that phosphorylation and dephosphorylation of NHP are catalyzed by nuclear protein kinase and phosphoprotein phosphatase. Their activities were assayed using the ^{32}P-labeling method. The specific activity of protein kinase in Hep. A cells was 2.11 times as high as that in normal cells, but that of phosphoprotein phosphatase was decreased, being about 58% of that in normal liver. The activity changes of these two enzymes might be responsible for the increase in phosphorylation of NHP in Hep. A cells. On the other hand, the increase of phosphorylation was lower than the increase in the number of NHP. This might be the main reason why phosphate groups per weight unit of nonhistone were lower than those of normal liver.

C. Electrophoretic Pattern of Nonhistone Proteins in Hepatoma

The NHP of hepatoma differ from those of normal liver cells, not only quantitatively but also qualitatively. The SDS-Page pattern of phosphorylated NHP of Hep. A cells showed an additional band of 47 000 daltons, which was invisible in the pattern of normal cells. Moreover, immunofluorescence and immunoperoxidase labeling of NHP in hepatoma cells induced by 3′-MeDAB demonstrated that antihepatoma chromatin immunoglobulin (Ig), when absorbed repeatedly by the nuclei of normal liver cells, reacted immunologically with chromatin of hepatoma other than with that of normal liver (Ding and He 1983 a; He et al. 1981). Similar reactions also took place during immunoelectrophoresis, double immunodiffusion, and immunorocket electrophoresis. Precipitate lines formed by the reaction of antihepatoma antibody with the chromatin of hepatoma were visible on the patterns of immunodiffusion, an indication that there were at least two kinds of immunologically specific protein in the chromatin of hepatoma. The immunological reaction of antihepatoma chromatin Ig to NHP which had been separated from the chromatin of hepatoma cells by ultracentrifugation also led to a positive result, and to a distinct precipitate line in immunoelectrophoresis, immunorocket electrophoresis, and double immunodiffusion.

All these facts proved that the specific immune material was present in the chromatin of hepatoma, and that the immunological characteristic of chromatin was due to the NHCP.

It can now be concluded that quantitative and qualitative changes of chromosomal protein are due mainly to NHP, and that its chemical modification is closely related to the development of hepatoma cells.

D. Nuclear Transcription Process in Hepatoma and in Normal Liver Cells

In recent years it has come to be recognized that different cancer inducers may act on different initial points, and that carcinogenesis may be due to the comprehensive action produced by multiple factors. According to the model of gene expression and its regulatory process, cancer inducers may cause changes in RNA and protein as well as abnormal gene regulation, which in turn leads to the abnormal division and differentiation of cells and then to the appearance of serious biological characteristics of cancer cells. Therefore, the role of transcription and its regulation is of practical significance in elucidating the mechanism of carcinogenesis.

Owing to the structural integrity of extracted nuclei and the insignificant loss of components participating in the transcription process, the experimental result becomes reliable and truly reflects transcriptional features in vivo. We compared the transcription process in hepatoma with that in normal liver nuclei after establishing the transcription system of nuclei with high enzyme activity (Zhao and He 1981); we discovered that the transcriptional activities of both Hep. A nuclei and BERH-2 hepatoma were significantly higher than those of normal liver by 80% and 54% respectively (Zhao and He 1982; Sun and He 1983). Further investigation showed that the increase of transcriptional activity in Hep. A nuclei was due mainly to the high enzyme activity of RNA polymerase II, being 2.3 times as high as that of normal liver (Table 3). As RNA polymerase II catalyzes the biosynthesis of mRNA precursor, the change in the enzyme activity of Hep. A cells is of great importance during abnormal gene expression. In contrast, the enzyme activity of RNA polymerase II remained unchanged in BERH-2 rat hepatoma, while either the specific activity or the content of RNA polymerase I was markedly increased. The variations in polymerase activity shown in different hepatoma implied the complexity of carcinogenesis.

The transcriptional products were also analyzed, while Hep. A nuclei were used as cancer model. The number of biosynthesized RNA chains in Hep. A cells was found to be nearly 4 times larger than that in normal cells. Though nuclear nuclease was also increased, it was higher than that of normal liver by about 50% only. The increase in the number of biosynthesized RNA chains is caused mainly by transcription. In addition, the elongation rate of RNA in Hep. A nuclei was increased

Table 3. Comparison of nuclear transcription activity between normal mouse liver and Hep. A

Nuclear transcription	Relative activity	
	Normal mouse liver	Hep. A
Transcription activity	100	180
RNase activity	100	150
RNA polymerase I	100	140
RNA polymerase II	100	230
RNA elongation rate	100	158
No. of RNA chains synthesized	100	380
Size of RNA synthesized	100	41

by 50%, which was much lower than the increase in the number of biosynthesized RNA chains. Therefore, the major cause of the change of transcriptional activity in Hep. A cells is the increase in its initiation rate (Zhao and He 1982).

When the transfer rates of newly synthesized RNAs from nuclei to cytosol were assayed, those of Hep. A nuclei were transferred at an increased rate as compared with those of normal liver nuclei. However, the ratio of transferred RNA to total synthesized RNA in both Hep. A and normal cells was almost the same, and the increase in RNA transfer in Hep. A cells might therefore be caused by the increased amount of the synthesized RNA.

E. Nuclear Digestion by Deoxyribonuclease I

In order to understand the relationship among the abnormality of transcriptional activity in hepatoma tissue, chromatin structure and NHCP, (Yan and He 1984) investigated the kinetics of deoxyribonuclease I (DNase I) digestion in BERH-2 hepatoma nuclei and normal liver nuclei, and the released high-mobility group of NHP (HMG proteins) was assayed quantitatively and qualitatively after limited DNase I digestion. Hepatoma nuclei were found to be more sensitive to DNase I digestion. When nuclei were treated by DNase I at 37 °C for 5 min, 45% of the DNA in hepatoma nuclei was digested, while in normal cell nuclei only 27% was digested (Yan and He 1984).

It is known that the active gene is more susceptible to DNase I digestion than the inactive one (Weintraub and Groudine 1976). The enhancement of nuclear DNA hydrolysis percentage in hepatoma cells after limited DNase I digestion indicates a structural change in chromatin, and that hepatoma chromatin possesses more transcriptionally active genes, which are more sensitive to DNase I than those of normal cells. It was also observed during the limited DNase I digestion that the HMG NHP released from hepatoma chromatin were 1.3 times higher than normal, but a qualitative difference of HMG NHP in the two types of cells was not observed. Because chromatin with transcriptionally active genes is liable to be degraded by DNase I, the chromosomal proteins attached to it may be released first during enzymatic digestion of the active gene. The enhancement in hepatoma cells of HMG proteins released indicates that the released HMG proteins are bound to the active gene. Since HMG protein is associated with the formation of active nucleosome, the increase in HMG proteins is considered to be a possible reason for the structural change of chromatin in hepatoma cells and for abnormal gene transcription.

In summary, both quantitative and qualitative changes take place during carcinogenesis, as does to chemical modification of NHP. The changed chromosomal proteins probably affect the structure and function of chromatin, causing abnormal gene expression and a series of biological abnormalities.

II. Cell Surface Membrane of Hepatoma

Under abnormal gene expression, the behavior of tumor cells differs significantly from that of normal cells. It is thought that the disappearance of cell contact inhibition may result in uncontrollable growth of the tumor cells, and that the decrease in cell-cell adhesion may be the cause of metastasis and infiltration of tumor cells into the peripheral tissues. All these types of cell behavior are closely related to the components of cell surface membrane, especially the glycoproteins and glycolipids. It is also reported that in many instances specific tumor antigens and oncofetal antigens are found in tumors, often located on the plasma membrane, and some of them (e.g., CEA and AFP) have already been used in clinical diagnosis. Some authors have even tried immunotherapy in the treatment of cancer (Weinstein et al. 1982). Therefore, a study of the components, receptors, and specific or oncofetal antigens on plasma membrane of hepatoma cells is important to illustrate the mechanism of carcinogenesis and to clarify the diagnosis and treatment of hepatoma.

A. Oncofetal Antigen on the Plasma Membrane of Hepatoma Cells

Human hepatoma tissue obtained from partial hepatectomy of hepatocellular cancer was used in preparing plasma membrane by means of sucrose density gradient centrifugation. After absorption with normal human liver powder, the antiserum against plasma membrane gave a positive reaction with the soluble product of the hepatoma cell plasma membrane in double immunodiffusion and CIEP, but a negative reaction with that of normal liver cell plasma membrane (Table 4; Department of Biochemistry, Shanghai First Medical College 1977). The immunofluorescent method demonstrated that this absorbed antiserum reacted specifically with the tissue slices from human hepatocellular hepatoma (six cases) and with a human hepatoma cell culture line (BEL 7402). It might be surmised that present on the plasma membrane of hepatoma cells is an antigen which is undetectable in normal liver cells. Further studies indicated that this antiserum could also react with the liver cell plasma membrane of 3- to 4-monthold fetuses. The antiserum against the plasma membrane of the fetus after absorption with the normal adult liver also reacted with the cancer cells; therefore, the antigen in hepatoma cells is an oncofetal antigen.

Table 4. Identification of oncofetal membrane antigen of hepatoma with double immunodiffusion and immunoelectrophoresis

Antigen	Antiserum[a] against membrane of fetal liver cells		Antiserum against membrane of hepatoma cells	
	DD[b]	CIEP[c]	DD	CIEP
Solution of membrane of hepatoma cells	+	+	+	+
Solution of membrane of fetal liver cells	+	+	+	+
Solution of membrane of adult human liver cells	−	−	−	−

[a] Antiserum absorbed with normal adult liver powder
[b] Double immunodiffusion
[c] Contercurrent immunoelectrophoresis

Membrane-associated embryonic antigen in hepatoma cells was also reported by Shi et al. (1977). Rabbit antiserum was prepared by injection of glutaraldehyde-treated fetal liver cells of 10- to 20-week-old human fetuses. After absorption by different kinds of normal human tissue it cross-reacted with three cell lines of hepatocellular carcinoma by the immunofluorescent method. This membrane-associated embryonic antigen has been extracted by 3M KCl (Shi and Cheng 1979).

B. Lectin Receptors on the Plasma Membrane of Hepatoma Cells

Lectins are carbohydrate-binging proteins which are ubiquitous in plants and animals. In the past 10 years or more many papers have reported that, in contrast to normal cells, tumor and embryonic cells can be agglutinated by lectins in very low concentration. In order to elucidate the biochemical basis of the difference in agglutinability between normal cells and cancer cells many factors have been investigated: the fluidity of plasma membrane, the function of microtubules and microfilaments in cell agglutination, and the number of lectin receptors. We used the radioreceptor method to examine the receptor number and the dissociation constant of lectin-receptor binding on hepatoma and normal liver cells. Lectin receptors (Con A and soy bean agglutining, SBA) were found to be almost equal in number on the two kinds of cells (Zhu and Gu 1982a; Ren et al. 1982), but the dissociation constant (or its reciprocal, association constant), as calculated from the Scatchard plot, revealed that there were two kinds of receptors on hepatoma cells. The scatchard plot of the hepatoma cell is an upward concave curve instead of the straight line of the normal adult liver cell (Zhu and Gu 1982b). There are two conditions in which the Scatchard plot presents as an upward concave curve: the presence of two different kinds of receptors or presence of negative cooperation among receptors. These can be identified by certain experiments, such as heat inactivation or dilution inhibitory dissociation tests. Our results revealed that there are two kinds (low- and high-affinity) of receptors on hepatoma cells but only one type (low-affinity) on normal liver cells (Table 5). It is possible that the high agglutinability of tumor cells by lectins is related to the presence of high-affinity receptors in these cells.

Table 5. Comparison between Con A receptors of normal liver cells and those of Hep. A cells

Cell membrane	Scatchard plot	Affinity constant (M^{-1})	No. of receptors	
			per cell	per μm²
Normal liver cell	Linear	$K = 7.89 \times 10^5$	4.10×10^5	2.45×10^5
Hep. A cell	Upward concave curve	$K_1 = 6.72 \times 10^6$ $K_2 = 5.00 \times 10^5$	$R_1 = 4.69 \times 10^6$ $R_2 = 2.13 \times 10^7$ $R_1 + R_2 = 2.60 \times 10^7$	5.68×10^4

C. Ganglioside Composition

Gangliosides are usually located at the plasma membrane of the cells. Recently, Magnani et al. (1981) reported that a unique ganglioside was present on the cells of colonic carcinoma. Here we report the discovery of a specific ganglioside component in human embryonic liver and hepatoma cells; the ganglioside was isolated and characterized according to the method of Ledeen and Yu (1982). The tissue was first extracted with 1:1 chloroform-methanol; the acidic and neutral lipids were then separated with DEAE-Sephadex A-25, and phospholipids were destroyed in mild alkaline solution. Finally, the gangliosides were further purified using Iatrobeads. The gangliosides obtained were identified on high-performance thin-layer chromatography (HPTLC), with brain white-matter gangliosides as the standard. The ganglioside component of the fetal liver was similar to that of the normal adult liver; the former, however, possessed an extra band (GM_4). The pattern of gangliosides from hepatoma was markedly different from those of normal and fetal liver (Table 6), more polar gangliosides being seen in hepatoma (Zhu et al. 1983).

The above-mentioned results clearly showed that there was considerable discrepancy between hepatoma cells and normal liver cells. Further studies of the properties of cancer cell membrane are important to the understanding of the behavior and abnormal gene expression of tumor cells, and will be helpful in developing new methods for cancer diagnosis and treatment.

III. Some Isozymes in Hepatoma

Isozyme is also a good index of cancer gene expression, and abnormal metabolism in cancer is closely correlated with the changes in some isozyme patterns. Therefore, studying isozymes in hepatoma can help us to understand the mechanism of carcinogenesis. We have studied pyruvate kinase (PK), arylamidase, and aldolase and their significance in Hep. A ascites hepatoma, laying emphasis on PK.

A. The Crabtree Effect of Hepatoma

The Crabtree effect is a well-known characteristic of abnormal metabolism in malignant tumor cells which show high glycolytic activities and whose respiration is inhibited by glycolysis under aerobic conditions; the mechanism, however, is not quite clear. There are several different theories at present (Warburg 1956; Koobs 1972; Sussman et al. 1980). It has been found that ADP, the substrate of PK and 3-phosphoglycerate kinase (3PGAK) in cytosol, can stimulate cell respiration in mitochondria, and that in malignant tumors the activity of PK is greatly increased (Ibsen 1977). In order to elucidate the mechanism of the Crabtree effect, our laboratory has further proved that there is a competition between PK and mitochondria for ADP (Shao and Chen 1982a).

Addition of fructose-1,6-diphosphate (FDP) to the homogenate of normal mouse liver did not cause the Crabtree effect, but a marked Crabtree effect resulted when it was added to the homogenate of Hep. A, probably owing to the increase in the gly-

Table 6. Comparison between ganglioside components of normal liver and those of hepatoma (in % of sialic acid)

Gangliosides	Normal mouse liver	Hep. A	Normal human liver	Human hepatoma
GM_4			1.42	0.12
GM_3	57.97	19.01	96.06	47.26
GM_2	42.03	50.44	0.62	17.87
GM_1				
GD_3		19.37	0.73	29.61
GD_{1a}		11.16	0.51	
GD_2+GT_{1a}				1.56
GD_{1b}				0.84
GT_{1b}				
GQ_{1b}			0.66	2.74
Total	100.0	99.98	100.0	100.0

Table 7. Crabtree effects with FDP or PEP as substrate, and activity of PK in normal liver and Hep. A of fasted mice

Tissue origin	No. of Exp.	O_2 uptake (µl/h/mg protein)			Crabtree effect (a) − (b) / (a) %
		− FDP (a)	+ FDP (b)	(a) − (b)	
Normal	14	20.6 ± 7.2[a]	28.7 ± 7.8	− 8.2 ± 5.1	− 46.4 ± 38.2
Hep. A	9	13.5 ± 2.4	10.7 ± 2.0	2.8 ± 1.3	+ 20.0 ± 9.3
		− PEP (c)	+ PEP (d)	(c) − (d)	(c) − (d) / (c) 5%
Normal	5	24.4 ± 3.7	23.1 ± 3.0	1.4 ± 0.8	+ 5.3 ± 2.1[b]
Hep. A	5	11.6 ± 1.2	9.2 ± 6.8	2.6 ± 0.6	+ 20.6 ± 3.8[b]
		Activity of PK (units/mg protein)			*P* value
Normal	5	0.177 ± 0.048			< 0.01
Hep. A	5	1.360 ± 0.210			

[a] Mean ± SD
[b] $P < 0.01$ FDP 10 m*M*, PEP 10 m*M*

colysis of FDP resulting in an inhibition of endogenous respiration (Table 7). Addition of phosphoenolpyruvate (PEP) to normal mouse liver homogenate, however, did cause the Crabtree effect. This suggests that PK – which takes PEP as its substrate – plays an important role in the production of the Crabtree effect, the possible mechanism of which is the afore-mentioned competition for ADP. The Crabtree effects induced by addition of FDP and PEP to Hep. A homogenate were similar, indicating that the emzymes which catalyzed the conversion of FDP to PEP were not important to causing the effect. The value of the effect caused by PEP in normal

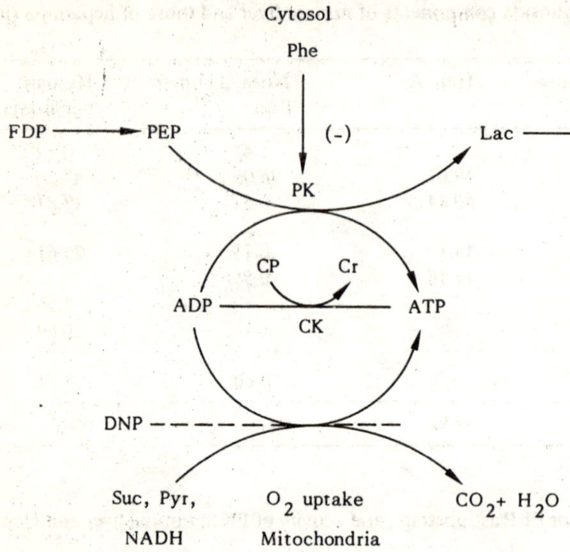

Fig. 1. Competition between PK and mitochondria for ADP. *Suc,* succinate; *Lac,* lactate; *Pyr,* pyruvate; *CP,* creatine phosphate; *Cr,* creatine; *CK,* creatine kinase

mouse liver was much lower than that in Hep. A ($P<0.01$), this diversity paralleling the difference of their PK actvities. Therefore, PK activity may be a major factor in causing the Crabtree effect.

It was found that addition of type-K PK, its substrate PEP, or decoupler 2,4-dinitrophenol (DNP) stimulated glycolysis but inhibited respiration in normal mouse liver, resulting in the Crabtree effect. The similar effect was seen when PEP was added to Hep. A homogenate. In contrast, addition of oxidative substrates (such as succinate, pyruvate and NADH), mitochondria, and the inhibitor of the type-K PK, L-phenylalanine (Phe), stimulated respiration but inhibited glycolysis. Exogenous ADP stimulated both respiration and glycolysis, and an ADP consumption system – creatine phosphate and creatine kinase – inhibited both processes. The above-mentioned results (see Fig. 1) have proved that the marked increase in type-K PK in Hep. A enhances the ability of cytosol to compete with mitochondria for ADP, and this might be an important mechanism of the Crabtree effect (Shao and Chen 1982b).

B. Pyruvate Kinase Isozyme Patterns

There are four types of PK isozymes. In normal mouse liver type-L PK is predominant, type-K PK being much less abundant. In Morris hepatoma the PK isozyme pattern is changed, with type L decreased and type K greatly increased (Ibsen 1977). Accordingly, we studied the relationship between the change of the PK isozyme pattern in Hep. A and the Crabtree effect.

Using the immunological method to determine the activity ratio of type-L and type-K PK, we found that the activity of type L in normal mouse liver was de-

Table 8. PK isozyme activity in supernatants of normal liver and Hep. A of fasted and unfasted mice

Tissue origin	No. of exp.	Type L (units/mg protein)	Type K (units/mg protein)	Type K (%)
Fasted				
Normal	5	0.122 ± 0.032[a]	0.056 ± 0.017	31.1 ± 1.8
Hep. A	5	0.082 ± 0.067	1.280 ± 0.210	93.7 ± 6.0
P value		< 0.01	< 0.01	< 0.01
Unfasted				
Normal	5	0.168 ± 0.029	0.045 ± 0.010	20.9 ± 3.2
Hep. A	4	0.097 ± 0.032	1.220 ± 0.030	92.5 ± 2.7
P value		< 0.05	< 0.01	< 0.01

[a] Mean ± SD

creased after fasting for 24 h; thus, the relative activity of type K was elevated, from 20% in unfasted mice to 31% in fasted ones. In Hep. A cells, regardless of whether the mice were fasted or not, the activity of type-L PK was only about 60% as high as that in normal mouse liver, but type-K PK was increased more than 20 times that of normal mouse liver, accounting for more than 90% of the total activity (Table 8). The change in the PK isozyme pattern in Hep. A is similar to that in fetal liver, indicating that there is a dedifferentiation of gene expression in Hep. A, as there is in Morris hepatoma of rats.

C. Kinetics of Type-L and Type-K Pyruvate Kinases

Some kinetic data of type-L PK in normal mouse liver and type-K PK in Hep. A were quite different. It has been found that type L showed Michaelis-Menten kinetics with respect to ADP – $K_m = 3.02$ m*M*, whereas type K showed positive cooperative allosteric kinetics – Hill's coefficient (η_H) = 1.40, and $K_{0.5s} = 0.658$ m*M*. Both enzymes showed positive cooperative allosteric kinetics with respect to PEP – $\eta_H = 1.30$ for type L and $\eta_H = 1.35$ for type K; $K_{0.5s}$ was 0.525 m*M* and 0.190 m*M* respectively. These results indicate that the affinity of type-K PK for both ADP and PEP was greater than that of type-L PK. Type L was also more sensitive than type K to the inhibition of ATP, the product of PK reaction (Table 9). Besides, as mentioned previously, the activity of type-K PK in Hep. A was more than 20 times that of type-K PK in normal mouse liver. In Hep. A, therefore, the competition of cytosol type-K PK with mitochondria for ADP was increased to a greater extent than it was in normal mouse liver. The changes in the PK isozyme pattern and the differences in kinetics between type-K and type-L PK may be another important mechanism of the Crabtree effect.

Table 9. Kinetic differences between type-L and type-K PK purified from normal mouse liver and Hep. A respectively

Substrate	Kinetic parameter	Type L	Type K
		Michaelis kinetics	Positive cooperative allosteric kinetics
ADP	η_H	1.05	1.40
	$K_{0.5s}$ (m*M*)	3.020	0.658
	$S_{0.5}$ (m*M*)	2.865	0.741
		Positive cooperative allosteric kinetics	Positive cooperative allosteric kinetics
PEP	η_H	1.30	1.35
	$K_{0.5s}$ (m*M*)	0.525	0.190
	$S_{0.5}$ (m*M*)	0.603	0.282
ATP	Concentration of 50% inhibition	3.4 m*M*	4.5 m*M*

D. Comparison of the properties of Type-K Pyruvate Kinase in Hepatoma and Normal Mouse Liver

Further studies of the differences in properties of the type-K PK in Hep. A and normal mouse liver make it possible to deduce whether there is a difference between the products of their gene expression (Chen et al. 1982). More than ten parameters of the properties of type-K PK from different origins were compared, including data from electrophoresis and chromatography, and on sensitivity to heat, pH activity curve, kinetics, molecular weight, and immunological specifity. As shown in Table 10, these parameters of the two type-K PKs were very similar or exactly the same, suggesting that the structures of both enzymes were probably identical, that the basic sequence in DNA coding for type-K PK in Hep. A was not different from that in normal mouse liver, and that the change in the PK isozyme pattern in Hep. A may be due to the disorder of gene expression regulation, which was responsible for the change in the synthesis of the proteins concerned. Of course, the final solution to the problem will depend on an analysis of the primary structures of both enzymes.

As the dedifferentiation of gene expression was responsible for the increase of type-K PK in hepatoma, (Weinhouse et al. 1972), the amount of type-K PK would be the same as that in fetal liver. In fact, much less information has been reported about the comparison of PKs in hepatoma and fetal liver. Balinsky et al. (1973) discovered that the kinetics of type-M_2 (K) PK from human hepatoma with respect to ADP was similar to that in fetal liver, showing the Michaelis kinetics; with respect to PEP it was different, the hepatoma enzyme showing an allosteric effect, but the fetal one the Michaelis kinetics. Further study is called for, on whether there are differences among the products of gene expression in normal adult tissue, cancerous tissue, and fetal tissue. This would be of significance to the understanding of the mechanism of carcinogenesis.

Table 10. Comparison of properties of type-K PK from normal mouse liver and those from Hep. A

Parameter		Normal	Hep. A
Elution peak on p-cellulose chromatography (KCl M)		0.30	0.29
Relative mobility on polyacrylamide gel electrophoresis		0.077	0.077
Half inactivation time at 50 °C (min)		11.5	11.5
Optimum pH		7.4	7.4
Inhibition by amino acids: Ala, Cys, Tyr (activities reserved after inhibition), %		49.1–54.6	48.9–57.3
Activation by Mg^{++}		+++	+++
by L-serine		+	+
by FDP		−	−
PEP	η_H	1.45	1.35
	$K_{0.5s}$ (m*M*)	0.196	0.191
	$S_{0.5}$ (m*M*)	0.325	0.292
ADP	η_H	1.45	1.45
	$K_{0.5s}$ (m*M*)	0.741	0.777
	$S_{0.5}$ (m*M*)	0.813	0.850
Phe	η_H	1.30	1.30
	$K_{0.5i}$ (m*M*)	1.97	2.00
ATP	η_H	Increase with ATP concentration	
	50% inhibition concentration (m*M*)	4.4	4.5
Molecular weight		224×10^3	210×10^3
Cross-reaction with anti-M serum		+	+

E. Other Isozymes

The arylamidases purified from normal mouse liver and Hep. A were also compared (Zha and Chen 1984). Their kinetic properties were similar, but some physicochemical characteristics, such as their behavior in polyacrylamide gel electrophoresis and DEAE-cellulose chromatography, were different. Since arylamidase is an enzyme of glycoprotein in nature, we found that the protein moieties of these isozymes are similar, whereas the sialic acid content of carbohydrate moieties are different. It was concluded that the arylamidase type difference between normal mouse liver and Hep. A cells belonged to post-translational isozyme.

In addition, there are two types of aldolase in normal mouse liver; type A (fetal) and type B (adult). It was found that type B was predominant in normal mouse liver, but type A was greatly increased and type B almost disappeared in Hep. A (Sheng and Chen 1983), indicating that there is a dedifferentiation of gene expression in Hep. A of mice as there is in in Morris hepatoma of rats (Ibsen 1977).

References

Balinsky D, Cayanis E, Bershon I (1975) Isozyme studies of human liver and hepatoma with particular reference to kinetic properties of hexokinase ans pyruvate kinase. In: Markert CL (ed) Isozyme III developmental biology. Academic, New York, pp 919–933

Bonner J (1975) Regulation of gene expression in high organisms: How it all works. In: The structure and function of chromatin. Ciba Found Symp 28: 315–335

Chen HL, Xu SZ, Zhou HR, et al. (1982) Studies on pyruvate kinase isoenzymes in hepatoma. III. Comparative studies on type-K pyruvate kinases purified from normal mouse liver and Hep. A ascites hepatoma. Acta Biochim Biophys Sinica 14: 189–198[1]

Department of Biochemistry, Shanghai First Medical College (1977) Studies on the fetal antigen of cell plasma membrane of human hepatoma cell. Acta Biochim Biophys Sinica 9: 339–346[1]

Ding RC, He KL (1983a) The study on phosphorylated chromosomal nonhistone protein of Hep. A hepatoma cells. I. Comparative study on phosphorylated chromosomal nonhistone protein of Hep. A cell and normal mouse liver cells. Acta Biochim Biophys Sinica 15 (4): 321–328[1]

Ding RC, He KL (1983b) The study on phosphorylated chromosomal nonhistone protein of Hep. A hepatoma cells. II. Study on chromatin-associated protein kinase and nuclear phosphoprotein phosphatase. Acte Biochim Biophys Sinica 15 (4): 339–347[1]

He KL, Li MS, Xu YD (1980) The quantitative changes of chromatin components in the experimental rat hepatoma. Acta Biol Exp Sinica 13: 79–85[1]

He KL, Shen HF, Chen KL (1981) Immunoidentification methods of chromosomal proteins. Acta Acad Med Primae Shanghai 8: 208–213[1]

Ibsen KH (1977) Interrelationships and functions of the pyruvate kinase isoenzymes and their variant forms – a review. Cancer Res 37: 341–353

Kleinsmith LJ (1978): Phosphorylation of nonhistone proteins. In: "Busch H (ed) The cell nucleus VI" Academic, New York, pp 221–261

Koobs DH (1972) Phosphate mediation of the Crabtree and Pasteur effects. Science 178: 127–133

Ledeen RW, Yu RK (1982) Ganglioside structure, isolation and analysis. Methods Enzymol 83: 139–199

Magnani JL, Brockhaus M, Smith DF, Ginsburg V, Blaszczyk M, Mitchell KF, Steplewski Z, Koprowaki H (1981) A monosialoganglioside is a monoclonal antibody-defined antigen of colon carcinoma. Science 212: 55–56

Ren SL, Lin JC, Gu TJ (1982) Comparison of soy bean agglutinin receptors on hepatoma and normal mouse liver cells. Tumor 2 (5): 4–8[1]

Shao MC, Chen HL (1982a) Studies on pyruvate kinase isoenzymes in hepatoma. I. Competition for ADP between pyruvate kinase and mitochondria. Acta Biochim Biophys Sinica 14: 171–180[1]

Shao MC, Chen HL (1982b) Studies on pyruvate kinase isoenzymes in hepatoma. II. Relationship between pyruvate kinase isoenzymes and the Crabtree effect. Acta Biochim Biophys Sinica 14: 181–188[1]

Sheng ZM, Chen HL (1983) Comparative study on the change of enzymes in H615 hepatoma and Hep. A ascites hepatoma. Acta Acad Med Primae Shanghai 10: 125–132[1]

Shi WK, Cheng CR (1979) Extraction of surface antigens from human fetal liver cells with hypertonic potassium chloride. Acta Biol Exp Sinica 12: 169–172[1]

Shi WK, Lu YL, Ye M, et al. (1977) Membrane-associated embryonic antigen in human hepatocellular carcinoma cells. Acta Zool Sinica 23: 337–343[1]

Stein GS, Spelsberg TC, Kleinsmith LJ (1974) Nonhistone chromosomal proteins and gene regulation. Science 183: 817–824

Stein GS, Stein JL, Thomson JA (1978) Chromosomal proteins in transformed and neoplastic cells – a review. Cancer Res 38: 1181–1201

Sun XJ, He KL (1983) A comparative study of the transcription in regenerating rat liver and BERH-2 hepatoma. Acta Acad Med Primae Shanghai 10 (3): 218–223[1]

Sussman I, Erecinska M, Wilson DF (1980) Regulation of cellular energy metabolism. The Crabtree effect. Biochim Biophys Acta 591: 209–223

Warburg O (1956) On the origin of cancer cells. Science 123: 309

Weinhouse S, Shatton JB, Criss WE, et al. (1972) Isozyme in regulation to differentiation in transplantable rat hepatoma. Gann Monograph 13: 1

Weinstein JN, Parker RJ, Keenan AM, et al. (1982) Monoclonal antibodies in the lymphatics toward the diagnosis and therapy of tumor metastasis. Science 218: 1334–1337

Weintraub H, Groudine M (1976) Chromosomal subunits in active gene have an altered comformation. Science 193: 848–856

Yan ZF, He KL (1984) Study on the role of HMG nonhistone chromosomal proteins in regulation of gene expression. I. The effect of HMG nonhistone on the transcription activity and DNase digestion of the mouse liver nuclei. Acta Biochim Biophys Sinica 16: 239–255[1]

Zha XL, Chen HL Purification and characteristics of normal mouse liver and Hep. A ascites hepatoma arylamidase. Acta Biochim Biophys Sinica (to be published)[1]

Zhao Q, Li MS, He KL (1981) Studies on the transcription system of isolated rat liver nuclei. Acta Biochem Biophys Sinica 13: 523–534[1]

Zhao Q, Li MS, He KL (1982) Effects of some anticancer drugs on transcription activity in nuclei. Acta Acad Med Primae Shanghai 9: 171–177[1]

Zhu ZM, Gu TJ (1982a) Concanavalin A receptor on normal liver and liver cancer cells determined with radioreceptor assay. Chin J Cell Biol 4: 21–24[1]

Zhu ZM, Gu TJ (1982b) Characterization of Con A receptors on hepatoma cells. Acta Biochem Biophys Sinica 14: 295–301[1]

Zhu ZM, Zheng DS, Yuan JD, Gu TJ (1983) The distribution pattern of gangliosides in normal embryonic and cancerous human liver. Acta Acad Med Primae Shanghai 10: 81–83[1]

[1] Chinese

28 Human Hepatocellular Carcinoma Cells Cultivated in Vitro

Shen Ding-wu, Chen Rui-ming

The tissue culture technique has been successfully employed in the establishment of a number of human cell lines derived from both normal and malignant tissues. A line of human uterine cervical carcinoma cells designated as HeLa, which was first established by Gey et al. early in 1952, is now being widely used in various laboratories all over the world. Since then, several other human cell lines have become available, such as those culitvated from mammary carcinoma by Lasfargues and Ozzello (1958). To our knowledge, however, lines from human liver carcinoma had not been established before 1960. Most of the work on liver carcinoma had been done with animal materials, in either ascitic or solid form, induced by carcinogens in vivo and/or cultivated in vitro. However, such material could hardly be expected to be exactly the same as human primary liver carcinomas. The establishment of a line of human liver carcinoma cells thus seemed highly desirable.

In 1960 we obtained 22 specimens of liver carcinomas from patients who had been operated on (Chen 1963). Part of one of the specimens had been successfully maintained in continuous proliferation in vitro for over 19 years, and another part preserved in a deep-frozen state for more than 15 years. This line of human hepatocellular carcinoma was designated as L-16 (It has now been renamed "BEL-16"). Since then, 12 such cell lines (shown in Table 1), have been established by various research groups. Among them were Chen et al. (1978) and Doi et al. (1975) who had independently cloned the lines of BEL-16 and HLE cells, and found that the bi-

Table 1. Twelve established cell lines of human hepatocellular carcinomas

Cell line	Year established	Investigator and reference	
BEL-16	1960	Chen et al.	(1963)
BEL-7402	1974	Chen et al.	(1975)
BEL-7404	1974	Chen et al.	(1980)
BEL-7405	1974	Chen et al.	(1980)
QGY-7703	1977	Wang et al.	(1981)
SMMC-7721	1977	Dong et al.	(1980)
HLE	1970	Doi et al.	(1975)
HLF	1970	Doi et al.	(1975)
SK-HEP	1971	Fogh	(1975)
Prozesky-1[a]	1972	Prozesky et al.	(1973)
Prozesky-2[a]	1972	Prozesky	(1973)
PLC/PRF/5	1973	Alexander et al.	(1977)

[a] No names were given in the original papers; the author's name was adopted

ological characteristics of these cloned cell populations were similar to those of their parental lines. The establishment of these cell lines supplied ideal materials for wide use in various investigations, such as studies on biomedical features, the regulation and control of cell division in relation to cell differentiation, the mode of action of anticancer drugs, the isolation of viruses, and other related subjects concerning the prevention and treatment of hepatocellular carcinomas.

I. Cultivation of Surgical Specimens

A. Source of Material

Among the 11 pathologically diagnosed patients, two were women and the rest men, while the two cases reported by Prozesky (1973) were not specified. The PLC/PRF/5 line was derived from the youngest patient, aged 24 years, the BEL-7404 from the oldest patient, aged 69 years. Only the SK-HEP-1 line (Fogh 1975) was derived from hepatoadenocarcinomas of ascitic form, and the rest were from solid forms of hepatocellular carcinoma. The seven cases tested for AFP were found to be positive. Two of the six cases tested for HB_sAg were found to be positive, while the remaining four cases were negative. Generally, cultivation was carried out as soon as the specimen was obtained.

B. Methods of Cultivation and Establishment of Cell Line

There are two different methods, starting either with tissue fragments or with dispersed cells, for the establishment of cell line.

1. Tissue-Fragment Culture Method

The first six lines (shown in Table 1) of human hepatocellular carcinoma cells were successfully established in our country by starting with fragments cultivated using the roll tube method.

Soon after the specimen was obtained, the portions which appeared softer, less fibrous, and not obviously necrotic were selected for use. They were washed several times with Hanks' BSS, cut into small fragments (1–1.5 mm^3), and cultivated by the chicken plasma-coated roll tube method at 37 °C. Generally, 50–60 fragments kept 5–8 mm apart were explanted in each tube. The culture medium employed was Eagle's MEM (or RPMI-1640 medium) containing 20%–40% fetal calf serum, inactivated at 56 °C for 45 min, and 200 units or penicillin plus 200 μg streptomycin per ml, pH 7.2–7.4, in addition. The roll drum was revolved at 37 °C at a rate of 10 rph. These were the primary cultures.

It was necessary to examine the condition of growth and the metabolism of cells daily with the light microscope. The medium was changed at intervals of 2–3 days, or longer if the growth proceeded slowly. The first transfer was made when a halo of cell outgrowth was observed in at least 60% of the explanted tissue fragments in each tube. The transfer procedure was carried out as follows: the culture medium was withdrawn from the tubes, and a sufficient quantity of Hanks' BSS added to wash the debris from the tissue cells. The washing was repeated once more, and Hanks' BSS containing 0.15% trypsin was introduced and allowed to act for 3–5 min at room temperature. The loosened cells and fragments were then dispersed by repeated pipetting back and forth with fresh medium to form a cell suspension of high density, which was then distributed into several 3 × 5 cm bottles and grown as stationary monolayer cultures. This was the first transfer; the time required for the first two transfers usually varied from specimen to specimen, the shortest time required being 7 days for the cells of BEL-16 line and the longest 107 days for BEL-7402 line. After the third transfer, and henceforth, as the rate of cell proliferation increased considerably, subsequent transfers could be made every 6 or 7 days. After the cells had undergone several transfers, the rate of cell proliferation sometimes became slow. The transfer was then delayed until the original rate of cell proliferation had resumed; thereafter the rate of proliferation remained fairly constant, and transfer could again be carried out every 6–7 days.

2. Monolayer Cell Culture Method

Monolayer cell culture is the general method used in foreign laboratories at present. The procedure is simpler but the probability of success is lower. The SK-HEP-1 line of cells was established directly from the ascites of a hepatocellular carcinoma patient as soon as the cells in the ascites had been isolated and grown as monolayer cultures. Prozesky (1973), Doi et al. (1975), and Alexander et al. (1977) all adopted the use of enzyme-dispersed cells from tissue fragments. The procedure for preparing a cell suspension from the specimen is as follows: Selected portions of specimen, as described by Alexander et al. (1977), are cut or chopped extremely fine with scissors or knives; enough fluid should be added during the chopping to keep the fragments well moistened. It is necessary to wash the tissues only when it seems desirable to free them of excess blood. Under these conditions, the washing in buffered saline solution should be done while the majority of the fragments are still 3 or 4 mm in diameter. The chopping may then be continued until the suspension is fine enough for the preparation of the cultures.

The discrete fragments are transferred to a small flask or centrifuge bottle, and the D-Hanks' solution (Ca^{++}–Mg^{++} free) containing 0.25% trypsin is added to act for 20 min at 37 °C. Then the tissue fragments are pipetted back and forth so as to disperse them into a cell suspension. This procedure is repeated until the fragments become whitish masses of connective tissue, and a small amount of serum is finally added to stop the trypsin action. After the cell suspension has been passed through a stainless-steel or nylon-gauze strainer (to remove the connective tissue) into a flask, it is transferred to a centrifuge tube and sedimented at 1000 rpm for 5 min. The supernatant is discarded and a known volume of nutrient medium added, and cell clumps, if any, are broken up by vigorous pipetting. The resulting cell suspension is ready to be inoculated into flasks and grown as stationary monolayer cell cultures, called "primary cultures." Prozesky found that the CO_2 incubater used for primary cultures gave good results.

The time duration allowed for growth of the primany cultures varied with different cell lines, from only 7 days for the SK-HEP-1 line to 114 days for the HLE line.

For subcultivation, trypsinization was generally sufficient, but Prozesky (1973) and Alexander et al. (1977) suggested that the trypsin-EDTA mixture was much better. The subsequent procedure of establishing cell lines was similar to that described by Alexander et al. (1977).

II. Biological Characteristics of Human HCC Cell Lines

It is necessary, first of all, to ascertain to what extent the human HCC cell lines established in vitro resemble those of the clinical specimens, in order to decide whether they can be considered ideal models for studies of human hepatoma. Three aspects of their cell biology, i.e., the structure, the function, and the behavior of human HCC cell lines were accordingly investigated and described below.

A. General Morphology, Submicroscopic Structure, and Karyotype Analysis

1. General Morphology

The human HCC cells generally appear as large, flattened polygonal epithelioid cells, except for the HLF line, established and cloned by Doi et al., which had spindle-shaped fibroblastic cells (Table 2). They were adherent to the glass surface and often laterally coherent to other cells of their kind, forming a sheet. Cells assumed a squamous arrangement and a piled-up growth pattern. Under the phase-contrast microscope, most of the mitochondria appeared spherical, but a few were filamentous. The majority of cells possessed one nucleus, very few of them were binuclear, and polynuclear giants were only occasionally observed. The number of nucleoli per cell varied from one to seven; more commonly there were three to four of irregular shape. Thus, even under the light microscope, they were observed to be malignant epithelioid cells (Fig. 1).

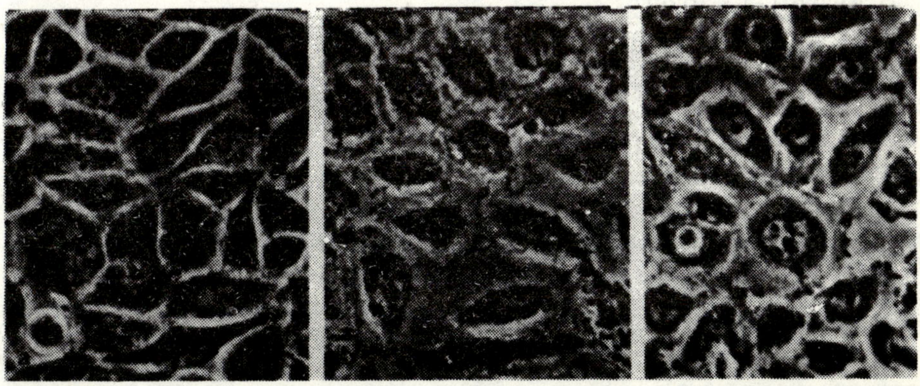

Fig. 1 a–c. Phase-contrast microscope photographs of living cultures, showing the morphology of three lines of cells. **a** BEL-7402 cells (× 560); **b** BEL-7404 cells (× 560); **c** BEL-7405 cells (× 560). (Reproduction by 20%)

2. Submicroscopic Structures

The submicroscopic structures of three lines of human HCC cells have been systematically examined by Chen et al. (1980) under the JEM-100B electron microscope. Numerous microvilli were seen on the surface of cells of these lines, and the desmosomes were present at certain areas on the plasma membranes of two adjoining cells. In the cytoplasm, tonofibrils and typical annulate lamellae, as well as scattered or aggregated glycogen granules were seen. These structures were typical of epithelial cells seen with electron microscopy. The nuclei were large and irregular in shape, so the N/C ratio was abnormally high. Nuclear indentations and invaginations were very pronounced and appeared as "pseudoinclusions" inside the nuclei as a result of sectioning. In fact, the pseudoinclusions consisted of a mass of cytoplasm enclosed by double-layered nuclear membrane. In addition, a great amount of coarse heterochromatin was found in the nucleus. The nucleoli, which vary in number and size, were compact and dense in appearance. Other organelles in the cytoplasm, such as the few mitochondria of different shapes and sizes were restricted to locations near the nucleus. Their internal structures were often altered, becoming swollen, with a matrix of lower electron density, or vacuolized, with or without short cristae. A small amount of rough endoplasmic reticulum was scattered throughout the cytoplasm in varying degrees of dilatation. Ribosomes were present in large numbers, and polysomes were more common in BEL-7404 and BEL-7405 cells, which also have better-developed Golgi complexes. Smooth endoplasmic reticulum was rarely seen. Lysosomes, normally concentrated near the Golgi complexes, were fairly abundant. Some had the simple structure of an electron-dense vesicle enclosed by a single layer of membrane, but more often they assumed the structure of secondary lysosomes in various stages, including myelinated bodies. In addition, small coated vesicles were often seen in the cytoplasmic region be neath the cell membrane. All these morphological and structural features of three lines of human HCC cells cultivated in vitro were very similar to those of the surgical specimens, and the results indicated that these cells were not very well differentiated malignant hepatoma cells.

3. Analysis of Karyotype

Aside from the structural abnormality, the extensive heteroploidy was another important feature of tumor cell populations. The analysis of the karyotype of 12 lines of human HCC cells showed that they were all heteroploid and that they generally exhibited a hypotriploid chromosomal mode (see Table 2). Interestingly, Chen et al. (1980) found that one abnormally large acrocentric chromosome (A_1) was present in 98% of BEL-7402 cells, 71% of BEL-7404 cells, and 26% of BEL-7405 cells. Morphologically, this marker chromosome is similar in length to the no. 1 chromosome of group A, and a faintly visible site of translocation can be detected on its long arm. In addition, BEL-7405 exhibited two other types of marker chromosomes: a minute acrocentric chromosome (A_2) and chromosome fragments (F_1), which appeared with a frequency of 62% and 78% respectively. The former was much smaller than the chromosome of group G, while there were usually two minute chromosome fragments. Karyotype analyses of the three lines of cells are shown in Fig. 2, and the features of other cell lines are listed in Table 2.

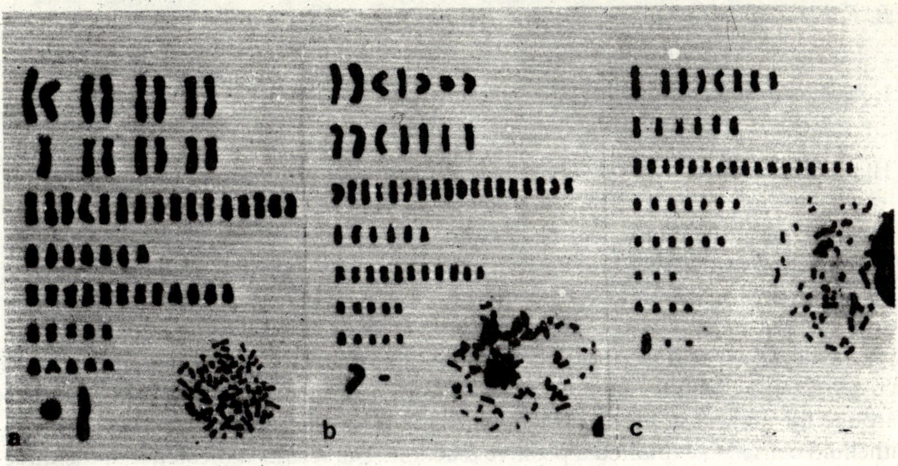

Fig. 2a–c. Karyotypes of three lines of human HCC cells. **a** BEL-7402 cell with 62 chromosomes; note the large acrocentric chromosome (last row, right). **b** BEL-7404 cell with 61 chromosomes. **c** BEL-7405 cell with 54 chromosomes (two minute)

Table 2. Morphology and karyotype of human hepatocellular carcinoma cell lines

Cell line	Morphology	Mode of chromosome number (%)	Abnormal chromosomes	
			Marker chromosome	Others
BEL-16	Epithelioid	56– 70 (62.72)	–	–
BEL-7402	Epithelioid	60– 63 (46.60)	A_1	–
BEL-7404	Epithelioid	58– 62 (88.00)	A_1	–
BEL-7405	Epithelioid	56– 60 (60.00)	A_2, F_1	A_1
QGY-7703	Epithelioid	111–117 (60.33)	–	D_1
SMMC-7721	Epithelioid	54– 58 (70.00)	M_3,	M_1, M_2, M_4
HLE	Epithelioid	3–4n	–	–
HLF	Fibroblastic	3–>4n	–	–
SK-HEP-1	Epithelioid	2n–>3n	S_1, A_4	–
Prozesky-1	Epithelioid	>2n	A_3	–
Prozesky-2	Epithelioid	>2n	–	–
PLC/PRF/5	Epithelioid	>2n	Lack D group of chromosomes Lack two, three, or four chromosomes of G group	–

Abbreviations: A_1 – large acrocentric chromosome, similar in length to that of no. 1 chromosome of A group; A_2 – minute acrocentric chromosome, smaller than that of G group; A_3 – extra-small acrocentric chromosome; A_4 – large acrocentric chromosome; D_1 – dicentric chromosome; F_1 – minute chromosome fragment; M_1 – large metacentric chromosome; M_2 – B subgroup, metacentric chromosome, long arm elongated; M_3 – C group, metacentric chromosome, median length; M_4 – D group, telocentric chromosome, long arm elongated; S_1 – large submetacentric chromosome

B. Functional Metabolism: Specific Protein Synthesis

1. Alpha-fetoprotein Detection

The presence of AFP in the serum is considered one of the significant phenotypic features of human HCC. The test of the serum AFP level can be applied not only to diagnose early hepatoma, but also to study the control of HCC gene expression. The question of whether human HCC cell lines cultivated and established in vitro would be able to continue AFP synthesis obviously required extensive investigation. In 1974, Chen et al. (1975) adopted the indirect immunofluorescence method for the detection of AFP in their three lines of human HCC cells. Fluorescence-microscopic examinations showed all three lines to be positive, with the cytoplasm around the nucleus appearing brightest (Fig. 3). Some cells other than polygonal epithelioid cells also exhibited a positive reaction. The results indicated that the three lines cultured in vitro for more than 2 years were still able to synthesize AFP intracellularly.

The detection of AFP in both the QGY-7703 and the SMMC-7721 lines showed similar results, while Doi et al. (1975), assaying the AFP content of the concentrated medium using the double agar-gel diffusion test, found that the HLE line was positive and the HLF negative, but that the HLE cells stopped secreting AFP on the 189th day of culture. As reasons for the stoppage of AFP secretion they postulated (a) long cultivation, leading to the predominance of the nonsecreting cells as a result of mutation or selection, or (b) inhibition by certain unknown factors. The results with short-term cultures may easily be taken as an indication that the hepatoma cells in vitro retain the ability to secrete AFP. But then one wonders why the long-term cultures failed to do so. The negative result may, of course, be due simply to a much lower rate of intracellular synthesis, so that the small amount of AFP secreted into the medium escaped detection. It may also be the result of a change in the functional properties of the cells under long-term cultivation with the loss of the ability to synthesize AFP. It is obvious that the most sensitive method of detection should be adopted on both the cultivated cells and their conditioned medium in order to

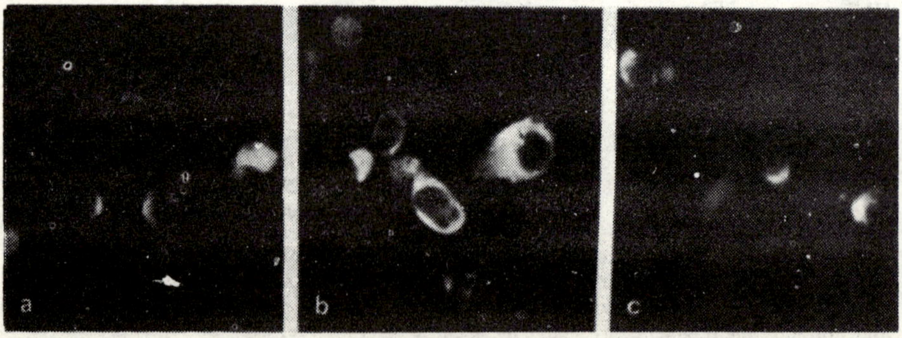

Fig. 3 a–c. Distribution of AFP in the cytoplasm of three cell lines of human hepatocellular carcinoma; indirect immunofluorescence, × 300. **a** BEL-7402 line; **b** BEL-7404 line; **c** BEL-7405 line

determine how long the cells can maintain their ability to synthesize AFP in vitro. To keep the cells AFP-positive it would be best to preserve them in a deep-frozen state before AFP synthesis disappears.

2. Analysis of LDH Isozyme

Resumed AFP synthesis by hepatoma cells is some of the most convincing evidence of a tendency toward "fetalism" in the rapidly growing and less well differentiated malignant tumors. Other proteins, such as LDH isozyme, also assumed their embryonic pattern (Schapira et al. 1974).

Using polyacrylamide gel electrophoresis and cytochemical assay methods, Chen et al. (1963, 1980) compared the LDH isozyme pattern of surgical specimens of human liver carcinomas, normal human adult liver and embryonic livers, and the three lines of human HCC cells. They found that type M (or A) was the major LDH isozyme in the normal adult liver and type H (or B) was very weak; H-type isozyme activity became more pronounced in human embryonic liver and hepatoma cells (Fig. 4).

It can also be seen from Table 3 that isozyme patterns for BEL-7404 and BEL-7405 cells were similar, i.e., the percentage of LDH-3 was highest. Although the activity of LDH-5 was slightly higher in the cells of BEL-7402 and SMMC-7721, the overall pictures were the same for all four lines of liver carcinoma cells. LDH-3 was the predominant form. In conclusion, the LDH isozyme patterns in four lines of human HCC cells were similar to those of surgical specimens of hepatoma.

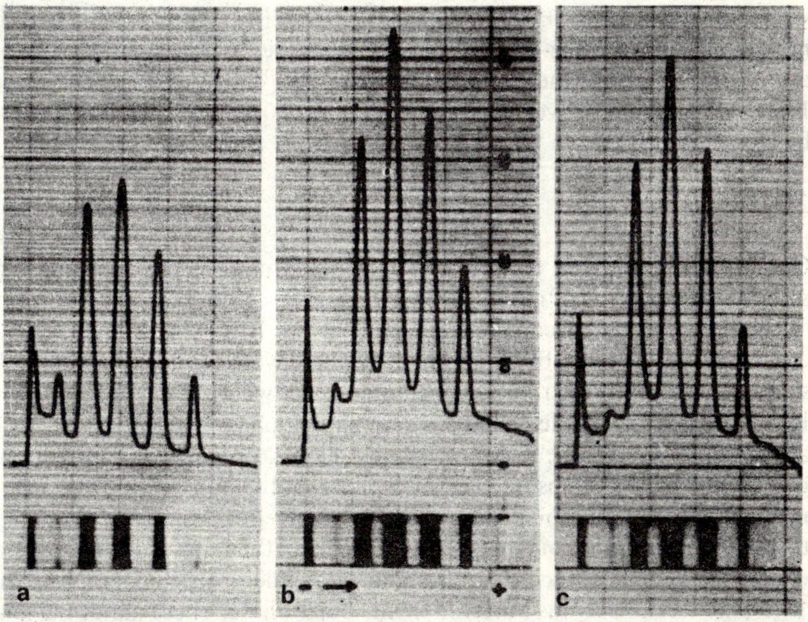

Fig. 4 a–c. Polyacrylamide gel electrophoretic assay of LDH isozyme of three lines of human HCC cells. **a** BEL-7402 line; **b** BEL-7404 line; **c** BEL-7405 line

Table 3. Gel electrophoretic analysis of LDH isozyme of four liver carcinoma cell lines and the densitometer scans of the gel stained with amido-black

Cell line	LDH (%)				
	LDH-5	LDH-4	LDH-3	LDH-2	LDH-1
BEL-7402	7.78	29.94	35.11	21.18	5.99
BEL-7404	1.70	22.95	37.76	27.21	10.38
BEL-7405	2.13	23.61	40.30	26.52	7.44
SMMC-7721	8.20	26.20	30.90	29.70	6.80

3. Others

The BEL-7402 cell line was tested for G-6-PD and TAT; Prozesky cell lines were tested for aspartic acid transferase; the PLC/PRF/5 cell line was tested for G-6-PD, LDH, hexokinase, and PK; the characteristics were similar to those of surgical specimens but different from those of human normal liver cells.

C. Growth Behavior

1. Doubling Times of Cell Population

The estimation of doub'.ng time (DT) or generation time (GT) of a cell line can reflect the growth rate of the cell population. The method adopted was pulse labeling with 1 μCi/ml mediun ^{3}H-thymidine (34 Ci/m*M*) for 1 h and examination by autoradiography. Among the ten lines of HCC cells, the DT for BEL-7402-line cells was estimated to be 20 h; the shortest DTs were 26 h and 23 h for the BEL-7404 and BEL-7405 lines respectively, and the longest was 70 h for the HLE line, as estimated by Doi et al. (1975).

2. Mitotic Activity

One of the pathological features of a malignant tumor is the appearance (expression) of various types of mitotic aberrations.

Upon careful microscopic examination of the BEL-7402 and BEL-16 lines of cells, various types of abnormal mitotic figures were found, and multipolar divisions and disorderly distribution of chromosomes were quite frequent. Other mitotic abnormalities include anaphase and/or telophase chromosome bridges, the asynchronized prophase of bi- or trinuclear cells, one or two multinucleate giant cells, individual chromosome lag, metaphase and telophase chromosome clumps, metaphase with multipolar figures, and amitosis. Besides, with "normal" mitosis, the number of cells during metaphase was greater than that in prophase or any other phase. As demonstrated clearly by time-lapse microcine-matography (Chen et al. 1978), the metaphase was longer than any other phase. These abnormal mitotic behaviour patterns of tumor cells may be closely related to the heteroploidy of malignant cells and to the abnormal regulation of the spindle mechanism.

3. Heterologous Transplantation

To test the cultured cells for their malignancy, heterologous transplantation was performed and microscopic examination made of the nodules formed at the site of inoculation.

Of the 12 lines of human HCC cells, seven lines – BEL-7402, BEL-7404, BEL-7405, QGY-7703, SMMC-7721, HLE, and HLF – were independently transplanted to conditioned animals. Only the HLE line failed to grow nodules in the cheek pouch of the Chinese hamster, while all others formed tumor nodules. Histological sections of the nodules showed massive cell clusters with intercalated distribution, no obvious intercellular fibrous network, and little lymphocyte infiltration. The tumor cells were variable in size, with a high N/C ratio and highly heteromorphous nuclei. Cells with two to four nuclei or with giant nuclei were fairly common. Nucleoli were prominent and irregular in shape, and were generally one or two, occasionally three in number. Mitotic figures were common but they had a high percentage of anomaly. These morphological features were in accordance with those of the original surgical specimens before cultivation.

III. Application of Hepatoma Cell Lines in Basic Cancer Research

The in vitro-cultured cell lines could serve as experimental models for various aspects of basic cancer research.

A. Immunology

The study of specific antigens associated with cancer cells has been of interest for both early diagnosis of cancer and the elucidation of the mechanism of tumorigenesis. The discovery of AFP helped greatly in massive screening for early diagnosis of hepatoma. Precancerous antigens other than AFP that persisted up to the late stage of hepatoma development have been found in chemically induced animal hepatomas (Farber 1976). Whether other types of antigens are present in human hepatoma cells, and whether there is any antigen common to different hepatomas, are questions of great interest.

Using indirect immunofluorescence for the detection of AFP in three lines of cells (BEL-7402, BEL-7404, and BEL-7405) Shi et al. (1977) found that their surface membranes were positive, with a greenish, continuous or discontinuous annular appearance. Liver cells of 3- to 5-month-old fetuses also showed a similar positive reaction, while those of adult liver, both freshly isolated and cultivated, were negative. This indicated that the surface membrane of three lines of human hepatoma cells still possessed some fetal antigens. Similar results were reported by the Biochemistry Department of the Shanghai First Medical College (1977). (Biochemistry Department of Shanghai First Medical College 1977).

The importance of cell-mediated immunity in the antitumor response of the body has already been confirmed. Zhang et al. (1978) labeled BEL-7402 cells with ^{125}I-UDR as a marker to assay peripheral lymphocyte microcytotoxicity in 33 hepatoma patients and found that the patients' lymphocytes against the microcytotoxicity of this line of cells were stronger than those of the normal controls. With lymphocytes from patients treated surgically or from patients in improved general health, the microcytotoxicity was stronger than in patients whose condition was getting worse. The results of the assay not only suggested that the state of cell-mediated immunity of the body mostly paralleled the development of disease, but also seemed to reveal the possible presence of a common tumor associated antigen (TAA) among tumors.

Yang et al. (1978) immunized a goat with BEL-7402 cells and isolated iRNA from the goat's lymphoid tissues. They observed that the BEL-7402 cells could be killed by iRNA-treated human lymphoidocytes. This indicated that the iRNA might be involved in cellular immunological response, ans suggested its possible trial use in the clinical treatment of cancer.

B. Virology

According to epidemiological surveys, hepatoma is closely associated with the occurrence of HB_sAg.

Macnab et al. (1976) found that the sera of patients from whom hepatoma cell lines were derived were HB_sAg positive. When the period of hepatoma cell culture was prolonged, the content HB_sAg of the supernatant of cell-cultured medium increased to an average of 500 ng/10^6 cells. Electron microscopy showed that viral granules were mostly oval and 16–24 nm (mostly 20 nm) in diameter. The tubular type, or Dane particles, was not seen. A test for the presence of HB_sAg in BEL-7405-line cells was positive. It would be of great significance to make further studies with cell lines on the relationship between HB_sAg and hepatomas. The Shanghai Epidemic Prevention Station and the Zhejiang Medical College have also used the BEL-16 line of cells in studies of viral multiplication and the isolation of virus. Prozesky (1973) found that hepatoma cell lines were very sensitive to human herpesvirus and Rift Valley fever virus.

C. Pharmacology

Cell lines established in vitro provide a simple system, independent of blood and nerve supply, in which the essential effect of an individual drug or agent and its mode of action can be studied under controlled experimental conditions.

Shen et al. (1977) examined the effect of P-QP (quinine-piperazine phosphate) on BEL-7402 and BEL-16 cells. They found that this drug intensively inhibited cell mitosis and damaged cell ultrastructures (such as nuclear chromatin, endoplasmic reticulum, mitochondria, and lysosomes) to varying extents. The damage appeared reversible if the dosage of drug administrated was low, but higher dosages might be lethal to cells.

Li et al. (1977) studied the effect of 2′,3′-oxy-adenosine dialdehyde on BEL-7402 cells. Using the cytokinetic technique, they found that this chemical inhibited cells at the S phase of the mitotic cycle; they suggested that it be used as an antitumor drug and that the results could a guideline for ehemotherapy. The effects of some traditional Chinese medicines and X-radiation have also been studied, with some promising results.

D. Pathogenesis

Whether tumorigenesis is monocellular or multicellular in origin has always been the subject of controversy. Cytogenetic analysis with BEL-7402, BEL-7404, and BEL-7405 lines of cells showed that there are two different situations. In karyotype analysis one abnormally large acrocentric chromosome appeared in 98% of BEL-7402 cells and in 71% of BEL-7404 cells, so they might be considered of monocellular origin, while in BEL-7405 cells three types (as shown in Table 2) – the large acrocentric chromosome, the minute acrocentric chromosome, and chromosome fragments – appeared with varying frequency, suggesting that they might be of multicellular origin. Apparently, both possibilities exist.

The existence of an abnormally large acrocentric chromosome seems to be a common feature of malignancy, since similar findings were reported (Lampert 1971) in other cancer cells, such as those from the lung, stomach, and colon as well as from cervical and ovarian cancer and Burkitt's lymphoma. Morphologically, they were similar. It is generally thought that the presence of this large abnormal acrocentric chromosome in tumors might be associated with human malignancy (Goh and Tenn 1968; Lube and Koller 1967).

An examination of pathological sections showed that multipolar mitotic figures and multinucleate giant cells were common. How were the multinucleate giants formed? Was there any relationship to multipolar mitosis? Chen et al. (1978) examined the BEL-7402 line of cells and their growth behavior with time-lapse microcinematography and carefully followed the sequence of multipolar mitosis. They found that many daughter cells were generated by multipolar division. The number of daughter cells was roughly in accordance with the number of polarities. These daughter cells, however, were not able to survive independently, but fused with each other to form a multinucleate giant cell. This could explain the presence of multinucleate cells in tumor specimens.

E. Reversion of Cancer Cells

The conventional treatment for cancer has been the killing of cancer cells by various combinations of chemotherapy, radiotherapy, traditional medicines, and surgery. Might there be any other way?

In 1974, the Shanghai Tumor Research Institute performed some experimental studies in an attempt to induce normal differentiation of liver cancer cells by normal liver cell RNA. The results showed that the hepatoma cells were functionally redifferentiated when treated with normal cell RNA, which could also inhibit the growth of tumor in animals. Later, (Biochemistry Department of Shanghai Tumour Research Institute 1977) they examined the effect of rat liver RNA on the BEL-7402 line of cells. They incubated cells with the RNA for 24 h and then added ^{14}C-leucine to assay the incorporation of the amino acid with serum albumin. The result showed that, when treated with RNA, human hepatoma cells could synthesize not only rat serum albumin but also human serum albumin with three to six times faster than untreated controls. In another experiment, Li et al. (1978) isolated liver mRNA and added it to cultured hepatoma cells (BEL-7402). They obtained a certain degree of reversibility of the neoplastic phenotype toward normality, as measured by the resumption of albumin synthesis. The agglutination of human hepatoma cells by concanavalin A was also weakened, and the changed characteristics persisted for three subpassages (through 10–20 GT or for 20 days), suggesting that the property of cancer cell membrane might also be reversed toward normality.

The effect of the exogenous RNA in reversing the functional differentiation of the cultured human hepatoma cells, however, did not seem to be species specific. Clarification of the mode of action of RNA awaits further studies.

In conclusion, the establishment of human HCC cell lines in vitro provides an ideal system for investigating liver cell carcinogenesis and for preventive research. The fields of application have broadened increasingly, and some of the preliminary results have been promising. At present, we use these cell lines for studying human liver carcinoma, with particular emphasis on gene expression and its regulation. We are also attempting to prepare the monoclonal antibody of liver carcinoma and to detect the presence of an oncogene.

References

Alexander J, Bey E, Macnab G (1977) Establishment of human hepatoma cell line which produces hepatitis B surface antigen (HB_sAg). In: Neiburgs HE (ed) Prevention and detection of cancer. Marcel Dekker, New York, pp 321

Biochemistry Department of Shanghai First Medical College (1977) Studies on embryonic membrane antigen of human hepatoma. Acta Biochim Biophys Sinica 9: 337[1]

Biochestry Department of Shanghai Tumor Research Institute (1977) Biological action of exogenous liver cytoplasmic RNA on human hepatoma cells and its distribution in the body. Acta Biochim Biophys Sinica 9: 237[1]

Chen RM (1963) The establishment of a strain of human liver cell carcinoma in vitro and some preliminary observations. Chin Med J 82: 228–237

Chen RM, Shen DW, Yang CH, et al. (1963) Studies on human liver cell carcinoma cultivated in vitro. I. Some cytological and histochemical observations. Acta Biol Exp Sinica 8: 423–446[1]

Chen RM, Chu TH, Yeh HJ, Shen DW et al. (1975) Establishment of human liver carcinoma cell line (BEL-7402) and its biological characteristics. Kexue Tongbao 20: 434–436[1]

Chen RM, Shen DW, Yang CH, Chang HC et al. (1978) Time-lapse microcinematographic observations of the growth behavior of human liver carcinoma cell line (BEL-7402) in vitro. Acta Biol Exp Sinica 11: 157–170[1]

Chen RM, Chu TH, Yeh HJ, Shen DW, Lu YH et al. (1980) Establishment of three human liver carcinoma cell lines and some of their biological characteristics in vitro. Scientia Sinica 23: 236–247

Doi I, Namba M, Sato J (1975) Establishment and some biological characteristics of human hepatoma cell lines. Gann monograph 66: 385–392

Dong RC, Shou YH, Lu FT et al. (1980) Establishment and some preliminary observations of human hepatoma cell line SMMC-7721. Acta Second Military Medical College of PLA 1: 5–9[1]

Farber E (1976) The pathology of experimental liver cell cancer. In: Cameron HM, Linsell DA, Warwick GP (eds) Liver cell cancer Elsevier, Amsterdam, pp 243–277

Fogh J (1975) Human tumor cells in vitro. Plenum, New York, p 142

Gey CO, Coffman WD, Kubicek MT et al. (1952) Tissue culture studies of the proliferative capacity of cervical carcinoma and normal epithelium. Cancer Res 12: 264–265

Lampert F (1971) Chromosome alteration in human carcinogenesis. Adv Cell Mol Biol 1: 185

Lasfargues EY, Ozzello L (1958) Cultivation of human breast carcinomas. J Natl Cancer Inst 12: 1131–1148

Li WY, Yeh HJ, Lu YH et al. (1977) Studies on the mechanism of 2′,3′-oxy-adenosine dialdehyde effect on hepatoma cells. Shanghai Cell Biol Inst (1973–1975) Sci Rec p 80[1]

Li WY, Wang PY, Li M et al. (1978) Translation of normal liver mRNA and its inducing activity on in vitro hepatoma cells. Acta Biol Exp Sinica 11: 109–124[1]

Lube JA, Koller S (1967) The prognostic significance of chromosome abnormalities in colon tumors. Ann Intern Med 67: 328

Macnab GM, Alexander J, Lecatsas G et al. (1976) Hepatitis B surface antigen produced by a human hepatoma cell line. Br J Cancer 34: 509–515

Prozesky OW (1973) In vitro culture of cell lines from Australia antigen-positive and -negative hepatoma patients. In: Saunders JJ, Terblanche J, (eds) Liver. Proceedings of an international liver conference, with special reference to Africa, held at the University of Cape Town Medical School. Pitman Medical, London p 358

Schapira F, et al. (1974) Fetal type of isozymes in cancer. XIth Internat Cancer Cong Abst 1: 123

Shen DW, Yang CH, Chen RM et al. (1977) Antitumor activity of P-QP. II. The effect of P-QP on the growth of human and rat hepatoma cells in vitro. Shanghai Cell Biol Inst (1973–1975) Sci Rec pp 92–96[1]

Shi WK, Lu YL, Yeh M, et al. (1977) Membrane-associated embryonic antigen in hepatocellular carcinoma cells. Acta Zool Sinica 23: 337–344[1]

Wang JB, Chu TH, Yeh HJ et al. (1981) Establishment and some characteristics of a hepatoma cell line (QGY-7703). Chin J Oncol 3: 241–244[1]

Yang SY, Wang QD, Zhang ZL et al. (1978) Immune cytolysis of human liver cancer cells mediated by xenogeneic "immune" RNA. Acta Biol Exp Sinica 11: 189–198[1]

Zhang ZL, Wang QD, Yang SY, et al. (1978) Microcytotoxicity assay of lymphocytes in hepatoma patients against 5-(^{125}I) iodo-2′-deoxyuridine-labeled hepatoma target cell. Kexue Tongbao 23: 185–188[1]

[1] Chinese

29 Storage and Analysis of Subclinical Hepatocellular Carcinoma: Comparision of Clinical Cases Using a Microcomputer

Ye Sheng-long, Tang Zhao-you

The computer, one of the greatest developments of this century in science and technology, has seen more and more extensive and intensive application in the field of biomedical research since its introduction. The appearance of the microcomputer, in particular, has allowed for striking success in the whole domain of science, including medicine.

For more than 4 years the microcomputer has been used in the laboratory of the authors' department for research in clinical medicine, such as differential diagnosis of PLC (Tang et al. 1981), prediction of surgical resectability and survival (Tang and Li 1981), storage and analysis of medical materials (Tang and Li 1982; Tang and Ye 1983), and calculation and statistics. It is evident that the utilization of the microcomputer by clinicians and researchers may noticeably improve efficiency and accuracy and solve a large number of medical research problems.

Tables 1–17 give the complete set of data obtained by comparison of SCHCC with CHCC in the authors' department; the microcomputer was used to store and analyze the data.

Type of Computer and Programming Language. An APPLE II PLUS microcomputer, with 64 K of random-access memory (RAM) and 16 K of read-only memory (ROM), was employed for the storage and analysis of clinical data. APPLESOFT II BASIC, an extended BASIC of APPLE II PLUS, was used as the programming language in analysis.

Data Storage. The clinical data on 566 PLC patients (559 cases were pathologically proven, the rest were confirmed by both AFP level determination and selective angiography) were collected and stored over 12 years, from January 1971 to December 1982. Of these, 100 cases were diagnosed as having subclinical (early stage) PLC and 466 as having clinical (moderate or late stage) PLC. The data were inputted on 5-in. diskettes, each of which can store as much as 124 KB of information via disk drive by means of random-access file. Every case comprised 61 items, recorded with Arabic numerals expressing the actual number or code of each item, including four on general data, seven on clinical findings, 17 on laboratory data, five on special examinations, 15 on treatment records, ten on pathological and operative findings, and three on follow-up studies.

Data Analysis. Detailed analyses of the data, focusing on subclinical PLC and comparing it with clinical PLC during the same period, were carried out (see Tables 1–17).

Table 1. Diagnosis and discovery of PLC patients

	Subclinical	Clinical
Total number of cases	100	466
Pathologically proven	95	464
AFP and angiogram (+)	5	2
Discovery approach		
Mass survey[a]	76 (76.0%)	34 (7.3%)
AFP monitoring[a]	22 (22.0%)	13 (2.8%)
Clinical finding[a]	2 (2.0%)	419 (89.9%)
Type of PLC[b]		
Simple	93 (93.0%)	340 (73.0%)
Cirrhotic	7 (7.0%)	115 (24.7%)
Inflammatory	0	11 (2.4%)
Stage of PLC[c]		
Early (subclinical)	100	0
Moderate	0	335 (71.9%)
Late	0	131 (28.1%)
Age of PLC patients (years)		
Range	20–65	13–82
Median	47.5	46
Tumor size of PLC (cm)[d]		
Range	0.8–16	1–35
Median	4.5	10
Male/female ratio	15.7:1	7.3:1

[a] $P < 0.001$

[b] Criteria for types of PLC:
Simple – without obvious clinical and laboratory evidence of cirrhosis
Cirrhotic – with obvious clinical and laboratory evidence of cirrhosis
Inflammatory – with rapid progress of the disease, persistent cancerous high fever or marked elevation of ALT

[c] Criteria of stages of PLC:
Subclinical (early) – without obvious symptoms or signs of liver cancer
Late – with obvious cachexia, jaundice, ascites or distant metastases
Moderate – between early and late stages

[d] Measured in maximum diameter of nodule

Table 2. AFP levels of PLC patients

	Subclinical	Clinical
Range of AFP level (ng/ml)	20–80000	20–700000
Median of AFP level (ng/ml)	2000	4750
No. of patients with AFP ≤ 20 ng/ml	2	135
No. of patients with AFP > 20 ng/ml	98	317
AFP < 500 ng/ml	22 (22.4%)	30 (9.5%)
AFP ≥ 500 ng/ml	76 (77.6%)	287 (90.5%)
Median level with different patterns of AFP change (ng/ml)		
Increasing from low level[a]	430	500
Moderate level[b]	400	370
High level[c]	2000	10000

[a] Increased gradually from low (around 50 ng/ml) to high.
[b] Persisted at between 200 ng/ml and 500 ng/ml
[c] Maintained at above 500 ng/ml

Table 3. Localization of PLC

Method used for positive localization	Subclinical		Clinical	
	n	(%)	*n*	(%)
Angiogram	32/37	(86.5)	19/ 22	(86.4)
A-mode ultrasonogram[a]	7/84	(8.3)	284/403	(70.5)
B-mode ultrasonogram[a]	22/37	(59.5)	98/104	(94.2)
Radionuclide scintigram[a]	31/97	(32.0)	382/430	(88.8)
X-ray diaphragm sign[a]	6/77	(7.8)	112/314	(35.7)

[a] $P<0.001$

Table 4. Laboratory findings and immunostatus

	Subclinical		Clinical	
	n	(%)	*n*	(%)
γ-GTP > 10 units[a]*	22/89	(24.7)	315/409	(77.0)
ALP > 13 units[b]*	20/89	(22.5)	235/413	(56.9)
5′-NPDase-V (+)[c]*	15/25	(60.0)	39/ 62	(62.9)
OT test (+)[d]**	64/81	(79.0)	184/308	(59.7)

* $P<0.001$
** $P<0.01$
[a] Modified Orlowski method
[b] King-Armstrong method
[c] Tsou method (Tsou et al. 1973), with some modification (Lu et al. 1980). Serum 5′-nucleotide phosphodiesterase (5′-NPDase)-V-positive was considered to contain five bands or to have an R_f value (migration coefficient) of the rapidly moving band of ≥0.58
[d] Results were measured 48–72 h after intradermal injection of 0.1 ml 1:2000 old tuberculin (OT). Nodules larger than 5 mm in diameter were considered OT positive (Lin et al. 1979)

Table 5. Background of liver disease in PLC

	Subclinical		Clinical	
	n	(%)	*n*	(%)
With hepatitis history*[a]	63/100	(63.0)	197/466	(42.3)
≤5 years	14/ 63	(22.2)	44/197	(22.3)
5.1–10 years	18/ 63	(28.6)	71/197	(36.0)
>10 years	31/ 63	(49.2)	82/197	(41.6)
Serum HB_sAg (+)[b]	51/ 87	(58.6)	124/253	(49.0)
Serum anti-HB_c (+)[c]	28/ 41	(68.3)	38/ 55	(69.1)
Serum ALT>40 units[d] **	10/100	(10.0)	96/464	(20.7)
Coexistent cirrhosis	78/ 91	(85.7)	231/287	(80.5)
No	13/ 91	(14.3)	56/287	(19.5)
Micronodular	19/ 91	(20.9)	54/287	(18.6)
Macronodular	59/ 91	(64.8)	177/287	(61.7)

* $P<0.001$
** $P<0.05$
[a] Median for entire series (260 cases) 10 years, range 1–25
[b] Either RPHA or CIEP
[c] Enzyme-linked immunosorbent assay
[d] Reitman method

Table 6. Treatment of PLC patients

	Subclinical		Clinical	
	n	(%)	*n*	(%)
Resected cases*	60/100	(60.0)	115/466	(24.7)
Local resection*	35	(58.3)	33	(28.7)
Left lateral segmentectomy	8	(13.3)	22	(19.1)
Left hemihepatectomy*	4	(6.7)	36	(31.3)
Extensive left hemihepatectomy	2	(3.3)	3	(2.6)
Right posterior lobectomy**	5	(8.3)	0	
Right hemihepatectomy***	3	(5.0)	18	(15.7)
Extensive right hemihepatectomy	0		1	(0.9)
Middle lobectomy	3	(5.0)	2	(1.7)
Unresected cases*	40/100	(40.0)	351/466	(75.3)
Cryosurgery	10	(25.0)	21	(6.0)
Laser	1	(2.5)	2	(0.6)
Ligation plus cannulation	3	(7.5)	18	(5.1)
Ligation	2	(5.0)	14	(4.0)
Cannulation	9	(22.5)	49	(14.0)
Radiotherapy	3	(7.5)	18	(5.1)
Chemotherapy plus Chinese herbs**	4	(10.0)	113	(32.2)
Chinese herbs	6	(15.0)	39	(11.1)
Chemotherapy	0		27	(7.7)
No treatment	2	(5.0)	50	(14.2)

* $P<0.001$
** $P<0.01$
*** $P<0.05$

Table 7. Operative findings and other surgical data

	Subclinical		Clinical	
	n	(%)	*n*	(%)
No. of tumor nodules				
One*	60/90	(66.7)	118/300	(39.3)
Two	15/90	(16.7)	28/300	(9.3)
Three or more*	15/90	(16.7)	154/300	(51.3)
Site of tumor				
Left lobe	15/93	(16.1)	68/307	(22.1)
Right lobe*	42/93	(45.2)	74/307	(24.1)
Portal*	22/93	(23.7)	22/307	(7.2)
Bilateral*	14/93	(15.0)	143/307	(46.6)
Resective mortality	1/60	(1.7)	7/115	(6.1)
Bloodless operation	5		0	
No. of reresections/reoperations	7/ 9		8/ 11	
No. of two-step resections/operations	3/ 3		3/ 5	

* $P<0.001$

Table 8. Pathological aspects of PLC

	Subclinical		Clinical	
	n	(%)	*n*	(%)
Histological classification				
Hepatocellular carcinoma**	94/95	(98.9)	435/464	(93.8)
Cholangiocarcinoma	0		13/464	(2.8)
Mixed carcinoma	1/95	(1.1)	16/464	(3.4)
Differentiative degrees of HCC				
Well	4/73	(5.5)	29/273	(10.6)
Moderate	59/73	(80.8)	193/273	(70.7)
Poor	10/73	(13.7)	51/273	(18.7)
Well encapsulated*	42/84	(50.0)	46/291	(15.8)
No tumor emboli*	57/59	(96.6)	78/146	(53.4)

* $P<0.001$
** $P<0.05$

Table 9. PLC patients whose AFP returned to normal after treatment

Subclinical cases	*n*	%
Resected cases[a]	48/57	84.2
Within 1–15 days	5/48	10.4
Within 16–30 days	14/48	29.2
Within 31–60 days	27/48	56.3
More than 60 days	2/48	4.2
Range of days returned to normal	8–152	
Median days returned to normal	35.5	
Unresected cases[b]	4/27	14.8
Median days with various original AFP levels		
<500 ng/ml		23.5
501– 5000 ng/ml		35.5
5001–50000 ng/ml		50
>50000 ng/ml		100.5

[a] Clinical PLC cases were 30/78 (38.5%), $P<0.001$
[b] Clinical PLC cases were 4/95 (4.2%), $P>0.05$

Table 10. Survival or PLC Patients

	Cases	No. of patients alive at					No. of months alive	
		1 yr	2 yrs	3 yrs	4 yrs	5 yrs	Longest	Median
Total group								
Subclinical	100	63	39	26	19	10	94	18
Clinical	466	85	32	21	14	8	130	4
Entire series	566	148	71	47	33	18	–	–
Resected group								
Subclinical	60	44	32	23	19	10	94	25.5
Clinical	115	51	23	17	12	8	130	10
Entire series	175	95	55	40	31	18	–	–
Unresected group								
Subclinical	40	19	7	3	0	0	42	11
Clinical	351	34	9	4	2	0	56	3
Entire series	391	53	16	7	2	0	–	–

Table 11. Survival rate of PLC patients

	No. of cases	Survival rate (%)[a]				
		1-yr	2-yr	3-yr	4-yr	5-yr
Total group						
Subclinical	100	75.5	54.5	47.7	43.9	43.9
Clinical	466	24.2	11.1	8.4	7.2	4.2
Entire series	566	33.3	19.0	16.0	13.9	11.6
Resected group						
Subclinical	60	85.0	76.2	72.9	72.9	72.9
Clinical	115	60.1	32.5	26.3	23.0	16.1
Entire series	175	69.5	48.5	44.5	41.1	37.3
Unresected group						
Subclinical	40	57.3	19.1	8.0		
Clinical	351	12.1	3.7	2.0	1.0	
Entire series	391	17.1	5.6	3.1	1.0	

[a] Life-table method

Table 12. Survival rates of unresected PLC cases with various treatments[a]

	Subclinical PLC				Clinical PLC			
	No. of cases	Survival (%)			No. of Cases	Survival (%)		
		1-yr	2-yr	3-yr		1-yr	2-yr	3-yr
Cryosurgery	10	60.0	20.0	10.0	21	35.4	8.8	0
Laser	1	–	–	–	2	–	–	–
Ligation plus cannulation	3	–	–	–	18	40.5	21.6	0
Ligation	2	–	–	–	14	9.4	0	–
Cannulation	9	44.4	0	–	49	22.5	3.4	–
Radiation	3	66.7	0	–	18	5.6	–	–
Chinese herbs plus chemotherapy	4	0	–	–	113	3.0	–	–
Chinese herbs	6	22.2	–	–	39	0	–	–
Chemotherapy	0	–	–	–	27	–	–	–
No treatment	2	–	–	–	50	–	–	–

[a] Life-table method

Table 13. Factors influencing survival of entire series of PLC patients

	No. of cases	Survival rate (%)[a]				
		1-yr	2-yr	3-yr	4-yr	5-yr
Age ⩽45 years	262	36.5	22.8	19.8	17.7	14.7
>45 years	304	30.0	15.0	11.8	10.3	7.1
Mass survey or AFP monitoring	145	64.4	45.2	40.2	34.7	34.7
Clinical discovery	421	22.8	10.1	7.3	6.9	3.7
Simple type	433	37.5	22.5	19.1	16.4	14.1
Cirrhotic type	122	19.2	4.8	4.8	2.4	2.4
Early stage	100	75.5	54.5	47.7	43.9	43.9
Moderate stage	335	32.6	15.5	11.8	10.1	5.9
Late stage	131	1.7	–	–	–	–
Original AFP <5000 ng/ml	301	42.9	25.7	20.6	17.4	15.2
⩾5000 ng/ml	249	21.2	11.5	10.6	10.6	6.2
Left lobe only	80	62.3	42.6	38.1	33.3	30.0
Other sites[b]	299	43.3	24.0	19.9	18.5	13.1
No cirrhosis or micronodular type	142	54.3	33.7	30.5	28.3	22.2
Macronodular cirrhosis	236	41.5	25.6	19.4	16.1	16.1
γ-GTP <20 units	243	55.0	34.7	29.5	25.1	21.8
⩾20 units	255	10.9	3.3	3.3	2.2	2.2
OT test (+)	248	43.1	23.1	20.5	18.3	15.8
(−)	141	24.9	17.5	12.0	12.0	12.0
Resection	175	69.5	48.5	44.5	41.1	37.3
Nonresection	391	17.1	5.6	3.1	1.0	–
Complete removal of tumor[c]	64	93.3	74.6	69.5	69.5	61.5
Palliative resection	111	55.5	32.5	27.0	22.5	22.5
Single nodule	172	68.4	45.4	40.5	36.0	32.3
Multiple nodules	200	30.0	12.9	8.0	8.0	5.4
Good encapsulation	86	82.3	67.4	60.3	54.7	49.0
Poor encapsulation	275	38.4	16.1	11.7	10.7	5.9
Postoperative AFP ⩽20 ng/ml	83	94.7	84.0	76.1	71.5	60.4
>20 ng/ml	200	28.8	7.0	4.3	–	–

[a] Using life table method.
[b] Including right, portal, and multiple
[c] With removal of well-encapsulated tumor, no tumor emboli in portal vein, and tumor residue in neither remaining liver tissue nor cut surface

Table 14. Comparison of resectability in subclinical PLC

	No. of cases	(%)
Age <30 years	8/10	80.0
30–49 years	35/54	64.8
⩾ 50 years	17/36	47.2
No cirrhosis, or micronodular type	25/32	78.1
Macronodular cirrhosis	35/59	59.3
Original AFP 31– 500 ng/ml	18/22	81.8
501–5000 ng/ml	28/53	52.8
>5000 ng/ml	13/23	56.5
γ-GTP <20 units	47/78	60.3
⩾20 units	4/11	36.4
Tumor site: left lobe	14/15	93.3
right lobe	31/42	73.8
portal	12/22	54.5
bilateral	3/14	21.4
A-mode ultrasonogram (+)	4/7	57.1
(−)	45/77	58.4
B-mode ultrasonogram (+)	15/22	68.2
(−)	9/15	60.0
X-ray diaphragm sign (+)	3/6	50.0
(−)	46/71	64.8
ALT >40 units	6/10	60.0
⩽40 units	54/90	60.0
OT test (+)	36/64	56.3
(−)	14/17	82.4
Cardinal red tongue (+)	27/51	52.9
(−)	27/37	73.0
Hepatitis history (+)	26/63	57.1
(−)	24/37	64.9

Table 15. Factors influencing survival after resection in subclinical PLC

	No. of cases	Survival rate (%)[a]				
		1-yr	2-yr	3-yr	4-yr	5-yr
Postoperative AFP ⩽20 ng/ml	48	93.2	85.7	82.0	82.0	82.0
>20 ng/ml	8	42.9	21.4	–	–	–
Tumor size ⩽5 cm	42	86.2	82.9	78.3	78.3	78.3
>5 cm	18	76.5	61.8	61.8	61.8	–
Single nodule	45	92.3	83.7	83.7	83.7	83.7
Multiple nodules	15	62.2	53.3	40.0	40.0	–
Local or left hepatectomy	49	86.4	80.9	76.4	76.4	76.4
Right hepatectomy	11	67.5	56.3	56.3	56.3	56.3
Age ⩽30 years	9	88.9	88.9	88.9	88.9	88.9
31–49 years	34	87.2	79.3	74.0	74.0	74.0
⩾50 years	17	69.6	60.9	60.9	60.9	60.9
no cirrhosis, or micronodular type	25	87.0	82.1	82.1	82.1	82.1
Macronodular cirrhosis	35	80.3	71.7	64.5	64.5	64.5

[a] Life-table method

Table 16. Factors influencing survival of subclinical PLC patients

	No. of cases	Survival rate (%)*				
		1-yr	2-yr	3-yr	4-yr	5-yr
Age < median[a]	50	74.2	61.9	55.4	51.7	51.7
⩾ median	50	74.2	46.5	35.3	35.3	35.3
Tumor site – left lobe	15	80.0	80.0	66.7	66.7	50.0
– other[b]	78	73.4	51.2	44.9	44.9	44.9
Single nodule	60	88.9	71.3	62.9	62.9	62.9
Multiple nodules	30	52.4	32.9	21.9	21.9	–
Tumor size ⩽ median[c]	45	88.2	79.9	69.6	69.6	69.6
> median	42	64.5	34.0	28.3	28.3	–
Cirrhosis – none or micronodular	32	82.8	71.6	66.5	66.5	66.5
– macronodular	59	74.0	51.4	38.9	35.4	35.4
Original AFP ⩽ median[d]	67	72.9	56.6	48.8	45.9	45.9
> median	33	77.0	50.4	40.1	40.1	40.1
Postoperative AFP ⩽31 ng/ml	52	93.7	86.7	80.4	80.4	80.4
>31 ng/ml	37	46.9	10.7	5.4	–	–

* Life-table method
[a] Median age 47.5 years
[b] Including right, portal and multiple sites
[c] Median size 4.5 cm
[d] Median AFP level 2000 ng/ml

Table 17. Comparison of PLC cases seen in two 6-year periods

Duration	1971–1976		1977–1982	
	No.	%	No.	%
Total cases	250		316	
Subclinical PLC*	23/250	9.2	77/316	24.4
Small HCC***	22/250	8.0	42/316	13.3
Resected cases**	61/250	24.4	114/316	36.1
Resective mortality	5/61	8.2	3/114	2.6
Survival rate for entire series (life-table method)				
1-year		26.5		38.5
2-year		13.3		24.3
3-year		10.4		21.7
4-year		8.3		20.6
5-year		6.5		20.6

* $P<0.001$
** $P<0.01$
*** $P<0.05$

References

Lin ZY, Tang ZY, Chen KJ, et al. (1979) Preliminary study on cell-mediated immunity in primary carcinoma of the liver. Acta Acad Med Primae Shanghai 6: 1–7[1]

Lu HM, Chen C, Sze PC, et al. (1980) The significance of 5′-nucleotide phosphodiesterase isozymes in the diagnosis of liver carcinoma. Int J Cancer 26: 31–35

Tang ZY, Li ZH (1981) Prediction of survival time with microcomputer after resection of primary hepatic cancer. Shanghai Med J 4: 470–473[1]

Tang ZY, Li ZH (1982) Storage and analysis of data from 46 cases of small hepatocellular carcinoma using microcomputer. Chin J Oncol 4: 287–289[1]

Tang ZY, Ye SL (1983) Using the microcomputer in storage and analysis of large amounts of clinical material. Acta Acad Med Primae Shanghai 10: 22–27[1]

Tang ZY, Li ZH, Yang BH, et al. (1981) Computer-aided differential diagnosis of liver cancer – analysis of 237 cases. Acta Acad Med Primae Shanghai 8: 143–147[1]

Tsou KC, Ledis S, McCoy MG (1973) 5′-Nucleotide phosphodiesterase isoenzyme pattern in the serum of human hepatoma. Cancer Res 33: 2215–2217

1 Chinese

Subject Index